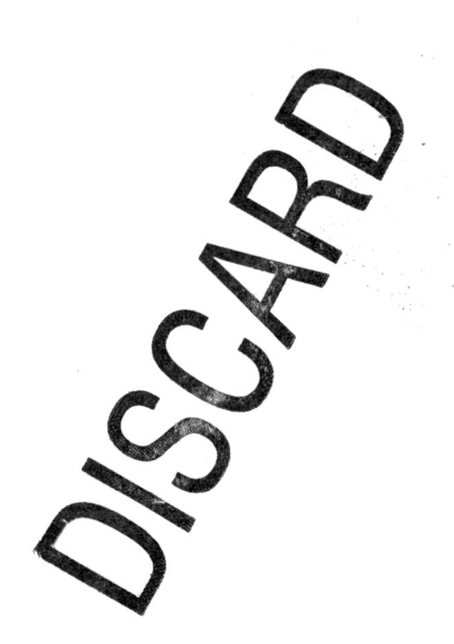
DISCARD

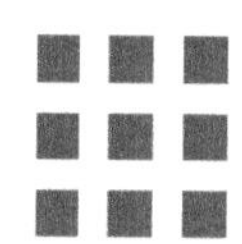

Biomaterials Nanoarchitectonics

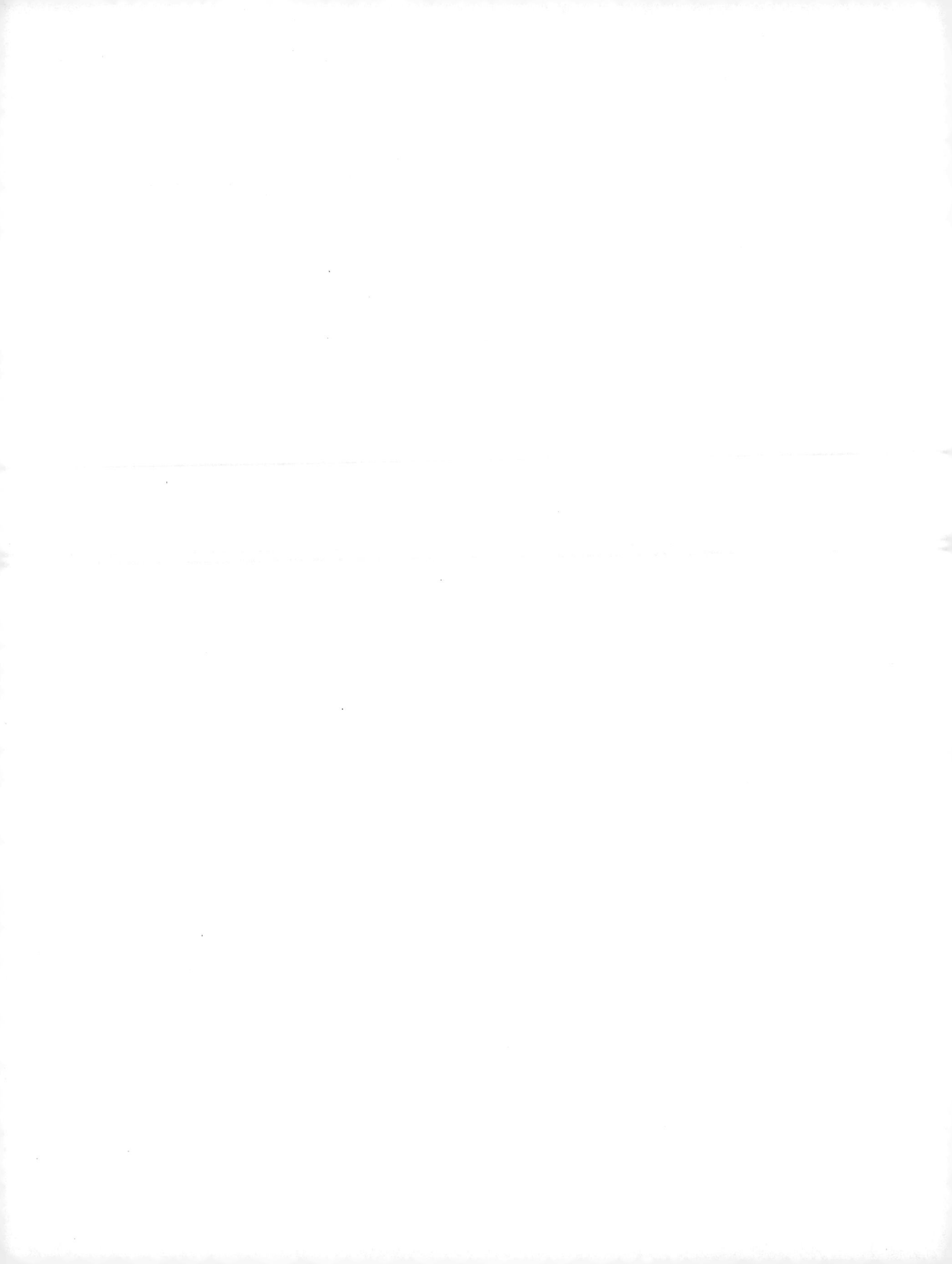

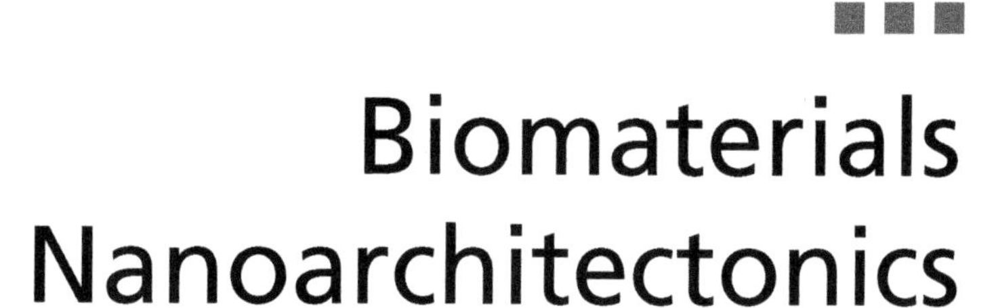

Biomaterials Nanoarchitectonics

Edited by

Mitsuhiro Ebara

International Center for Materials Nanoarchitectonics (MANA),
National Institute for Materials Science (NIMS),
Tsukuba, Japan

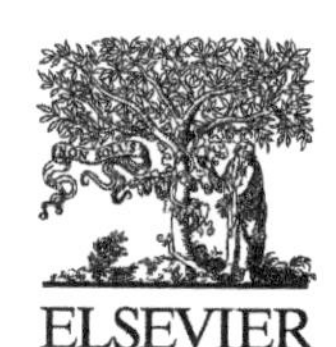

Amsterdam • Boston • Heidelberg • London
New York • Oxford • Paris • San Diego
San Francisco • Singapore • Sydney • Tokyo
William Andrew is an imprint of Elsevier

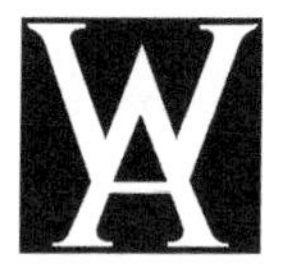

William Andrew is an imprint of Elsevier
The Boulevard, Langford Lane, Kidlington, Oxford, OX5 1GB, UK
50 Hampshire Street, 5th Floor, Cambridge, MA 02139, USA

British Library Cataloguing-in-Publication Data
A catalogue record for this book is available from the British Library

Library of Congress Cataloging-in-Publication Data
A catalog record for this book is available from the Library of Congress

ISBN: 978-0-323-37127-8

For information on all William Andrew publications
visit our website at http://store.elsevier.com/

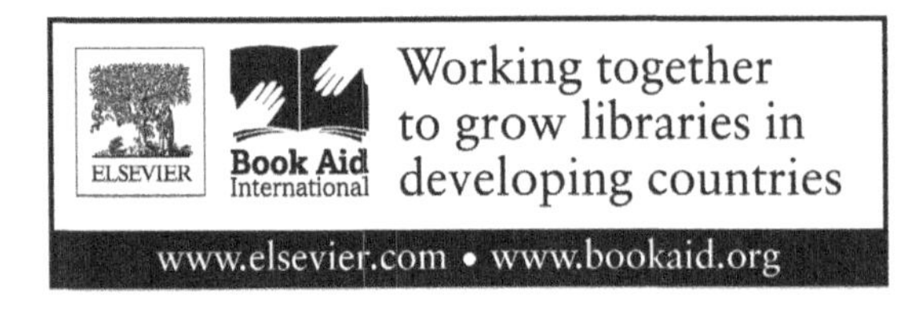

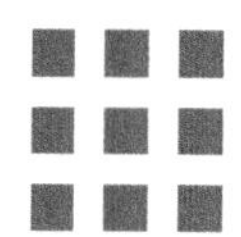

Contents

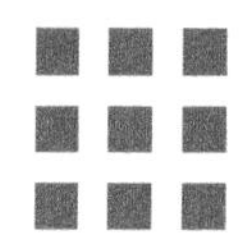

List of Contributors

Aya Mizutani Akimoto

Department of Materials Engineering, School of Engineering, The University of Tokyo, Tokyo, Japan

Katsuhiko Ariga

International Center for Materials Nanoarchitectonics (MANA), National Institute for Materials Science (NIMS), Tsukuba, Japan

Guoping Chen

Tissue Regeneration Materials Unit, International Center for Materials Nanoarchitectonics (MANA), National Institute for Materials Science (NIMS), Tsukuba, Japan

Chong-Su Cho

Department of Agricultural Biotechnology and Research Institute for Agriculture and Life Sciences, Seoul National University, Seoul, South Korea

Cole A. DeForest

Department of Bioengineering, University of Washington, Seattle, WA, USA

Mitsuhiro Ebara

International Center for Materials Nanoarchitectonics (MANA), National Institute for Materials Science (NIMS), Tsukuba, Japan

Naokazu Idota

Kagami Memorial Research Institute for Materials Science and Technology, Waseda University, Shinjuku, Tokyo, Japan

Gaku Imamura

International Center for Young Scientists (ICYS) & International Center for Materials Nanoarchitectonics (MANA), National Institute for Materials Science (NIMS), Tsukuba, Japan

Yasuhiko Iwasaki

Department of Chemistry and Materials Engineering, Faculty of Chemistry, Materials and Bioengineering, Kansai University, Osaka, Japan

Rajendrakumar Santhosh Kalash

Department of Biomedical Sciences, BK21 PLUS Center for Creative Biomedical Scientists at Chonnam National University, Research Institute of Medical Sciences, Chonnam National University Medical School, Gwangju, South Korea

Akifumi Kawamura

Department of Chemistry and Materials Engineering, Kansai University, Osaka, Japan

Naoki Kawazoe

Tissue Regeneration Materials Unit, International Center for Materials Nanoarchitectonics (MANA), National Institute for Materials Science (NIMS), Tsukuba, Japan

Deok-Ho Kim

Department of Bioengineering, University of Washington, Seattle, WA, USA

Jun Kobayashi

Institute of Advanced Biomedical Engineering and Science, Tokyo Women's Medical University (TWIns), Tokyo, Japan

Yohei Kotsuchibashi

International Center for Young Scientists (ICYS) and International Center for Materials Nanoarchitectonics (MANA), National Institute for Materials Science (NIMS), Tsukuba, Japan

Rio Kurimoto

International Center for Materials Nanoarchitectonics (MANA), National Institute for Materials Science (NIMS), Tsukuba, Japan

James J. Lai

Department of Bioengineering, University of Washington, Seattle, WA, USA

Vinoth Kumar Lakshmanan

Department of Biomedical Sciences, BK21 PLUS Center for Creative Biomedical Scientists at Chonnam National University, Research Institute of Medical Sciences, Chonnam National University Medical School, Gwangju, South Korea

Tsukuru Masuda

Department of Materials Engineering, School of Engineering, The University of Tokyo, Tokyo, Japan

Takashi Miyata

Department of Chemistry and Materials Engineering, Kansai University, Osaka, Japan

Yasuhiro Nakagawa

International Center for Materials Nanoarchitectonics (MANA), National Institute for Materials Science (NIMS), Tsukuba, Japan; Graduate School of Pure and Applied Sciences, University of Tsukuba, Tsukuba, Japan

Jun Nakanishi

International Center for Materials Nanoarchitectonics (MANA), National Institute for Materials Science (NIMS), Tsukuba, Japan

Ravin Narain

Department of Chemical and Materials Engineering, University of Alberta, Edmonton, AB, Canada

Eri Niiyama

International Center for Materials Nanoarchitectonics (MANA), National Institute for Materials Science (NIMS), Tsukuba, Japan

Yuichi Ohya

Department of Chemistry and Materials Engineering, Faculty of Chemistry, Materials and Bioengineering; Organization for Research and Development of Innovative Science and Technology (ORDIST), Kansai University, Suita, Osaka, Japan

Teruo Okano

Institute of Advanced Biomedical Engineering and Science, Tokyo Women's Medical University (TWIns), Tokyo, Japan

Nuttada Panpradist

Department of Bioengineering, University of Washington, Seattle, WA, USA

In-Kyu Park

Department of Biomedical Sciences, BK21 PLUS Center for Creative Biomedical Scientists at Chonnam National University, Research Institute of Medical Sciences, Chonnam National University Medical School, Gwangju, South Korea

Kota Shiba

International Center for Young Scientists (ICYS) & International Center for Materials Nanoarchitectonics (MANA), National Institute for Materials Science (NIMS), Tsukuba, Japan

Koichiro Uto

Department of Bioengineering, University of Washington, Seattle, WA, USA

Ryo Yoshida

Department of Materials Engineering, School of Engineering, The University of Tokyo, Tokyo, Japan

Genki Yoshikawa

International Center for Materials Nanoarchitectonics (MANA), National Institute for Materials Science (NIMS), Tsukuba, Japan

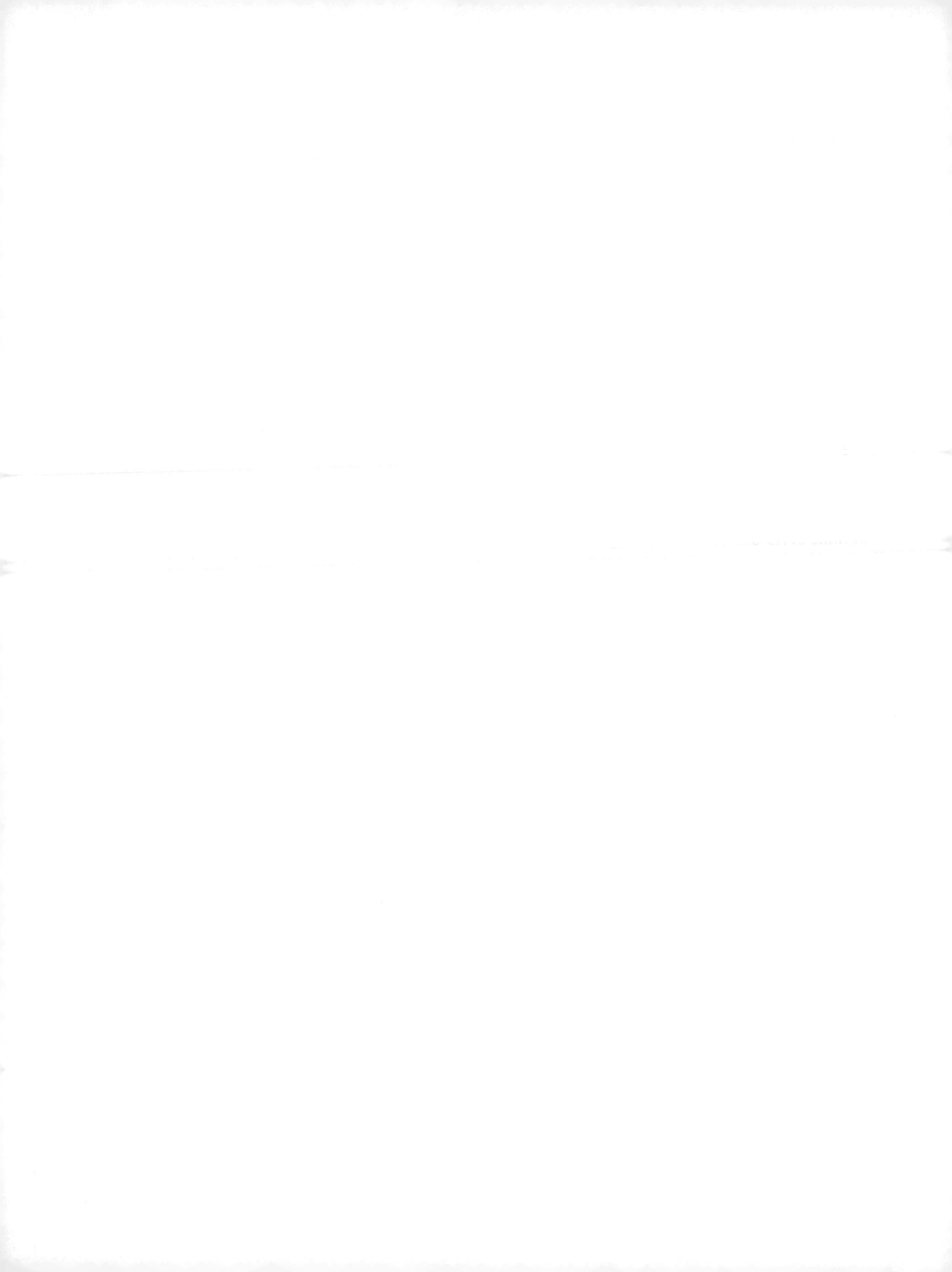

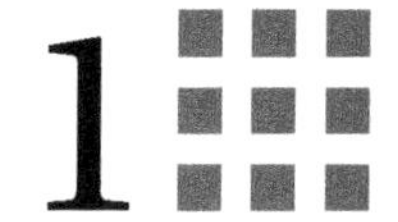

Introductory Guide to Nanoarchitectonics

Mitsuhiro Ebara

INTERNATIONAL CENTER FOR MATERIALS NANOARCHITECTONICS (MANA), NATIONAL INSTITUTE FOR MATERIALS SCIENCE (NIMS), TSUKUBA, JAPAN

CHAPTER OUTLINE

1.1 From Nanotechnology to Nanoarchitectonics

Even long before the start of the "nanotechnology era," people were using various nano-sized objects without realizing that they were dealing with the world of "nano" technology. For example, ancient civilizations used natural fabrics such as flax, cotton, wool, and silk that had pores the size of nanometers. In ancient Egypt, people were able to make hair dyeing paste react with sulfur and produce galenite particles a few nanometers in size, which provided even and steady dyeing. In Europe in the Middle Ages, the engineering of multicolored church stained-glass windows achieved a high quality because of the use of additives of gold or other metal nanoparticles. It was also revealed that the steel of Damascus blades, which were first encountered by the Crusaders in the war against the Muslims, contained carbon nanotubes as well as cementite nanowires [1]. The idea of nanotechnology first came about from the well-known lecture of Richard Feynman at an American Physical Society meeting in 1959 [2]. It was the great inventions in microscopy (the scanning tunneling microscope and the atomic force microscope) in the 1980s that allowed researchers to see single atoms and then manipulate them on a surface. Both these instruments were invented by Binning, Rohrer, and Ruska from IBM Zurich [3]. In 1985, Smalley, Kroto, and Curl discovered a new form of the element carbon: a molecule consisting of 60 atoms of carbon assembled in a form similar to a football [4]. In 1991, the first nanotechnological program of the National Scientific Fund began to operate in the United States. In 2001, the National Nanotechnological Initiative of the United States was approved, which was to become the basis for the economy and national security of the United States in the first half of the twenty-first century. Today, nanotechnology can offer the promise of new products to improve energy efficiency, clean up toxic chemicals, and flight disease.

Although nanotechnology research has already produced many technologies with potential applications, it may be possible to go even further and design more sophisticated structures such as pseudoliving organisms. In terms of materials design, "nano" is not a direct extension of "micro," and an architectonic concept is thus required rather than a fabrication technology. At nanoscale dimensions, for example, the properties of materials no longer depend solely on composition and structure in the usual sense, and thus nanomaterials display new phenomena associated with the preponderance of surfaces and interfaces. From this regard, a new paradigm shift in nanomaterials science was required. In fact, the central concept is now changing from nanotechnology to nanoarchitectonics. The terminology of nanoarchitectonics was first proposed by Masakazu Aono at the First International Symposium on Nanoarchitectonics using Suprainteractions in 2000 [5]. Nanoarchitectonics is a technology system where the aim is to arrange nanoscale structural units, which are a group of atoms or molecules or a nanoscale functional component, in an intended configuration that creates a novel functionality through mutual interactions among those units. Therefore, materials nanoarchitectonics targets two hierarchical classes of materials development: nanomaterial creation and nanosystem organization (Fig. 1.1) [6–8].

1.2 Challenges in Biomaterials Research

Biomaterials are becoming increasingly important in biomedical practice, particularly as the population ages [9]. Because the human body is made up of hierarchies of nanostructures of biological molecules, cells, and tissues; it is clear that biological responses to materials depend on structural properties of the material at the nanometer scale [10]. To cite an example that emphasizes the importance of gaining control of "nanostructures and properties of biomaterials, surfaces of implanted materials have been designed to control adsorption of biological molecules onto them." Interestingly, introduction of implanted materials into the human body was noted far back in prehistory. A spear point was embedded in the hip of human remains found in United States in 1996. It had apparently healed in and did not significantly impede activity. This unintended implant illustrates the body's capacity to deal with implanted foreign materials. Thus, to control material properties at the nanoscale is a very important challenge in biomaterials science. Although materials with multiscale organization should be more advantageous in biomedical applications, general methods for controlling material properties at the nanoscale are lacking. For example, traditional materials used as *in vitro* cell culture substrates have rigid and flat surfaces that lack the exquisite nanoscale features of the *in vivo* extracellular environment. Therefore, a new methodology to produce architectures organized on multiple length scales, which bear a closer resemblance to biological matrices than those with single-scale features, has been required [11].

How can the nanoarchitectures of biomaterials be controlled, then? The following chapters present a point of view on this question (Fig. 1.2). In Chapter 2, we focus on the synthesis and characterization of nanoparticles, supramolecules, hydrogels, and

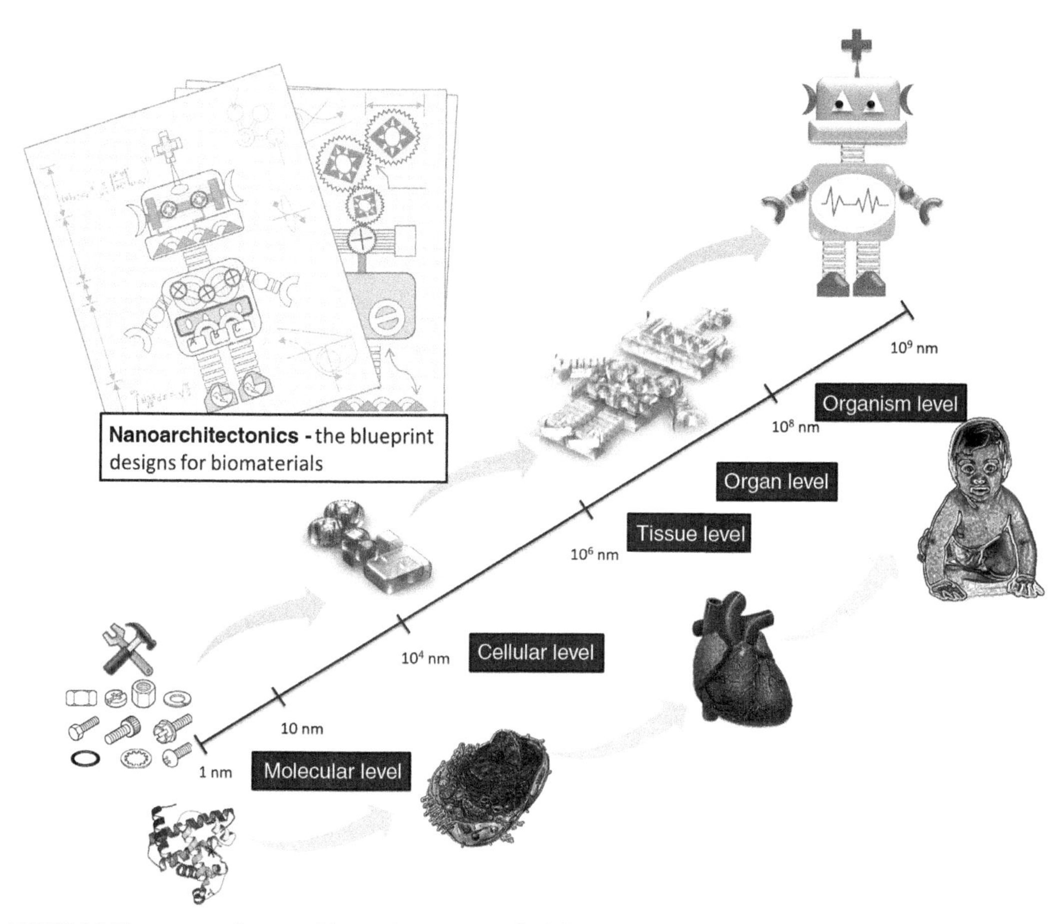

FIGURE 1.1 The concept of nanoarchitectonics: a new methodology to produce architectures organized on multiple length scales, which bear a closer resemblance to the human body made up of hierarchies of nanostructures of biological molecules, cells, and tissue.

nature-inspired polymers toward drug and gene delivery applications. Because nanosized particles demonstrate unique properties, they can provide a particularly useful platform for wide-ranging therapeutic applications. In Chapter 3, we present rationally designed surfaces especially for regenerative medicines including tissue engineering, cell sheet technologies, and cell manipulation technologies. In Chapter 4, we focus on diagnostic technologies including point-of-care diagnostics, biosensors, nanomechanical sensors, as well as theranostics. In Chapter 5, we describe recent advances in the next generation biomaterials including self-oscillating materials, shape-memory materials, cell membrane engineering, fibrous materials, and switchable interfaces. As stated previously, we hope that the following chapters will stimulate further research and generate unexpected novel ideas.

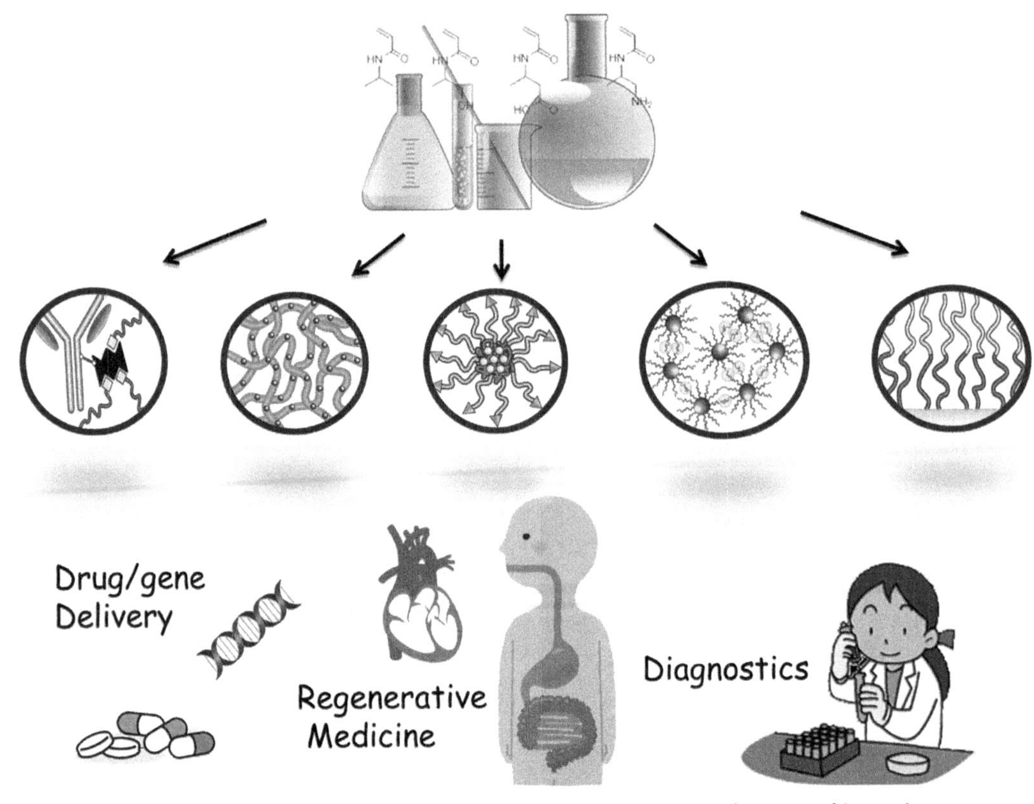

FIGURE 1.2 Unlike conventional biomaterials, the biomaterials designed based on the nanoarchitectonic concept possess highly functional abilities, which make them particularly attractive for a variety of biomedical applications, such as drug/gene delivery, regenerative medicine, and diagnostic technologies.

References

[1] M. Reibold, P. Paufler, A.A. Levin, W. Kochmann, N. Pätzke, D.C. Meyer, Nature 444 (2006) 286.

[2] R. Feynman, There's plenty of room at the bottom: an invitation to enter a new field of physics, Eng. Sci. V 23 (5) (1960) 22–36.

[3] G. Binning, H. Rohrer, Surface Sci. 126 (1983) 236.

[4] H.W. Kroto, J.R. Heath, S.C. O'Brien, R.F. Curl, R.E. Smalley, Nature 318 (1985) 162.

[5] M. Aono, Sci. Technol. Adv. Mater. 12 (2011) 040301.

[6] K. Ariga, T. Mori, J.P. Hill, Adv. Mater. 24 (2012) 158.

[7] M. Osada, T. Sasaki, Adv. Mater. 24 (2012) 210.

[8] T. Hasegawa, K. Terabe, T. Tsuruoka, M. Aono, Adv. Mater. 24 (2012) 252.

[9] B.D. Ratner, A.S. Hoffman, F.J. Schoen, J.E. Lemons, Biomaterials Science, third ed., Academic Press, Inc, Boston, (2012).

[10] K. Ariga, K. Kawakami, M. Ebara, Y. Kotsuchibashi, Q. Ji, J.P. Hill, New J. Chem. 38 (2014) 5149.

[11] M. Ebara, Y. Kotsuchibashi, R. Narain, N. Idota, Y.-J. Kim, J.M. Hoffman, K. Uto, T. Aoyagi, Smart Biomaterials, NIMS Monographs, Springer, New York, (2014).

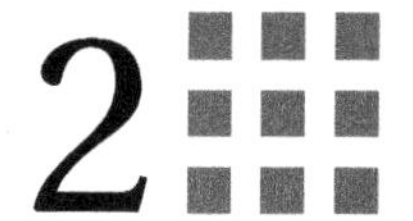

Drug and Gene Delivery Technologies

2.1

Nanoparticles

Yohei Kotsuchibashi*, Yasuhiro Nakagawa**,†, Mitsuhiro Ebara**

*INTERNATIONAL CENTER FOR YOUNG SCIENTISTS (ICYS) AND INTERNATIONAL CENTER FOR MATERIALS NANOARCHITECTONICS (MANA), NATIONAL INSTITUTE FOR MATERIALS SCIENCE (NIMS), TSUKUBA, JAPAN; **INTERNATIONAL CENTER FOR MATERIALS NANOARCHITECTONICS (MANA), NATIONAL INSTITUTE FOR MATERIALS SCIENCE (NIMS), TSUKUBA, JAPAN; †GRADUATE SCHOOL OF PURE AND APPLIED SCIENCES, UNIVERSITY OF TSUKUBA, TSUKUBA, JAPAN

CHAPTER OUTLINE

2.1.1 Introduction

Drug and gene delivery technologies possess great potential for various types of disease treatments. However, simple drugs and genes have certain disadvantages in the human body such as nonspecific adsorption due to the hydrophobic and/or electrostatic interaction, rapid biodegradability, and rapid clearance from blood circulation. To overcome these problems, the drugs/genes have been encapsulated in polymeric biomaterials. The origin of a controlled drug delivery system (DDS) using polymeric biomaterials dates back to the 1960s, and the material sizes have been continuously decreasing (macrosize in the 1970s, microsize in the 1980s, and nanosize in the 1990s) with the development of technologies [1,2]. On the basis of the Ringsdorf model for polymer drugs [3], various types of nanoparticles have been produced in the 2000s. The development of nanoparticles was mainly supported by three key technologies: (1) PEGylation, (2) passive targeting (solid tumor accumulation via the enhanced permeability and retention [EPR] effect), and (3) active targeting (specific cell interaction by ligand-conjugated polymeric materials) (Fig. 2.1.1a). PEGylation is a covalent attachment between poly(ethylene glycol) (PEG) and molecules, which decreases their immunogenicity and increases their blood circulation time [4]. In 1977, Abuchowski et al.

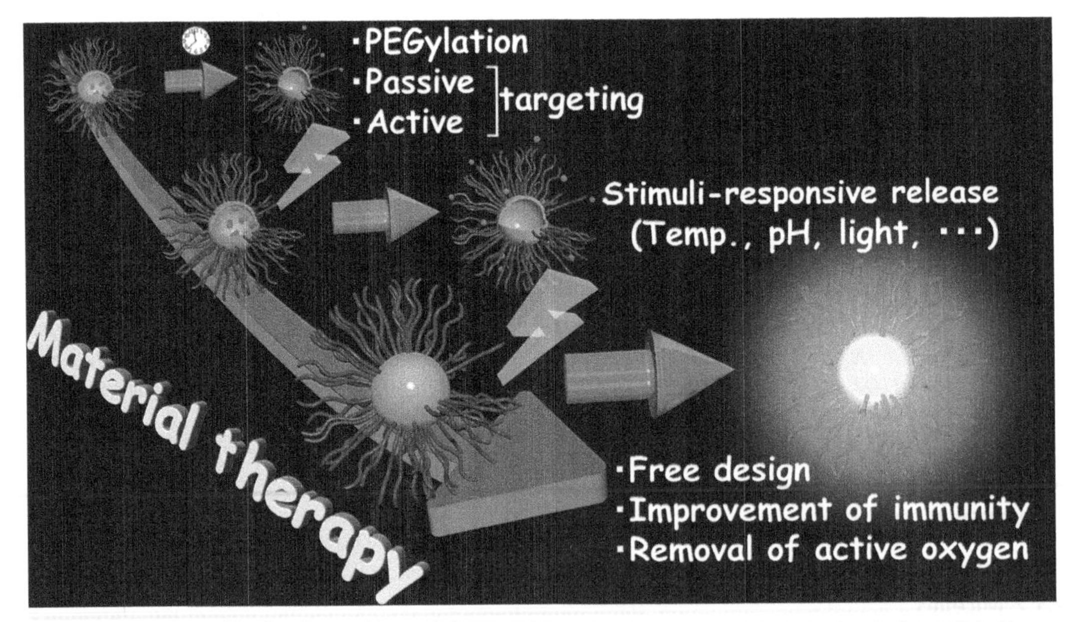

FIGURE 2.1.1 Nanoparticles for drug and gene delivery system.

reported that the covalent attachment of PEG to albumin reduced its immunogenicity [5]. Subsequently, they also found that PEGylated biomolecules had a longer blood circulation time than the corresponding normal biomolecules [6]. Various types of molecules have been PEGylated, such as small molecules [7–12], peptides [13,14], proteins [15–20], antibodies, and their fragments [21,22] and oligonucleotides [23,24]. The EPR effect was found by Maeda et al., which is a phenomenon whereby nanoparticles tend to accumulate in tumor tissue for the gap of the blood vessel around the tumor caused by the rapid growth of cancer cells, and their underdeveloped lymph vessel [25]. Moreover, these drug carriers must also be designed with appropriate sizes to overcome living barriers, for instance, the reticuloendothelial system, and so on. The system of nanocarriers accumulated in a tumor by the EPR effect is known as passive targeting. On the other hand, for more effective accumulation, nanocarriers with an affinity site on the surface have been reported to interact with target cells; this system is called active targeting. Cancer cells usually express superabundant receptors such as low-molecular-weight compounds and antibodies, as compared with normal cells. In active targeting, the receptors are used as targeting sites for the injected nanocarriers. However, these cancer cells are usually located outside of blood vessels. Therefore, nanocarriers for active targeting first experience the EPR effect, and the diameter plays an important factor in this targeting. Table 2.1.1 summarizes the approved or under clinical trial DDS pharmaceuticals based on passive or active targeting [26].

Drug release from nanoparticles was mainly triggered by biodegradability and drug diffusion. To achieve an "on/off" switchable drug release, the excellent DDS nanoparticles have been combined with stimuli-responsive (or smart) polymers (Fig. 2.1.1b). The stimuli-responsive polymers can recognize the slight change in their external environment,

Table 2.1.1 Pharmaceuticals Based on Passive or Active Targeting [26]

Passive Targeting			
Name	**Platform**	**Compound**	**Clinical Stage**
NK105	Micelles	Paclitaxel	P3
NC-6004	Micelles	Cisplatin	P2
NK012	Micelles	SN-38	P2
Smancs	Polymer conjugate	Neocarzinostatin	Approved
Doxil	Liposome	Doxorubicin	Approved
Abraxane	Albumin particle	Paclitaxel	Approved
Xyotax	Polymer conjugate	Paclitaxel	P3
CT-2106	Polymer conjugate	Camptothecin	P2
EndoTAG	Cationic liposome	Paclitaxel	P2
MAG-CPT	Polymer conjugate	Camptothecin	P1
LE-SN-38	Liposome	SN-38	P2
PK1	Polymer conjugate	Doxorubicin	P2
IT-101	Polymer conjugate	Camptothecin	P2
SP1049C	Micelles	Doxorubicin	P3
CPX-1	Liposome	CPT-11, floxuridine	P2
Active Targeting			
Name	**Platform**	**Compound**	**Clinical Stage**
Mylotarg	Anti-CD33-Ab	Calicheamicin	Approved
Zevalin	Anti-CD20-Ab	^{90}Y	Approved
Bexxar	Anti-CD20-Ab	^{131}I	Approved
PK2	Galactose-polymer	Doxorubicin	P1
MCC465	Ab-liposome	Doxorubicin	P1
MBP-426	Transferrin-liposome	Oxaliplatin	P1
CALAA-01	Transferrin-polymer	siRNA	P1
T-DM1	Anti-HER2-Ab	CM1	Approved

such as temperature, pH, light, magnetic field, and molecular concentration. For example, pH-responsive polymers have been used as the carriers for anionic/cationic drugs, nucleic acids, polymers, and metal ions via electrostatic interaction [27–33]. Moreover, the nanoparticles have the potential to be a drug themselves, for example, they can improve immunity, remove active oxygen, and be used in radiation therapy and thermotherapy [34,35]. Material therapy is expected to be the next generation of DDS (Fig. 2.1.1c). In this chapter, we focus on the recent nanoparticles for drug/gene delivery systems. The chapter is divided into three parts: micelles, liposomes, and conjugated nanoparticles.

2.1.2 Micelles

An amphiphilic block copolymer with a precisely hydrophilic/hydrophobic balance can form a core–shell micelle structure in an aqueous solution. The hydrophobic inner core can encapsulate the hydrophobic drugs and the high drug-loading capacity has been applied to an excellent drug carrier (Fig. 2.1.2) [36–38]. Kataoka et al. have reported various

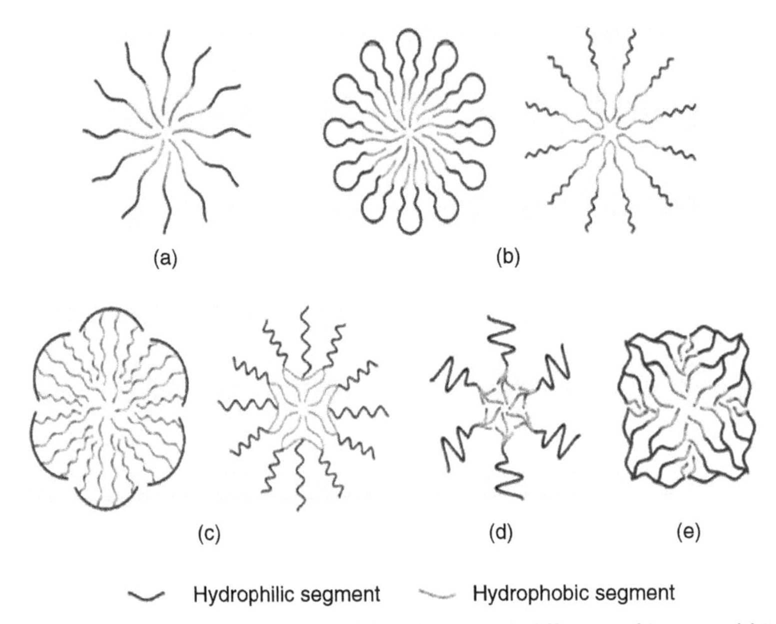

FIGURE 2.1.2 Polymer self-assemblies based on amphiphilic polymers with different architectures. (a) Diblock copolymer, (b) triblock copolymer, (c) graft copolymer, (d) star copolymer, and (e) hyperbranched copolymer [38].

types of self-assembled micelle consisting of biocompatible block copolymers. A block copolymer of PEG-*b*-poly(α,β-aspartic acid) was prepared, and the α,β-aspartic acid unit was used as a reactive to combine the anticancer drug doxorubicin (DOX) by covalent bonds. The hydrophobic DOX-modified segments formed a micelle core, and the combined DOX units also accelerated a loading capacity of free DOX via the π–π interaction [39,40]. The poly(α,β-aspartic acid) segments can also interact with cationic polymers by electrostatic interaction. Using the interaction, Harada et al. prepared unique micelles called polyion complex micelles by a simple mixing of PEG-*b*-poly(α,β-aspartic acid) and PEG-*b*-poly(L-lysine) [41]. The anionic charged nucleic acids are also encapsulated into the poly(L-lysine) micelle core [42]. As a biomaterial, micelle also has to possess biodegradability. A disulfide bond (S–S) is one of the most studied breakable covalent bonds, and a micelle core cross-linked via the S–S bonds can be collapsed to locate in an endocytotic reducing environment after uptake into the cell [43]. On the other hand, temperature-responsive polymers can show reversible micelle formation/collapse by changing solution temperature without adding any materials. Moreover, the core and/or shell functionalities are easily customized via a mixture of copolymers before the temperature rises.

We have focused on the design of multistimuli-responsive nanoparticles using a mixture of block copolymers having a common temperature-responsive segment. The shell-mixed nanoparticles (shell: poly(*N*-isopropylacrylamide) (poly(NIPAAm)) and PEO segments) have been prepared via hydrophobic–hydrophobic interaction [44], stereocomplex interaction [45], and electrostatic interaction [46]. We used the temperature-responsive poly(NIPAAm) segment for the shell-mixed nanoparticles. Poly(NIPAAm)-*b*-poly(NIPAAm-*co*-HMAAm)s

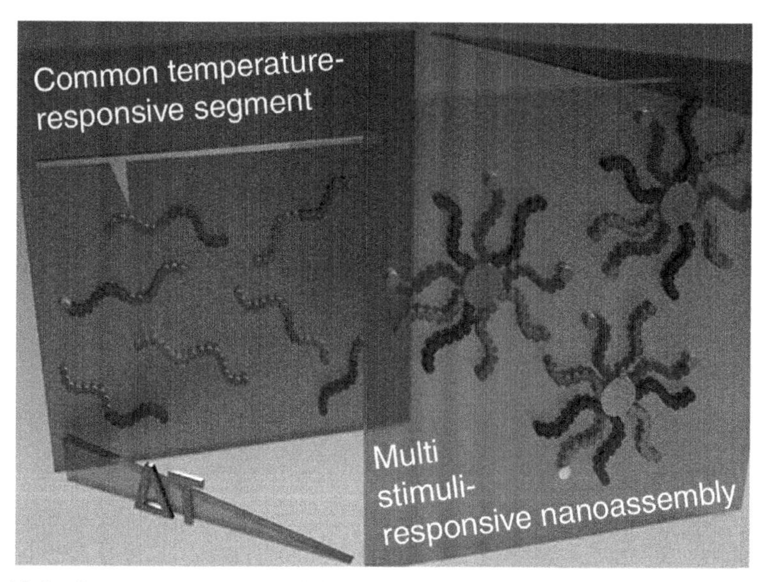

FIGURE 2.1.3 Multistimuli-responsive nanoassembly by mixing of selected block copolymers with the common temperature-responsive segment [48].

were mixed with polyNIPAAm-*b*-poly(NIPAAm-*co*-AMPS) [47]. A mixture of the block copolymers was easily dissolved in water at below the lower critical solution temperature (LCST) of the poly(NIPAAm) segment. The diameters of the mixed nanoparticles were controlled by the mixture ratios (e.g., the diameter was 178 ± 53 nm at mixture ratios of 1:1 weight). Moreover, nanoparticle aggregations were observed above another LCST of the poly(NIPAAm-*co*-HMAAm) shell. Interestingly, the aggregations showed high stability similarly with a narrow size distribution due to electrostatic repulsion of the poly(NIPAAm-*co*-AMPS) shell. On the basis of the concept, we also prepared a nanoparticle having three types of segments in the shell (Fig. 2.1.3) [48]. A poly(NIPAAm-*co*-BMAAm) segment (LCST 17°C) was prepared as a common temperature-responsive segment. As another segment in the block copolymers, a temperature-responsive poly(NIPAAm-*co*-HMAAm) segment (LCST 35°C), a biocompatible PEG segment, and a poly(NIPAAm-*co*-HMAAm) (LCST 70°C)-*b*-poly(2-lactobionamidoethyl methacrylate [LAMA]) segment were prepared. The poly(LAMA) segment was for specific interaction with the target cancer cells via a carbohydrate receptor. On the other hand, temperature-responsive segment was for creating the particle core. A typical temperature-responsive core, however, has a disadvantage in that it has a low drug loading as compared to that of amphiphilic block copolymer nanoparticles (the hydrophobic drug loading < 1 wt%). We found that temperature-responsive statistical copolymers were efficiently encapsulated in the temperature-responsive block copolymer as a core-mixed nanoparticle [49]. The loading amount was over 50 wt%. The encapsulation phenomena were observed using dynamic light scattering (DLS) and fluorescence resonance energy transfer. Interestingly, there was a selectivity on the encapsulatable statistical copolymers in the nanoparticle core. In other words, temperature-responsive block

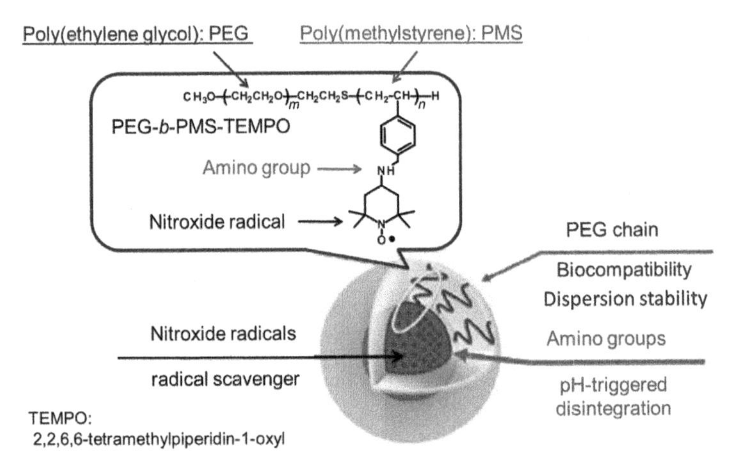

FIGURE 2.1.4 Schematic of nitroxide radical-containing nanoparticle (RNP) [70].

copolymers can recognize its optimum statistical copolymers when they form mixed core nanoparticles. For example, according to calculations, a drug loading of paclitaxel (PTX), which is an anticancer drug, reaches 11 wt% in the core-mixed nanoparticles, when two PTX molecules are combined with the temperature-responsive statistical copolymer. The drug loading value is in no way inferior to the nanoparticles consisting of typical amphiphilic block copolymers.

Nanoparticles can work not only as drug carrier but also as drugs themselves, that is, improvement of immunity, adsorption of active oxygen, as an adjuvant material, and in virus neutralization [34,35,50,51]. Excess reactive oxygen species (ROS), which is a trigger of oxidative stress, is well known for having a relationship with not only aging but also various types of diseases, such as cancers, myocardial infarction, inflammatory bowel disease, kidney failure, arteriosclerosis, diabetes, rheumatoid arthritis, Parkinson's disease, and Alzheimer's disease [52–62]. One of the most plausible ways to prevent these oxidative stress injuries is the administration of an exogenous ROS scavenger. Recently, the ROS scavengers, including synthetic and/or of natural low molecular weight, have been reported [63–66]. However, there are problems due to the preferential renal clearance as well as the adverse effects, such as mitochondrial dysfunction and antihypertensive activity [67,68]. Recently, Yoshitomi et al. have been focusing on a new design of nanoparticles for a stress nanotherapy using self-assembled polymers with nitroxide radicals [69–72] (Fig. 2.1.4). The nitroxide radical is combined with a micelle core as a ROS scavenger, which is surrounded by the biocompatible PEG chains. The ROS scavenger micelles have been applied in the treatment of various types of diseases. A drug resistance of cancer tissue is one of the serious problems on cancer treatments. Chronic inflammation of the cancer microenvironment has been reported to influence such drug resistance [73,74]. Moreover, generated ROS activate transcription factors such as nuclear factor-kappa B (NF-κB), which is known to promote cancer development and drug resistance [75,76]. Therefore, the suppression of inflammation in cancer tissue is expected

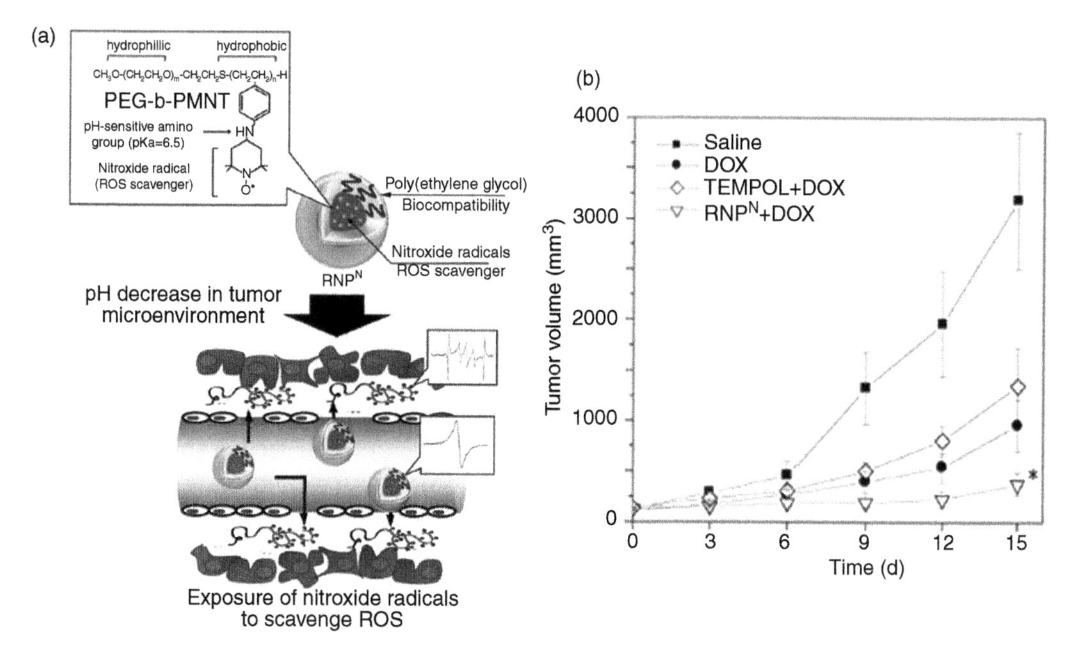

FIGURE 2.1.5 (a) Schematic illustration of pH sensitive RNP and the effective accumulation and disintegration of RNP in the tumor area. (b) Effect of RNP pretreatment on the anticancer activity of DOX in BALB/c mice bearing colon-26 tumors [77].

to overcome the drug resistance. As the ROS scavenger, pH-sensitive redox nanoparticle (RNP) was prepared for drug resistance cancer treatment (Fig. 2.1.5) [77]. The RNP can be disintegrated under acidic conditions (such as cancer tissue) and the nitroxide radicals are exposed, leading to strongly scavenging ROS. In fact, the RNPs showed the suppression of both inflammation and activation of NF-κB. The anticancer drug DOX was encapsulated into the RNP for the synergistic cancer treatment in BALA/c mice bearing colon-26. The RNP/DOX dramatically restrained the growth of the cancer tissue as compared with the control group. The RNP series is also applied in the relief of acute kidney injury [78]. In this case, the RNP could be disintegrated in renal acidic lesion for exposing ROS scavengers. Moreover, orally administered RNPs were prepared for suppression of indomethacin (IND)-induced small intestinal inflammation [79]. IND is commonly a drug for antipyretic, analgesic, and anti-inflammatory use. However, IND also has a risk of small intestinal injuries. The accumulation of RNPs in small intestines by oral administration was observed using fluorescent intensity and electrospin resonance, and the value of accumulated RNPs in both the jejunum and ileum tissues was 40 times higher than that of low-molecular-weight nitroxide radical molecules. In an *in vivo* test, mice were treated with IND and IND/RNP as a survival experiment. The daily administration of IND seriously damaged small intestines, and the survival rate was 28.6% after 7 days. On the other hand, the survival rate of IND/RNP was improved to 57.1% due to the high accumulation and long retention in small intestines.

2.1.3 Vesicles

The polymer vesicle (or polymersome) is a micrometer to nanometer-order hollow particle that has a bilayer membrane consisting of amphiphilic copolymers [80–82]. In contrast to micelles having the hydrophobic core, polymer vesicles can encapsulate water and hydrophilic molecules into the hollow core. Hydrophobic molecules can be also encapsulated in the hydrophobic bilayer membrane. Moreover, functionalities such as stimuli-responsive, cellar targeting, and molecular recognition are easily added to the polymer vesicle via inserting the functional copolymers in the bilayer membrane, which is applied in carriers for drug and gene delivery. The condition to form a vesicle structure is decided by the hydrophilic/hydrophobic balance of the amphiphilic molecules. Amphiphilic block copolymers, particularly, follow an equation of the "packing parameter": p', that is, $p = (v/a_o) \times l_c$ (v, volume of the hydrophobic chains; a_o, optimal area of the head group; and l_c, length of the hydrophobic tail), and the assembled nanostructures are predicted by the calculated p value (micelles: $p \leq 1/3$, cylindrical micelles: $1/3 \leq p \leq 1/2$, and vesicles/polymersomes: $1/2 \leq p \leq 1$) [83]. Ladmiral et al. directly prepared nanoassembled materials in polymerization solution with a high concentration using a polymerization-induced self-assembly method [84]. A mixture solution of hydrophilic macrochain transfer agents of polyglycerol monomethacrylate and galactose-based polymer was polymerized to grow hydrophobic poly(2-hydroxypropyl methacrylate) block in water at 70°C. The structures of nanoassemblies were controlled to be in the form of spheres, worm-like micelles, and vesicles by the polymer compositions. Stimuli-responsive copolymers can be switchable to the nanoassembly structures via the changing external environment (e.g., temperature, pH, light, magnetic field, and molecules). Wei et al. prepared a dual temperature-responsive triblock copolymer (poly(ethylene glycol)(PEG)$_{45}$-*b*-poly(*N*-isopropylacrylamide) (poly(NIPAAm)$_{380}$)-*b*-poly(NIPAAm$_{423}$-*co*-*N*-hydroxyethyl acrylamide (HEAAm)$_{42}$) [85]. The hydrophobic region in the triblock copolymer was controlled by the continuous dehydration of the PNIPAAm and poly(NIPAAm-*co*-HEAAm) segments that showed LCST at 37 and 48°C, respectively. In fact, the assembled structures were converted between micelle (37~45°C, around 260 nm) and vesicle (over 50°C, ~420 nm). Pietsch et al. prepared a charge-controlled block copolymer consisting of poly(2-(dimethylamino)ethyl methacrylate (DMAEMA)) and poly(di(ethyleneglycol)methyl ether methacrylate (DEGMA)) segments [86]. The poly(DMAEMA) (cloud point ~49°C) and poly(DEGMA) (cloud point ~33°C) segments were charged with positive and negative charges, respectively. The charge density was changed resulting in temperature-responsive dehydration, which led to unique assembled structures of the multilamellar vesicular aggregates and unilamellar vesicle structures at 33 and 55°C.

In this way, structure-switchable nanoassemblies can control the drug loading/release, and the structure changes are also expected to affect the cell biology such as cell toxicity, improvement of immunity, and cell differentiation. Bellomo et al. prepared a polymer vesicle consisting of diblock copolymer peptides, and the encapsulated drug release was controlled via solution pH [87]. The copolymer peptides allow the construction of a complex three-dimensional structure such as α-helices and β-sheet, which is usually difficult to achieve using typical synthetic copolymers [88–90]. The diblock copolymer peptide has L-lysine residues in the structure. At high pH, the uncharged poly(L-lysine) domain is not water soluble, and preferentially adopts the α-helical conformation, resulting in the vesicle structure. On the other hand, at low pH (pH 3), the helix-to-coil conformation led to a structural change from vesicle to mesoporous and this structural change became a trigger for the drug release.

These polymer vesicles have been also applied in biomimetic systems. For example, cell membrane is usually modified with various types of sugars that have a deep relationship with the biological functions such as cell recognition, inflammation, infection, and cancer metastasis. The nanomaterials that possess the artificial cell membrane are expected to be a unique DDS. For example, dendritic glycopolymers have been actively studied in order to better understand their interactions with proteins and carbohydrates, as these studies can shed further light on their biological properties. Martos-Maldonado et al. prepared polyamino amine-based mannose–glycodendrimers, which were used for the detection of concanavalin A [91]. Percec et al. prepared glycodendrimersomes by self-assembly [92]. The dendritic vesicle materials (with D-mannose or D-galactose) were composed of a hydrophilic glycosite and hydrophobic alkyl chains of different chain lengths and were used in the detection and antibacteria. The enzyme-catalyzed synthetic pathway is one of the most important biological systems. Phospholipid liposomes have been used to mimic the biological systems; however, their relative thermodynamic and mechanical instability are problems [93–96]. To overcome the problems, Vriezema et al. focused on polymer vesicles that were composed of amphiphilic block copolymers. Polymer vesicles have high structural stability as compared with that of phospholipid liposomes, and the bilayer membrane is easily decorated with channel proteins and proton pumps [97,98]. Three types of enzymes (*Candida antarctica* lipase B [CALB], horseradish peroxidase [HRP], and glucose oxidase [GOX]) were combined with the polymer vesicle system as a nanoreactor to reproduce a cascade reaction [99]. As a model substrate, 1,2,3,4-tetra-O-acetyl-*b*-glucopyranose (GAc4) was selected. The CALB, HRP, and GOX are located in the outside of vesicle (CALB), bilayer membrane (HRP), and inside of vesicle (GOX), respectively. The acetate groups of substrate GAc4 were hydrolyzed to glucose via the CALB. The glucose was immediately incorporated into the water pool of polymer vesicle, and was transformed to lactone, resulting in the generation of H_2O_2. The H_2O_2 was used via HRP to convert from the ABTS to $ABTS^{\bullet+}$. The conversion of $ABTS^{\bullet+}$ was around 22% for 1500 min when all enzymes were in the vesicle system. On the other hand, in the absence of CALB, the $ABTS^{\bullet+}$ conversion was <0.5%. These results suggest that the reactions were achieved as a cascade reaction via the combination of vesicles and enzymes. Choi et al. proposed a polymer vesicle system for ATP generation (Fig. 2.1.6) [100]. ATP is an energy source for biological reaction, which occurs in mitochondria or chloroplast [101–104]. The bacteriorhodosin (BR: a light-driven proton pump) and F_0F_1-ATPsynthase motor protein were incorporated into the polymer vesicle membrane. The activated BR by light irradiation led protons into the vesicle, which was a trigger for driving the F_0F_1-ATPsynthase motor protein, resulting in ATP generation.

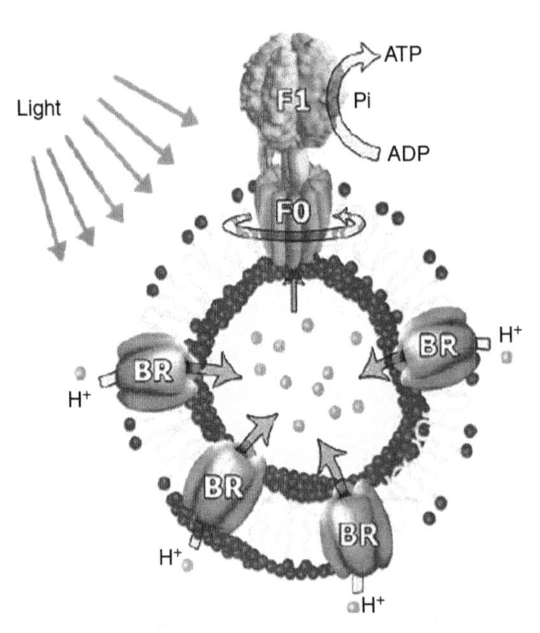

FIGURE 2.1.6 Schematic representation of proteopolymersomes reconstituted with both bacteriorhodosin (BR) and F0F1-ATP synthase. Adenosine triphosphate (ATP) synthase uses an electrochemical proton gradient generated by BR to synthesize ATP from adenosine diphosphate (ADP) and inorganic phosphate (Pi) [100].

This system is expected to apply in artificial cell engineering. Takakura et al. reported a self-reproducible polymer vesicle that inspired the cell division phenomenon (Fig. 2.1.7) [105,106]. There are mainly three gradual processes for artificial cell division: (1) encapsulation of the precursor molecules into the vesicle, (2) conversion from the precursors to vesicle components, and (3) enlargement/division by increasing vesicle components in the vesicle. The precursor molecules were converted to cationic amphiphilic molecules in the vesicle via the processes. Using this system, it was observed that a vesicle generated at least the third generation of the vesicle (i.e., grandchild vesicle). The same group also encapsulated the DNA into the self-reproducible cationic giant vesicle system [107]. The amplified DNA in the vesicle was succeeded by the generated vesicle (daughter vesicle) from the original one (mother vesicle).

It is usually difficult to add functionalities (i.e., to insert other amphiphilic molecules into a bilayer membrane) to self-assemble a bilayer nanoparticle after its self-assembly in solvents because the assembled bilayer membrane is a thermodynamically stable. If one can controlled the self-assemble phenomena, more complexed nanostrucutres can be achieved, and it will open a new stage of drug/gene delivery system. Bui et al. prepared a bilayer membrane nanoparticle via two-step self-assemblies using a solubility of amphiphilic block copolymer (Fig. 2.1.8) [108]. The nanoparticles were composed of a positively charged complex core (siRNA and polyethyleneimine [PEI]) and a capsid-like (bilayer) shell. The preparation processes were divided into two steps: (1) an electrostatic

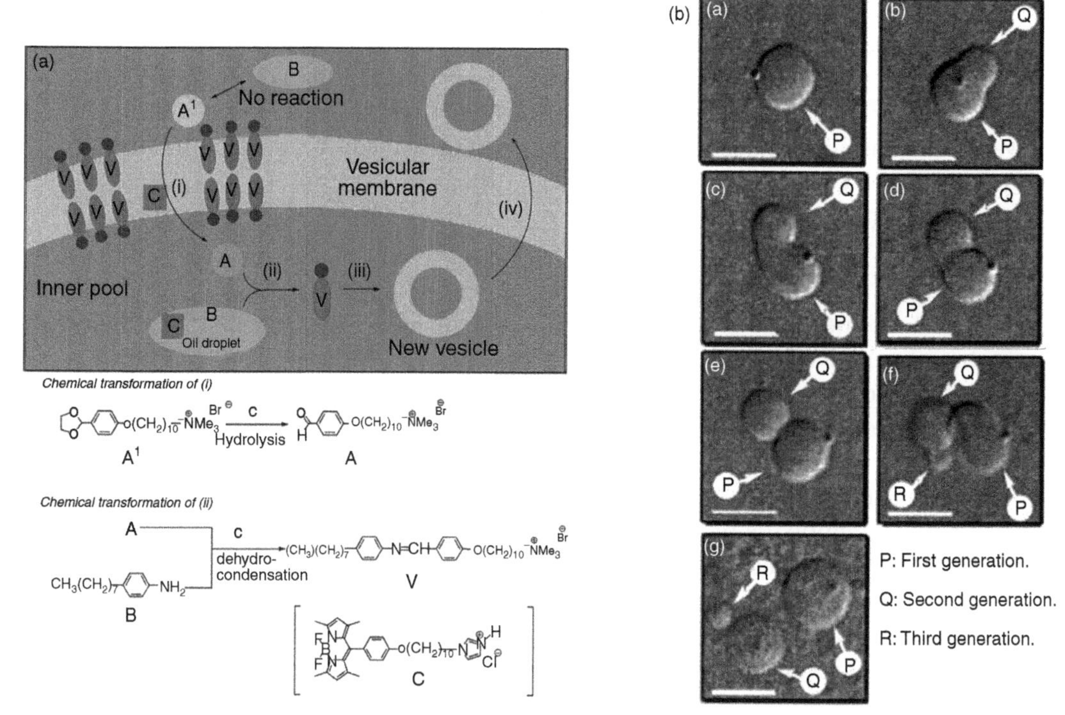

FIGURE 2.1.7 (a) Schematic illustration of the self-reproducing giant vesicles: (i) locked precursor A′ is incorporated into a vesicle composed of V and catalyst C and is unlocked to produce reactive precursor A; (ii) A reacts with lipophilic precursor B inside the vesicle to form vesicular molecule V; (iii) new vesicles are generated as V is produced; (iv) generated vesicles are extruded through the membrane to the bulk water. (b) Self-reproducing system of multilamellar vesicle [105,106].

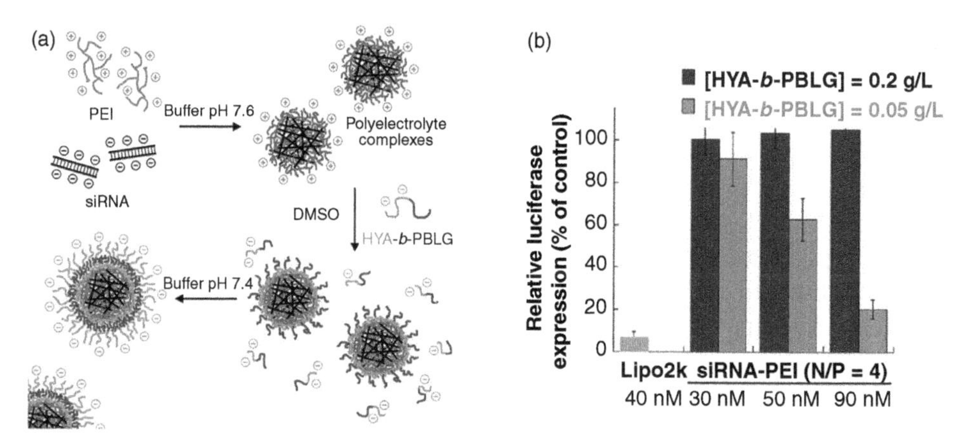

FIGURE 2.1.8 (a) Design of virus-like polymer particles by self-assembling amphiphilic block copolymer molecules around RNA-based polyelectrolyte complexes. (b) Uptake and intracellular distribution of bilayer siRNA–polyethylenimine (PEI) complexes prepared at different concentrations of copolymer into HeLa cells after 24 h of incubation ([siRNA] = 50 nM). Copolymer and siRNA molecules are labeled with fluorescein and Cy5, respectively. Last column: Overlay of DIC (differential interference contrast) and fluorescence images (blue: nuclei stained with DAPI [4′,6-diamidino-2-phenylindole]) [108].

interaction between the amphiphilic block copolymer and a positively charged complex nanoparticle in dimethyl sulfoxide, and (2) construction of a bilayer membrane on the (1)-nanoparticle via a hydrophobic interaction with free amphiphilic block copolymers by increasing water content. The siRNA–polyelectrolyte complexes with bilayer membrane showed high gene silencing activity as compared to that of complexes alone.

2.1.4 Conjugated Nanoparticles

Bioconjugations with synthetic polymers is a versatile way to add new value, advanced features, and unique properties to biomolecules. Especially, smart polymer–protein conjugates have been investigated over the past 30 years. Since the conjugation of smart polymer to single molecule can generate a nanoscale switch, many researchers have conjugated smart polymers to proteins for a great variety of applications in affinity separations, enzyme bioprocesses, drug delivery, diagnostics and biosensors, cell culture processes including tissue engineering, and DNA motors. Biomolecules that can be conjugated with smart polymers include not only proteins but also peptides, polysaccharides, DNA, lipids, etc. Kulkarni et al. observed reversible particle formation and dissolution kinetics of mesoscale PNIPAAm/streptavidin conjugates by DLS [109]. The transition from soluble conjugates to particles was found to be rapid and to occur in a narrow temperature range at the critical point. After reversal of the temperature stimulus, the scattering intensity decreased by more than 90% within 2 min. The particle formation and dissolution kinetics of smart bioconjugates also depends on the concentration. Interestingly, the particles were stable once formed (>16 h) and further dilution at the elevated temperatures did not significantly affect the size of the particles. Particle sizes were comparable for the 25.9, 14.9, and 4.8 kDa conjugates, with no significant change in size with a change in molecular weight. The particle sizes also depend on the molecular weight of the PNIPAm used for conjugation. Conjugates of higher molecular weight polymers form more uniform particles. Smaller particles were formed at higher heating rates, and nanoparticles of fixed sizes could be formed by varying the heating rate. The particles had a wider distribution when formed at lower heating rates. On the other hand, the final temperature did not affect the particle size significantly. These results indicate that the particle size is largely governed by the kinetics of aggregation at defined concentrations and polymer molecular weights.

The switchability of smart polymer conjugates also opens the door to potential uses in microfluidic formats where the differential diffusive and physical properties might be exploited for separation, analyte concentration, and signal generation. Microfluidic platforms have shown promise for conducting diagnostic measurements in both clinical and point-of-care settings. While great strides have been made, the potential of this technology has not yet been fully realized and several challenges remain. One important outstanding need is the handling of dilute antigens and biomarkers, particularly their purification and enrichment from complex biological fluids. A reversible microchannel surface capture system has been further developed for bioanalytical samples [110–112]. The capture/release efficiency and enrichment of PNIPAAm–antibody conjugates in PNIPAAm-grafted poly(dimethylsiloxane) microchannels have been investigated using a helical flow, circular microreactor. The conjugate's immobilization and release were limited by mass transport to and from the functionalized PNIPAAm surface. Transport and adsorption efficiencies were dependent on the aggregate size of the PNIPAAm–streptavidin conjugate above the LCST as well as on whether the conjugates were heated in the presence of the stimuli-responsive surface or preaggregated and then flowed across the surface. Mixing and recirculation substantially increase the conjugate release rate and sharpness once the temperature has dropped below the phase transition temperature. The concentration of protein–polymer conjugates could be achieved by a continuous conjugate flow into the heated recirculator, allowing nearly linear enrichment of the conjugate reagent from larger volumes. This capability was shown with anti-p24 HIV monoclonal antibody reagents that were enriched over five-fold by using this protocol. pH-responsive surface traps have also been constructed in the channel wall by the same methods. These studies provide insight into the mechanism of smart polymer–protein conjugate capture and release in grafted channels and show the potential of this purification and enrichment module for processing diagnostic samples.

2.1.5 Conclusions and Future Trends

This chapter focused on nanoparticles as biomaterials using current reports. Recently, several types of nanoparticle have been developed using new preparation and analysis techniques as unique drug carriers for biomedical fields. These drug carriers possess unique properties, namely, biocompatibilities, long circulation time, active targeting, controlled drug release, and biodegradation for a desirable carrier system. The development of multifunctional nanomaterials using structural designs, controlled self-assemblies, and a few types of raw material is one of our challenges. However, we are convinced that these revolutionary material designs open a new stage in the nanoparticles field.

References

[1] A.S. Hoffman, J. Control. Release 132 (2008) 153.

[2] N. Nishiyama, K. Kataoka, Adv. Polym. Sci. 193 (2006) 67.

[3] H. Ringsdorf, J. Polym. Sci. 51 (1975) 135.

[4] Y. Ikeda, Y. Nagasaki, J. Appl. Polym. Sci. 131 (2014) 40293.

[5] A. Abuchowski, T. Es, N.C. Palczuk, F.F. Davis, J. Biol. Chem. 252 (1977) 3578.

[6] A. Abuchowski, J.R. McCoy, N.C. Palczuk, T. van Es, F.F. Davis, J. Biol. Chem. 252 (1977) 3582.

[7] H. Zhao, B. Rubio, P. Sapra, D. Wu, P. Reddy, P. Sai, A. Martinez, Y. Gao, Y. Lozanguiez, C. Longley, L.M. Greenberger, I.D. Horak, Bioconjug. Chem. 19 (2008) 849.

[8] F. Pastorino, M. Loi, P. Sapra, P. Becherini, M. Cilli, L. Emionite, D. Ribatti, L.M. Greenberger, I.D. Horak, M. Ponzoni, Clin. Cancer Res. 156 (2010) 4809.

[9] E.K. Rowinsky, J. Rizzo, L. Ochoa, C.H. Takimoto, B. Forouzesh, G. Schwartz, L.A. Hammond, A. Patnaik, J. Kwiatek, A. Goetz, L. Denis, J. McGuire, A.W. Tolcher, J. Clin. Oncol. 20 (2003) 148.

[10] L.C. Scott, J.C. Yao, A.B. Benson III, A.L. Thomas, S. Falk, R.R. Mena, J. Picus, J. Wright, M.F. Mulcahy, J.A. Ajani, T.R. Evans, Cancer Chemother. Pharmacol. 63 (2009) 363.

[11] F.M. Veronese, O. Schiavon, G. Pasut, R. Mendichi, L. Andersson, A. Tsirk, J. Ford, G. Wu, S. Kneller, J. Davies, R. Duncan, Bioconjug. Chem. 16 (2005) 775.

[12] G. Pasut, F.M. Veronese, Prog. Polym. Sci. 32 (2007) 933.

[13] E.M. Kopecky, S. Greinstetter, I. Pabinger, A. Buchacher, J. Romisch, A. Jungbauer, Biotechnol. Bioeng. 93 (2006) 647.

[14] K.W. Woodburn, C.P. Holmes, S.D. Wilson, K.L. Fong, R.J. Press, Y. Moriya, Y. Tagawa, Xenobiotica 42 (2012) 660–670.

[15] U.K. Narta, S.S. Kanwar, W. Azmi, Crit. Rev. Oncol. Hematol. 61 (2007) 208.

[16] C.M. Ensor, F.M. Holtsberg, J.S. Bomalaski, M.A. Clark, Cancer Res. 62 (2002) 5443.

[17] F.W. Holtsberg, C.M. Ensor, M.R. Steiner, J.S. Bomalaski, M.A. Clark, J. Control. Release 80 (2002) 259.

[18] P.N. Cheng, T. Lam, W. Lam, S. Tsui, A.W. Cheng, W. Lo, Y. Leung, Cancer Res. 67 (2007) 309.

[19] Y.S. Wang, S. Youngster, M. Grace, J. Bausch, R. Bordens, D.F. Wyss, Adv. Drug Deliv. Rev. 54 (2002) 547.

[20] X.Q. Li, J.D. Lei, A.G. Su, G.H. Ma, Process Biochem. 42 (2007) 1625.

[21] K. Yang, A. Basu, M. Wang, R. Chintala, M.C. Hsieh, S. Liu, J. Hua, Z. Zhang, J. Zhou, M. Li, H. Phyu, G. Petti, M. Mendez, H. Janjua, P. Peng, C. Longley, V. Borowski, M. Mehlig, D. Filpula, Protein Eng. 16 (2003) 761.

[22] A.P. Chapman, Adv. Drug Deliv. Rev. 54 (2002) 531.

[23] E.W. Ng, D.T. Shima, P. Calias, E.T. Cunningham Jr., D.R. Guyer, A.P. Adamis, Nat. Rev. Drug Discov. 5 (2006) 123.

[24] J. Ruckman, L.S. Green, J. Beeson, S. Waugh, W.L. Gillette, D.D. Henninger, L. Claesson-Welsh, N. Janjic, J. Biol. Chem. 273 (1998) 20556.

[25] H. Maeda, J. Wu, T. Sawa, Y. Matsumura, K. Hori, J. Control. Release 65 (2000) 271.

[26] Y. Matsumura, Drug Deliv. Sys. 28 (2013) 215.

[27] D. Schmaljohann, Adv. Drug Deliv. Rev. 58 (2006) 1655.

[28] C.L. Lo, C.K. Huang, K.M. Lin, G.H. Hsiue, Biomaterials 28 (2007) 1225.

[29] Y. Kakizawa, K. Kataoka, Adv. Drug Deliv. Rev. 54 (2002) 203.

[30] S. Fukushima, K. Miyata, N. Nishiyama, N. Kanayama, Y. Yamasaki, K. Kataoka, J. Am. Chem. Soc. 127 (2005) 2810.

[31] M. Oishi, Y. Nagasaki, K. Itaka, N. Nishiyama, K. Kataoka, J. Am. Chem. Soc. 127 (2005) 1624.

[32] S. Guragain, B.P. Bastakoti, S. Yusa, K. Nakashima, Polymer 51 (2010) 3181.

[33] M. Ahmed, Z. Deng, R. Narain, ACS Appl. Mater. Interfaces 9 (2009) 1980.

[34] J. Leleux, R. Krishnendu, Adv. Healthc. Mater. 2 (2013) 72.

[35] T. Yoshitomi, Y. Nagasaki, Adv. Healthc. Mater. 3 (2014) 1149.

[36] K. Kataokaa, A. Haradaa, Y. Nagasaki, Adv. Drug Deliv. Rev. 47 (2001) 113.

[37] G.S. Kwon, T. Okano, Adv. Drug Deliv. Rev. 21 (1996) 107.

[38] S. Chen, S.-X. Cheng, R.-X. Zhuo, Macromol. Biosci. 11 (2011) 576.

[39] M. Yokoyama, T. Okano, Y. Sakurai, K. Kataoka, J. Control. Release 32 (1994) 269.

[40] M. Yokoyama, S. Fukushima, R. Uehara, K. Okamoto, K. Kataoka, Y. Sakurai, T. Okano, J. Control. Release 50 (1998) 79.

[41] A. Harada, K. Kataoka, Macromolecules 28 (1995) 5294.
[42] S. Katayose, K. Kataoka, Bioconjug. Chem. 8 (1997) 702.
[43] S. Takae, K. Miyata, M. Oba, T. Ishii, N. Nishiyama, K. Itaka, Y. Yamasaki, H. Koyama, K. Kataoka, J. Am. Chem. Soc. 130 (2008) 6001.
[44] X. Ye, J. Fei, K. Xu, R. Bai, J. Polym. Sci. Polym. Phys. 48 (2010) 1168.
[45] S.H. Kim, J.P.K. Tan, F. Nederberg, K. Fukushima, Y.Y. Yang, R.M. Waymouth, J.L. Hedrick, Macromolecules 42 (2009) 25.
[46] S.D. Santis, R.D. Ladogana, M. Diociaiuti, G. Masci, Macromolecules 43 (2010) 1992.
[47] Y. Kotsuchibashi, M. Ebara, K. Yamamoto, T. Aoyagi, Polym. Chem. 2 (2011) 1362.
[48] Y. Kotsuchibashi, M. Ebara, N. Idota, R. Narain, T. Aoyagi, Polym. Chem. 3 (2012) 1150.
[49] Y. Kotsuchibashi, M. Ebara, A.S. Hoffman, R. Narain, T. Aoyagi, Polym. Chem. 6 (2015) 1693.
[50] M.O. Oyewumi, A. Kumar, A. Cui, Expert Rev. Vaccines 9 (2010) 1095.
[51] A.A. McCormick, K.E. Palmer, Expert Rev. Vaccines 7 (2008) 33.
[52] D. Harman, J. Gerontol. 11 (1956) 298.
[53] P. Karihtala, Y. Soini, APMIS 115 (2007) 81.
[54] M.C. McDonald, K. Zacharowski, J. Bowes, S. Cuzzocrea, C. Thiemermann, Free Radical Biol. Med. 27 (1999) 493.
[55] N.J. Simmonds, D.S. Rampton, Gut 34 (1993) 865.
[56] D. Singh, K. Chopra, Pharmacol. Res. 50 (2004) 187.
[57] B. Halliwell, Br. J. Exp. Pathol. 70 (1989) 737.
[58] S. Muhammad, A. Bierhaus, M. Schwaninger, J. Alzheimers Dis. 16 (2009) 775.
[59] T. Ishibashi, Curr. Pharm. Des. 19 (2013) 6375.
[60] Q. Liang, A.D. Smith, S. Pan, V.A. Tyurin, V.E. Kagan, T.G. Hastings, N.F. Schor, Biochem. Pharmacol. 70 (2005) 1371.
[61] G. Multhaup, T. Ruppert, A. Schlicksupp, L. Hesse, D. Beher, C.L. Masters, K. Beyreuther, Biochem. Pharmacol. 54 (1997) 533.
[62] B. Halliwell, Free Radical Biol. Med. 46 (2009) 531.
[63] N.C. Park, H.J. Park, K.M. Lee, D.G. Shin, Asian J. Androl. 5 (2003) 195.
[64] Y. Higashi, D. Jitsuiki, K. Chayama, M. Yoshizumi, Recent Pat. Cardiovasc. Drug Discov. 1 (2006) 85.
[65] J.M. Loeffler, R. Ringer, M. Hablutzel, M.G. Tauber, S.L. Leib, J. Infect. Dis. 183 (2001) 247.
[66] L.Y. Dong, J. Jin, G. Lu, X.L. Kang, Mar. Drugs 11 (2013) 960.
[67] E. Monti, R. Supino, M. Colleoni, B. Costa, R. Ravizza, M.B. Gariboldi, J. Cell Biochem. 82 (2001) 271.
[68] C.S. Wilcox, A. Pearlman, Pharmacol. Rev. 60 (2008) 418.
[69] Y. Nagasaki, Therap. Deliv. 3 (2012) 1.
[70] T. Yoshitomi, Y. Nagasaki, Adv. Healthc. Mater. 3 (2014) 1149.
[71] T. Yoshitomi, R. Suzuki, T. Mamiya, H. Matsui, A. Hiryama, Y. Nagasaki, Bioconjug. Chem. 20 (2009) 1792.
[72] K. Toh, T. Yoshitomi, Y. Ikeda, Y. Nagasaki, Sci. Technol. Adv. Mater. 12 (2011) 065001.
[73] A. Mantovani, P. Allavena, A. Sica, F. Balkwill, Nature 454 (2008) 436.
[74] M. Jinushi, S. Chiba, H. Yoshiyama, K. Masutomi, I. Kinoshita, H. Dosaka-Akita, H. Yagita, A. Takaoka, H. Tahara, Proc. Natl. Acad. Sci. USA 108 (2011) 12425.

[75] M. Bentires-Alj, V. Barbu, M. Fillet, A. Chariot, B. Relic, N. Jacobs, J. Gielen, M.P. Merville, V. Bours, Oncogene 22 (2003) 90.

[76] S. Oiso, R. Ikeda, K. Nakamura, Y. Takeda, S. Akiyama, H. Kariyazono, Oncol. Rep. 28 (2012) 27.

[77] T. Yoshitomi, Y. Ozaki, S. Thangavel, Y. Nagasaki, J. Control. Release 172 (2013) 137.

[78] T. Yoshitomi, A. Hirayama, Y. Nagasaki, Biomaterials 32 (2011) 8021.

[79] S. Sha, L.B. Vong, P. Chonpathompikunlert, T. Yoshitomi, H. Matsui, Y. Nagasaki, Biomaterials 34 (2013) 8393.

[80] D.E. Disher, A. Eisenberg, Science 297 (2002) 967.

[81] J. Du, R.K. O'Reilly, Soft Matter 5 (2009) 3544.

[82] B.M. Disher, Y. Won, D.S. Ege, J.C. Lee, F.S. Bates, D.E. Disher, D.A. Hammer, Science 284 (1999) 1143.

[83] A. Blanazs, S.P. Armes, A.J. Ryan, Macromol. Rapid Commun. 30 (2009) 267.

[84] V. Ladmiral, M. Semsarilar, I. Canton, S.P. Armes, J. Am. Chem. Soc. 135 (2013) 13574.

[85] H. Wei, S. Perrier, S. Dehn, R. Ravariana, F. Dehghani, Soft Matter 8 (2012) 9526.

[86] C. Pietsch, U. Mansfeld, Macromolecules 45 (2012) 9292.

[87] E.G. Bellomo, M.D. Wyrsta, L. Pakstis, D.J. Pochan, T.J. Deming, Nat. Mater. 3 (2004) 244.

[88] T.J. Deming, J. Polym. Sci. Polym. Chem. Ed. 38 (2000) 3011.

[89] A.P. Nowak, V. Breedveld, L. Pakstis, B. Ozbas, D.J. Pine, D. Pochan, T.J. Deming, Nature 417 (2002) 424.

[90] J.N. Cha, G.D. Stucky, D.E. Morse, T.J. Deming, Nature 403 (2000) 289.

[91] M.C. Martos-Maldonado, J.M. Casas-Solvas, I. Quesada-Soriano, L. García-Fuentes, A. Vargas-Berenguel, Langmuir 29 (4) (2013) 1318.

[92] V. Percec, P. Leowanawat, H.-J. Sun, O. Kulikov, C.D. Nusbaum, T.M. Tran, A. Bertin, D.A. Wilson, M. Peterca, S. Zhang, N.P. Kamat, K. Vargo, D. Moock, E.D. Johnston, D.A. Hammer, D.J. Pochan, Y. Chen, Y.M. Chabre, T.C. Shiao, M. Bergeron-Brlek, S. André, R. Roy, H.-J. Gabius, P.A. Heiney, J. Am. Chem. Soc. 135 (2013) 9055.

[93] G. Weissman, G. Sessa, M. Standish, A.D. Bangham, J. Clin. Invest. 44 (1965) 1109.

[94] T. Oberholzer, K.H. Nierhaus, P.L. Luisi, Biochem. Biophys. Res. Commun. 261 (1999) 238.

[95] A. Fischer, A. Franco, T. Oberholzer, Chem. Biol. Chem. 3 (2002) 409.

[96] S.M. Nomura, K. Tsumoto, T. Hamada, K. Akiyoshi, Y. Nakatani, K. Yoshikawa, Chem. Biol. Chem. 4 (2003) 1172.

[97] M. Nallani, S. Benito, O. Onaca, A. Graff, M. Lindemann, M. Winterhalter, W. Meier, U. Schwaneberg, J. Biotechnol. 123 (2006) 50.

[98] H.-J. Choi, C.D. Montemagno, Nano Lett. 5 (2005) 2538.

[99] D.M. Vriezema, P.M.L. Garcia, N.S. Oltra, N.S. Hatzakis, S.M. Kuiper, R.J.M. Nolte, A.E. Rowan, J.C.M. Hest, Angew. Chem. Int. Ed. 46 (2007) 7378.

[100] H.J. Choi, C.D. Montemagno, Nano Lett. 5 (2005) 2538.

[101] P. Mitchell, Nature 191 (1961) 144.

[102] R.L. Cross, Annu. Rev. Biochem. 50 (1981) 681.

[103] J.H. Wang, Annu. Rev. Biophys. Bioeng. 12 (1983) 21.

[104] P.D. Boyer, Annu. Rev. Biochem. 66 (1997) 717.

[105] K. Takakura, T. Toyota, T. Sugawara, J. Am. Chem. Soc. 125 (2003) 8134.

[106] K. Takakura, T. Sugawara, Langmuir 20 (2004) 3832.

[107] K. Kurihara, M. Tamura, K. Shohda, T. Toyota, K. Suzuki, T. Sugawara, Nat. Chem. 3 (2011) 775.

[108] L. Bui, S. Abbou, E. Ibarboure, N. Guidolin, C. Staedel, J.J. Toulmé, S. Lecommandoux, C. Schatz, J. Am. Chem. Soc. 134 (2012) 20189.

[109] S. Kulkarni, C. Schilli, A.H.E. Müller, A.S. Hoffman, P.S. Stayton, Bioconjug. Chem. 15 (2004) 747.

[110] M. Ebara, J.M. Hoffman, A.S. Hoffman, P.S. Stayton, Lab Chip 6 (2006) 843.

[111] M. Ebara, J.M. Hoffman, P.S. Stayton, A.S. Hoffman, Radiat. Phys. Chem. 76 (2007) 1409.

[112] M. Ebara, A.S. Hoffman, P.S. Stayton, J.J. Lai, Langmuir 29 (2013) 5388.

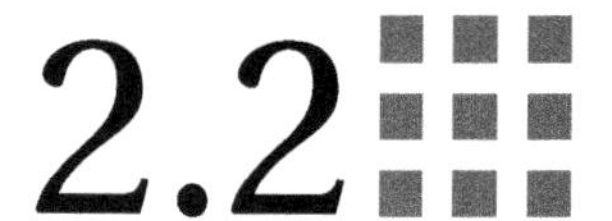

Supermolecules

Katsuhiko Ariga

INTERNATIONAL CENTER FOR MATERIALS NANOARCHITECTONICS (MANA), NATIONAL INSTITUTE FOR MATERIALS SCIENCE (NIMS), TSUKUBA, JAPAN

CHAPTER OUTLINE

2.2.1 Introduction: Basics of Supramolecular Chemistry

Supramolecular chemistry is defined as chemistry beyond the molecule. This research field was initialized in the last century by many researchers in combined research fields, including Nobel Prize winners Lehn, Cram, and Pedersen [1–4]. One of them, Lehn, invented the word supermolecule, whereby supramolecular chemistry is chemistry beyond the molecule bearing on the organized entities of higher complexity that result from the association of two or more chemical species held together by intermolecular forces. Supramolecular structures are a result of various noncovalent interactions, including van der Waals interaction, electrostatic interaction, hydrogen bonding, hydrophobic interaction, coordination, etc., some of which are often cooperatively working in one supramolecular complex. More importantly, properties of the formed supramolecular complexes are far beyond summation of the individual components.

Since supramolecular complexes are based upon various interactions, the sizes of supermolecules differ widely from molecular size to macroscopic size (Fig. 2.2.1). The smallest category of supermolecules is the so-called host–guest complex. Host–guest complexes are pairs of molecules and/or ions that are specifically associated through molecular recognition. Molecular recognition was discussed to some extent in the middle of the nineteenth century. A clear milestone for the origin of molecular recognition is considered to be the proposal of the lock and key principle by Emil Fischer in 1894. Similarly, it was known in 1950s that natural products can recognize particular molecules, including the

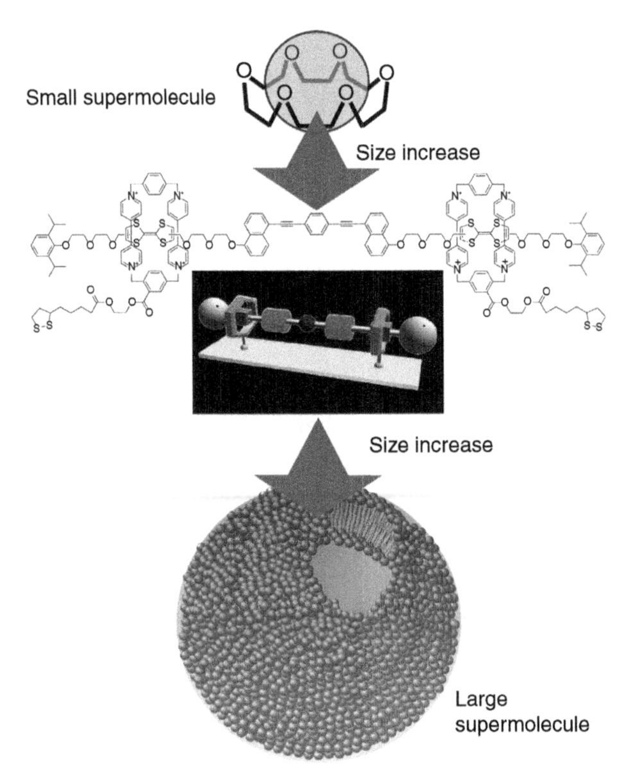

FIGURE 2.2.1 Various supramolecular systems from small host–guest complex to large molecular assembly.

recognition capability of cyclic oligosaccharide cyclodextrin and cyclic oligopeptide valinomycin. Charles Pedersen discovered crown ether to be the first artificial host molecule capable of molecular recognition in 1967. Donald Cram established a new field of chemistry, host–guest chemistry, through developing this concept to wide range of molecular systems. Finally, in 1978, Jean-Marie Lehn combined related chemical fields, including host–guest chemistry and molecular assembly chemistry into supramolecular chemistry.

Molecular association is not limited to two or three molecules. The extension of specific molecular recognition to open structural formation induces molecular association with infinite numbers of molecules to make materials with regular internal structures. Formation of hydrogen bonding and/or coordination linkage at multiple sites of component molecules results in important supramolecular materials such as regularly structured crystals, metal–organic frameworks, and porous coordination polymers. These types of strict molecular association create molecular assemblies with defined structures, which are sometimes called programmed assemblies.

On the other hand, molecular association with rather ambiguous molecular interaction such as hydrophobic interactions in aqueous media lead to the formation of flexible and soft assemblies. Typical examples are assemblies of surfactants and amphiphiles. Molecules with an amphiphilic nature possess a hydrophilic part and a hydrophobic part in one molecule, which induces formation of rather ambiguous molecular assemblies in aqueous media. Their simplest form is micelle, where amphiphiles self-assemble to expose their hydrophilic part to water and shield the other part from water according to minimization of total energy. Similarly, lipid bilayer structures can be spontaneously formed to be spherical hollow capsules with huge numbers of component molecules. Since these assemblies are usually very flexible and capable of accommodation of certain kinds of drug molecules, they are often used as carriers for drug delivery systems (DDS). This kind of science of molecular assemblies was started from findings by A.D. Bangham in 1964. Dispersion of lipid molecules extracted from cells in water spontaneously forms a cell-like assembly, the so-called liposome. Later, Kunitake and Okahata demonstrated the formation of similar assembly from various artificial amphiphiles in 1977 [5]. The latter assembly is often called vesicle. Liposomes and vesicles have essentially the same structural features.

These spontaneous processes of molecular assemblies are often combined with intentional processes of nanostructure formation. Representative techniques and methods are fabrications of self-assembled monolayers, Langmuir–Blodgett (LB) films, and layer-by-layer (LbL) assemblies [6]. As described later in this chapter, these methods are powerful for the modification and decoration of material surfaces and constructing hierarchic structures. This combined approach creates a strong tool to make functional materials useful for certain kinds of biorelated applications, including drug delivery.

In addition, many biological systems share common working principles with supramolecular chemistry because both biological systems and supramolecular systems rely heavily on molecular interactions. Therefore, artificial supramolecular systems mimicking biological systems have been extensively researched, as seen in molecular transport, information transmission and conversion, energy conversion, and molecular conversion (enzymatic function). In other words, we can say that the best supramolecular system is the living being, that is, the ultimately successful supramolecular assemblies are ourselves. Therefore, strategies relying on supramolecular chemistry for development of biomedical applications are reasonable.

With these backgrounds, we can understand the critical importance of supramolecular chemistry in biomaterials nanoarchitectonics. In this chapter, we focus on supramolecular strategies for drug delivery functions as typical examples of biorelated and/or biomolecule-included examples. In addition to DDS and related functions using standard host–guest complexes and molecular assemblies, drug release controls from supramolecular materials by mechanical stimuli are included as forefront examples.

2.2.2 Drug Delivery Systems With Host–Guest Systems

The formation of a host–guest complex based on molecular recognition is a reversible process that is highly appropriate for drug accommodation and release. Therefore, control of molecular interactions between hosts and guest resulted in regulated drug release function.

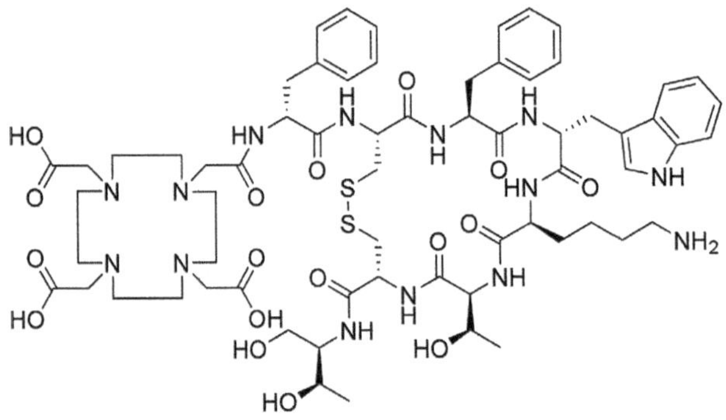

FIGURE 2.2.2 Host molecule for medical diagnostics and tumor targeting.

For molecular recognition, various molecular interactions play crucial roles as seen in electrostatic interactions between charged molecules. Even in the absence of net charges, dipole–dipole and dipole–ion interactions have an unavoidable contribution. In many biological systems, hydrogen bonding sometimes plays the most important role in the discrimination of specific molecules. Hydrogen bonding is a kind of dipole–dipole interaction where positively polarized hydrogen atoms in hydroxyl (OH) groups or amino groups ($-NH_2-$) interact strongly with other electron-rich atoms (O in C=O, N in CN). Such an interaction is unfavorable in polar media like aqueous solutions, because the strength of charge–charge interactions is in inverse proportion to the dielectric constant of the surrounding medium. Therefore, placing host–guest systems in rather nonpolar hydrophobic media such as the interior of a lipid membrane and polymers becomes an advantageous strategy. In addition, it has been proved that the interfacial environment of hydrophobic media enhances these charge-based and/or dipole-based interactions. Therefore, considerations on surrounding environments for host–guest systems are important. In addition to these interactions, van der Waals interactions, coordinate interactions, hydrophobic interactions, π–π interactions, and halogen bonding are frequently used for the design of host–guest systems.

Typical host molecules for molecular entrapments are certain kinds of cyclic molecules. For example, cyclodextrins are natural products with the capability of accommodating guest drugs in their interior cavity. Chemical modification of cyclodextrins' hosts often improved their usefulness by altering their solubility with enhancing capacity for the guest drugs. Therefore, cyclodextrin deliveries are regarded as useful host molecules in DDS. Not limited to such natural cyclic host molecules, various cyclic molecules based on organic syntheses have been used for medial uses. As shown in Fig. 2.2.2, Mäcke and coworkers proposed use of (tetraazacyclododecane-1,4,7,10-tetraacetic acid)-functionalized somatostatin (an abundant neuropeptide) analog for medical diagnostics and tumor targeting [7]. This host molecule can entrap a variety of transition metal cations as magnetic resonance imaging-active elements. Such metal-included host–guest complexes have a rich diversity of methods for encoding both structural and dynamic molecular information. Sadler and coworkers used the bis-tetraazamacrocycle xylyl-bicyclam for entrapment of

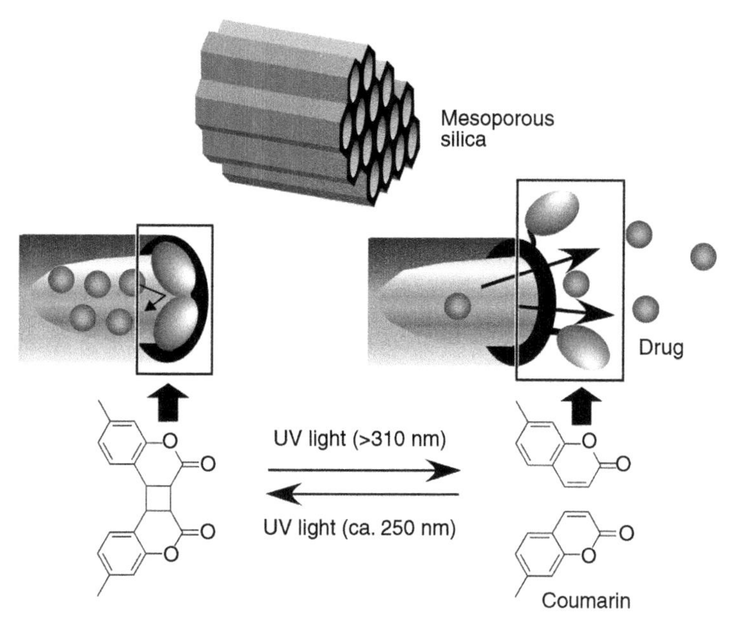

FIGURE 2.2.3 Control of drug release from mesopore channel by coumarin supramolecular gate.

transition metal cations, especially Zn(II), as a potent anti-HIV agent [8]. The obtained results on anti-HIV activities of these xylyl-bicyclam complexes having various metal ions indicated the importance of several factors including affinity for carboxylates, configurational flexibility, and kinetic factors.

Coupling of host–guest molecular systems with drug-carrier materials would create efficient controlled release systems of drugs. Attaching supramolecular elements as gates at the surfaces of carrier materials induces controlled release of target drugs from inside the carrier materials based on host–guest interaction. As carrier materials for this strategy, nanoporous materials with large surface areas and pore volumes can be appropriate candidates for this purpose. For example, mesoporous silica materials have been investigated as drug-carrier materials. Mesopore channels of mesoporous silica materials possess defined diameters over the length range from nanometers to tens of nanometers, which are appropriate for drug accommodation. Huge pore volumes per unit mass of mesoporous material are surely advantageous for drug storage. Through modification of inlets of channels with host–guest gate functional groups, the decorated materials may become ideal carriers for controlled release by external stimuli.

As pioneering work, Fujiwara and coworkers demonstrated photo-controlled regulation of drug storage and release from mesoporous silica functionalized with photoactive coumarin functional group at the pore outlet (Fig. 2.2.3) [9]. Guest drugs such as cholestane can be entrapped into the mesopores that are kept in the mesoporous carriers with closed gates upon formation of coumarin dimers by irradiation of ultraviolet (UV) light. Irradiation of UV light results in cleavage of the coumarin dimers and induces release of cholestane drugs from mesopores inside. Lin and coworkers proposed a controlled-release delivery system using colloid capping methods on mesoporous silica materials [10]. Gates of the proposed systems consist of a 2-(propyldisulfanyl)ethylamine functional group on a mesoporous silica nanosphere. The modified surface can capture and release the water-soluble mercaptoacetic acid-derivatized cadmium sulfide nanocrystals upon formation of disulfide linkages and their chemical cleavage. Controlled delivery of a neurotransmitter drug was successfully demonstrated as well as *in vitro* biocompatibility with neuroglial cells (astrocytes).

Martínez-Máñez and coworkers immobilized polyamines on mesoporous solid support-controlled entrapment and release of guest ions and ions [11]. Release of guest molecules depends greatly on protonation of polyamines, adjusted by sounding pH values, and supramolecular complex formation with stimuli molecules. In the latter mode, addition of aqueous adenosine triphosphate (ATP), adenosine diphosphate (ADP), and guanosine monophosphate (GMP) induces effective pore blockage. Efficiency of the pore blockage was observed depending on the strength of supramolecular interactions between polyamines and nucleotides (ATP > ADP > GMP). Stoddart and coworkers used pseudorotaxanes as gates at the entrances of the cylindrical pores in mesostructured silica materials [12] (Fig. 2.2.4). The [2]pseudorotaxane in the form of a tethered 1,5-dioxynaphthalene-containing derivative, acting as the gatepost, and cyclobis(paraquat-*p*-phenylene), which recognizes dioxynaphthalene, controls access in and out of the nanopores. Addition of external reducing reagents such as sodium cyanoborohydride can open the nanovalve inducing release of guest molecules from mesopores inside to external medium.

2.2.3 Drug Delivery Systems With Supramolecular Assemblies

Soft and flexible molecular assemblies are regarded as powerful carriers of drug delivery. Micelles are the simplest of molecular assemblies that can accommodate hydrophobic drugs. Especially, polymer micelles without using toxic small surfactants have been paid much attention from the viewpoints of their practical uses. As more advanced assemblies, liposomes and lipid vesicles with bilayer shell structures can accommodate both hydrophilic within an interior aqueous phase and hydrophobic drugs in their lipid bilayer shells. Usages of these supramolecular assemblies for drug delivery functions are extensively described elsewhere.

As a powerful methodology to assemble various components into soft supramolecular organizations, the LbL assembly method shows continuous progresses in the fields of drug delivery under the supramolecular concept (Fig. 2.2.5). The LbL method has excellent versatility for the assembly of various kinds of substances [13]. This method covers a wide range of available materials including proteins, nucleic acids, saccharides, virus particles micelles, vesicles, LB films, and other lipid membranes as well as conventional polyelectrolytes, conductive polymers, inorganic nanomaterials, nanocarbons, and dye

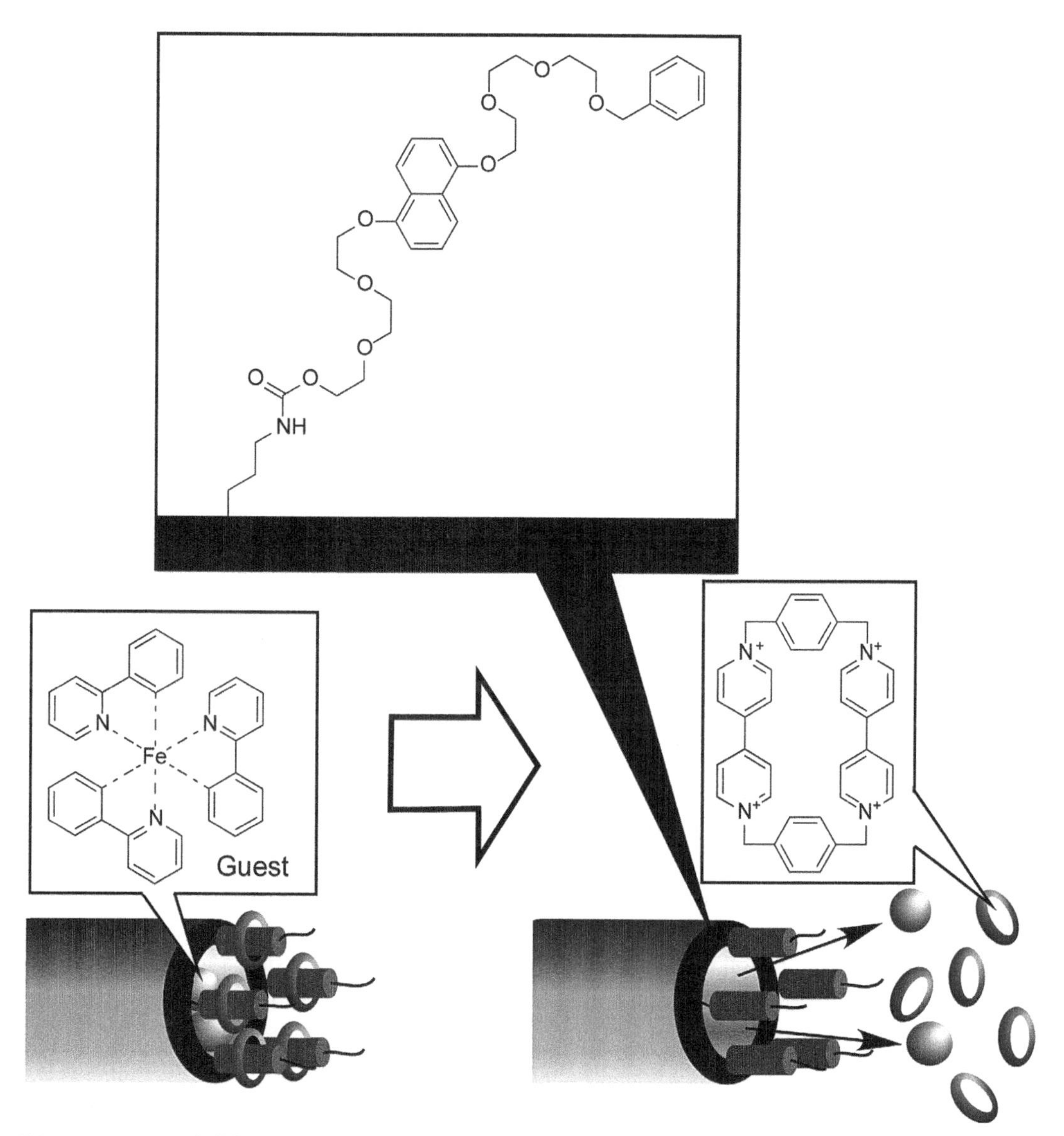

FIGURE 2.2.4 Control of drug release from mesopore channel by rotaxane supramolecular gate.

aggregates. It can be regarded as one of the most powerful methods for fabrication of supermolecular assemblies. Electrostatic attraction is most frequently used as a driving force of LbL processes. Not limited to typical electrostatic interaction, various interactions such as hydrogen bonding, metal coordination, charge transfer, stereo-complex formation, supramolecular inclusion, and biospecific recognition can be applied to LbL assembly. In most cases, LbL assembly can be performed using a low-cost experimental set-up using only beakers and tweezers. Spin coating, spraying, and automatic processes are also

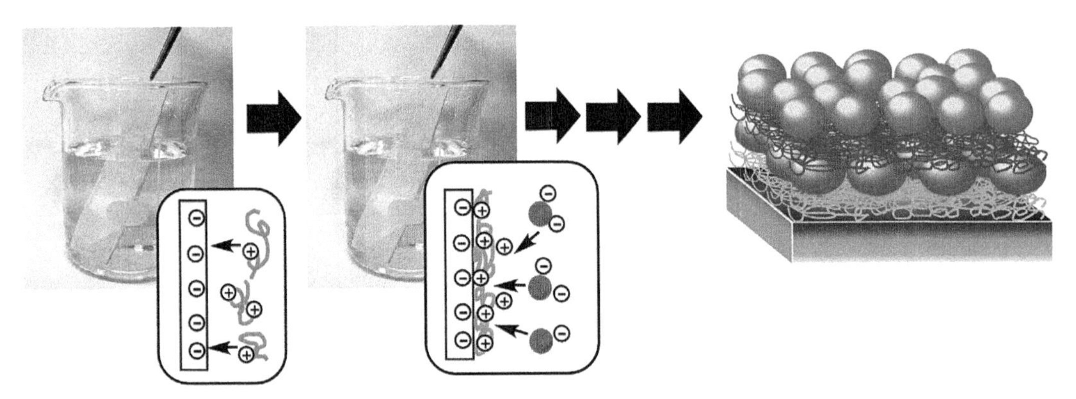

FIGURE 2.2.5 Outline of LbL assembly.

possible. Since LbL processes require only mild conditions for film construction, structural disturbances during assembling processes can be minimized, even the direct use of biomaterials. This LbL method can provide ultrathin films with designable layer sequence through costless and simple procedures.

LbL assembly is a powerful method to fabricate hierarchic assemblies, too. Ji and coworkers demonstrated the construction of a capsule in layer structures through LbL assemblies of mesoporous silica capsules with organic polyelectrolytes with the aid of coassembly of silica nanoparticles (Fig. 2.2.6) [14]. In the presented systems, mesoporous hollow silica capsules possessing capsule interiors (1000 × 700 × 300 nm) and mesopores of average diameter 2.2 nm at the shells were assembled into layered structures. Water and liquid guest molecules can be entrapped within mesopore capsules. Release of entrapped materials to the air was quantitatively investigated using quartz crystal microbalance to provide unusual guest release profiles where on/off-type stepwise release profiles were observed even upon application of no external stimuli. In the initial step, guest molecules entrapped in mesopore channels at the external shell were preferentially released to the outside. Only after most of the guest molecules were released from the mesopore channels did supply of water from the capsule interior into the mesopores become possible. This process is driven through rapid capillary penetration. These processes are repeated resulting in the on/off-type stepwise release of guest molecules. This type of stimulus-free controlled release system has never been well explored. However, this concept would be of great utility for the development of energy less and clean stimuli-free drug release applications.

Use of the LbL assembly is not limited to fabrication of thin films on flat substrates. It can be applied to a microsized colloidal particle core to prepare hollow capsules, which are expected to be highly useful for DDS applications. In this innovative strategy, LbL films are assembled sequentially on a colloidal core similar to the conventional LbL assemblies on a flat substrate. Destruction of the central particle core after completion of the LbL assembly results in formation of hollow capsule structures. Figure 2.2.7 illustrates one example to prepare a biocompatible polyelectrolyte microcapsule with DNA encapsulation by Lvov and coworkers [15]. In their approach, water-insoluble DNA/spermidine complexes were

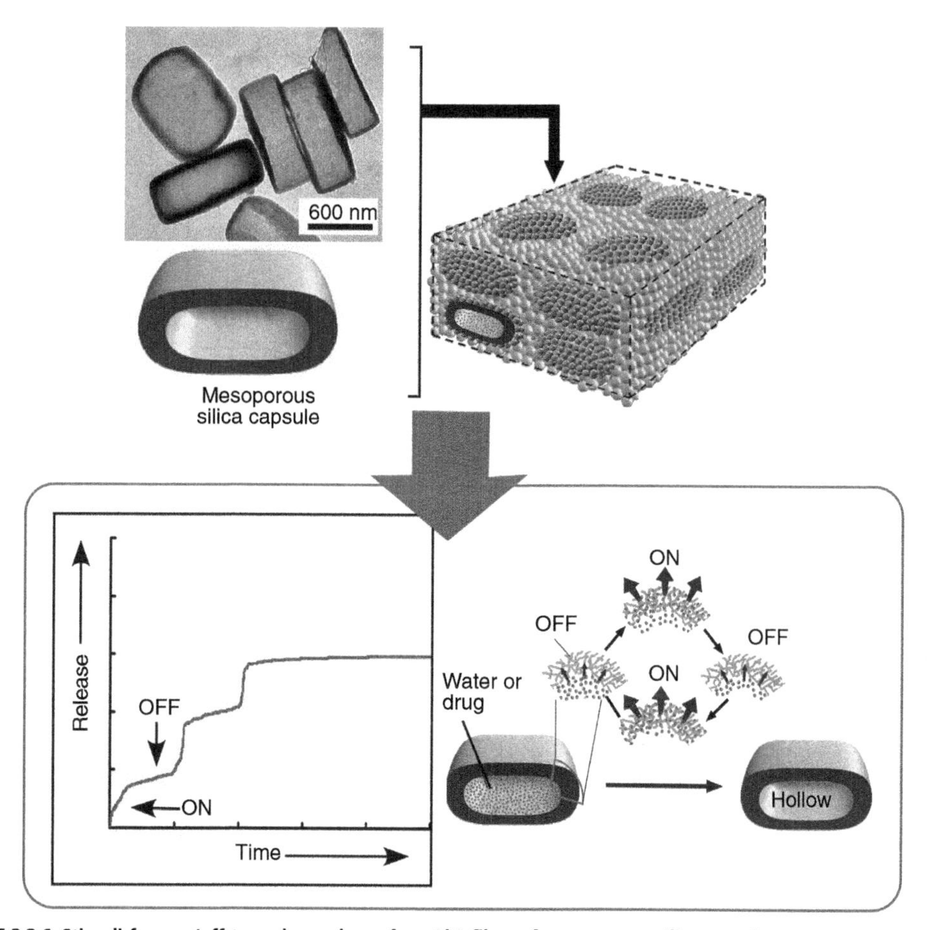

FIGURE 2.2.6 Stimuli-free on/off-type drug release from LbL films of mesoporous silica capsule.

first precipitated onto manganese (II) carbonate ($MnCO_3$) template core particles on which LbL assemblies of biocompatible polyarginine and chondroitin sulfate were next conducted. Destruction and dissolution of the central $MnCO_3$ core particle led to formation of a hollow capsule with biocompatible shells with DNA/spermidine complex inside the capsule. Further dissociation of the DNA/spermidine complex resulted in selective release of low-molecular-weight spermidine and selective entrapment of DNA.

Since the hollow capsule form of LbL assemblies has high potential in DDS application, research efforts to develop LbL functional capsules for DDS applications have been continuously performed. Raichur and coworkers fabricated hydrogen-bonded LbL microcapsules of poly(vinyl pyrrolidone) and poly(methacrylic acid) for encapsulation and release of the antituberculosis drug rifampicin using [16]. A burst type of drug release was observed above pH 7 upon rapid disintegration of the capsule structures. Control of drug release upon application of external stimulus has been extensively investigated. For example, Zhang and coworkers fabricated magnetically sensitive alginate-templated

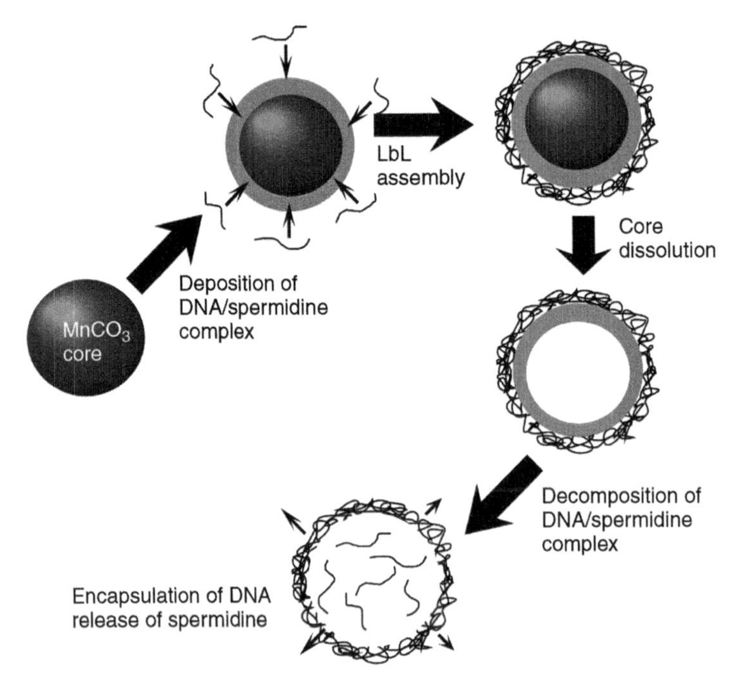

FIGURE 2.2.7 LbL assembly on a colloidal core to prepare hollow capsules and entrapment of DNA.

polyelectrolyte LbL microcapsules [17]. Release of doxorubicin drug from the prepared capsules was significantly accelerated upon application of a high-frequency magnetic field. Choi and coworkers prepared photosensitive LbL microcapsules based on inclusion photoacid generators in the capsule shells. Irradiation to UV light of the capsules led to activation of photoacid generators, inducing protons release from the shells. The resulting pH drops triggered a swelling of the microcapsules. Alternate processes between UV light irradiation and washing with neutral water resulted in control of drug release. When UV light was irradiated for a long time, decomposition of the microcapsules caused accelerated release of the entrapped drugs.

However, LbL microcapsules usually have their diameters in the ranges from micron to submicron size, although injection of drug carriers requires much smaller diameters of drug carriers. There is currently only a limited number of nanoscale delivery systems established for the continuous sustained release of drugs. Therefore, nanoformulation of insoluble drugs, such as paclitaxel, tamoxifen, dexamethasone, and camptothecin, is in demand for practical drug delivery. Lvov and coworkers developed a methodology for the preparation of LbL nanocapsules for cancer drugs. In their approach, powerful ultrasonic treatment is applied to aqueous suspensions of insoluble drugs to prepare nanosized cores [18]. Successful assemblies of ultra-thin polyelectrolyte shells onto the nanosized drug particles were performed through sequential addition of polycations and polyanions to the particle solution. This method resulted in preparation of multilayer nanocapsules with thicknesses of 5–50 nm and requisite composition.

They also realized the fabrication of stable nanocolloids of tamoxifen and paclitaxel with high drug content (up to 90 wt%) covered with LbL multilayer shells [19]. In this case, sustainable release of the drug with a release rate in the range of 10–20 h can be regulated though varying thicknesses of multilayer shells. As another method of nanoparticle formulation for low water-soluble drugs, they reported encapsulation of curcumin and paclitaxel that were first dissolved in a water-miscible organic solvent such as ethanol and acetone, and drug nucleation was initiated by the addition of aqueous polyelectrolyte under powerful ultrasonication [20]. Then, the resulting nanoparticles were coated with biocompatible polyelectrolytes in an LbL manner. This system realized sustained drug release over 25 h.

2.2.4 Interfacial Supramolecular Systems for Mechanically Controlled Drug Delivery Systems

Stimuli-responsive supramolecular systems have realized various successful results of DDS applications with on-demand control with external signals such as thermal, photonic, magnetic, and sonic stimuli. These systems often request usages of special facilities and/or instrumentation. It may limit availability of DDS systems under unsatisfied conditions including uses in economically developing countries and in emergency situations. Therefore, materials that respond to simple or commonly available stimuli for DDS applications have to be developed. One of the easiest and common stimuli to apply would be manual mechanical forces. For example, we use actions of pushing, pulling, bending, pressing, and twisting all the time. Developing materials systems for DDS based on these simple stimuli is important.

Incorporation of supramolecular functions into soft deformable materials would realize mechanically controllable supramolecular behaviors for DDS functions. Among various materials, gels are soft and structurally flexible materials with a specific feature of highly developed covalent and/or noncovalent networks at their interiors. Such gel materials could be ideal materials for mechanical stimuli-responsive release of target drugs because of their large changes in volume and morphology with mechanical stress. In order to construct materials for mechanical control of specific host–guest systems within gel structures, Kawakami and coworkers fabricated alginate gel materials cross-linked with β-cyclodextrin (Fig. 2.2.8) [21]. Cyclodextrin is a typical host structure to accommodate the guest molecule in a shape- and size-specific fashion. In their strategy, guest-included cyclodextrin moieties are used as joints of cross-linking points of the gel. Mechanical deformation of the entire gel induces perturbation of host–guest interaction with cyclodextrin and a drug guest.

To demonstrate this, a selected drug, ondansetron, was first included within the cyclodextrin cores embedded in the alginate gel. Release profiles of the ondansetron drug were then investigated upon compression of the gel with gentle pressures in various sequences and frequencies. Repeated single compression action after intervals of 1, 4, 7, and

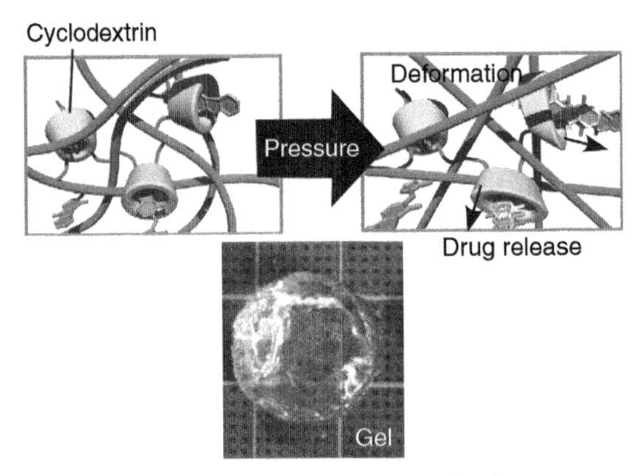

FIGURE 2.2.8 Mechanical control of drug release from cyclodextrin-based gel.

10 h accelerates drug release, where drug release was observed only at the moments of pressure application. On the other hand, application of five-cycle compression actions after 25, 28, 31, 34, 49, and 52 h resulted in pulsatile releases in response to the compression cycles. Binding constants for the supramolecular complex formation within the alginate gel showed clear correlation with the stress–strain curve. The binding constants decrease dramatically under strains above 50%, while these constants remain constant upon application of strains up to 30%. As a future goal, intravenous injection of the proposed system would lead to the development of materials with which patients themselves can control drug release by using their own hands. This strategy can be regarded as a novel dosing strategy for improvement of patient compliance.

As the final topic of this chapter, the future-oriented approach of mechanically controlled DDS and sensing using molecular machines is presented. Molecular machines are certain kinds of state-of-the-art objects in current organic chemistry, supramolecular chemistry, and nanotechnology. A single molecule and/or a complex formed with a couple of molecules work as a machine in ultrasmall dimensions. However, most research efforts on molecular machines stay within the fine science level, and practical uses of molecular machines are still at the dream level. If we can control functions of molecular machines by conventional mechanical actions such as hand motions, it would open the way to common uses of molecular machines in daily life. In order to realize mechanical control of molecular machines, it would be required to couple two kinds of motions over very different length scales, that is, mechanical motions in meter or centimeter size and molecular motions in nanometer scale have to be combined. It can be rationally done if we use a two-dimensional medium where in-plane directions possess macroscopically visible dimensions and their thicknesses are maintained in the nanometer region [22]. Manual control of molecular machines can be accomplished at dynamic two-dimensional media.

As a pioneering model, one kind of molecular machine, steroid cyclophane, was embedded at the air–water interface as a dynamic interface, to demonstrate capture and release of a target guest molecule through macroscopic mechanical motions (Fig. 2.2.9) [23]. The steroid cyclophane machine possesses a cyclic core consisting of a 1,6,20,25-tetraaza[6.1.6.1]

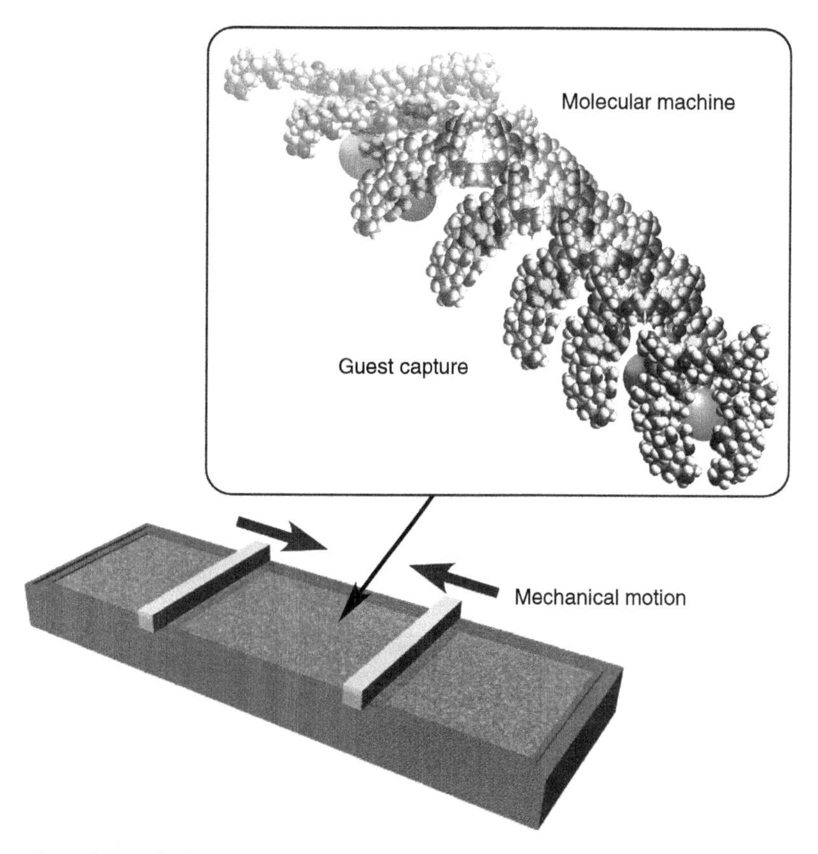

FIGURE 2.2.9 Mechanical control of guest capture and release by molecular machine at interfacial medium.

paracyclophane connected to four steroid (cholic acid) moieties via a flexible L-lysine spacer. Since the molecular plane of cholic acid has a hydrophilic face and a hydrophobic face, the steroid cyclophane machine adopts its open conformation at low pressures though favorably contacting its hydrophilic face to the water surface. Application of lateral pressures induces conformational change of the steroid cyclophane machine from open form to cavity form upon flexible bending of spacer moieties. Since the formed cavity is capable of accommodating specific molecules such as naphthalene derivatives, target molecules can be captured into the cavity of the steroid cyclophane machine upon macroscopic mechanical motions. Furthermore, capture and release can be reversibly repeated upon conversion of machine conformation between open and cavity under controlled macroscopic mechanical motions. Using this concept, it would become possible to regulate delivery and capture of drugs along with molecular machine operations by visible-size mechanical motions such as hand motions.

Not limited to molecular capture and release, the similar concept can be applied for mechanical control of drug discrimination. For example, mechanical control of chiral discrimination of amino acids was demonstrated using a polycholesteryl-substituted

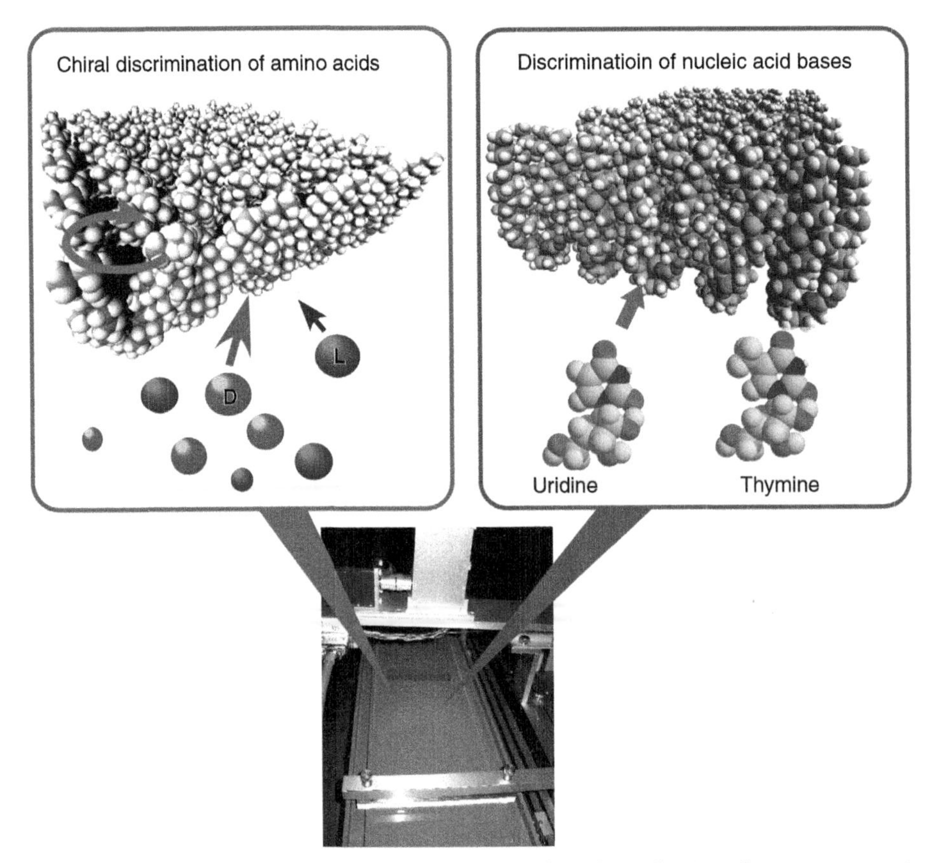

FIGURE 2.2.10 Control of fine discrimination of biomolecules through mechanical tuning of receptor-type molecular machines.

cyclen as a molecular machine at the air–water interface (Fig. 2.2.10) [24]. This molecular machine adopts twisting motions with two possible quadruple helicate structures that can be tuned by macroscopic lateral mechanical motions. Upon mechanical compression of the monolayer of the polycholesteryl-substituted cyclen machine, detection selectivity converted from D- to L-form in the case of valine. Similarly, by using a cholesterol-armed triazacyclononane as a molecular machine component, sensitive discrimination between thymine and uracil was realized [25] although natural DNA and RNA cannot discriminate between these two nucleic acid bases.

In most cases of molecular recognition, stable crystal structures are only considered and therefore one host molecule basically has one type of recognition capability. Switching between several metastable states to modulate molecular recognition behaviors has been also reported. Unlike these past examples, the presented mechanical control of molecular recognition can be regarded as operating in tuning modes where purposed recognition can be optimized among numerous conformational candidates based on mechanical tuning of soft molecular structures.

2.2.5 Conclusions and Future Perspectives

This chapter explained contributions of supramolecular chemistry to biomaterials nanoarchitectonics mainly based on DDS functions. Supramolecular chemistry deals with noncovalent interactions that support specific host–guest molecular recognition and the dynamic nature of molecular assemblies. These features are advantageous in designs of smart responsive controlled release systems of drug molecules. These spontaneous assembling systems are sometimes combined with techniques for intentional materials organization such as LbL assemblies. As a recently emerging approach, mechanically controllable drug release systems were introduced in the final part of the chapter. Considering the interfacial environment, macroscopic mechanical motions can be coupled with molecular motions. Therefore, controls of host–guest interaction and molecular machine functions by conventional actions such as hand motions become possible based on interracial supramolecular designs. These emerging strategies could be called hand-operating nanotechnology as a symbolized concept to express the importance on regulation of nanosystems by conventional common actions [26,27].

References

[1] K. Ariga, T. Kunitake, Supramolecular Chemistry: Fundamentals and Applications, Springer-Verlag, Berlin, 2006.

[2] C.J. Pedersen, Angew. Chem. Int. Ed. Engl. 27 (1988) 1021.

[3] J.-M. Lehn, Angew. Chem. Int. Ed. Engl. 27 (1988) 89.

[4] D.J. Cram, Angew. Chem. Int. Ed. Engl. 27 (1988) 1009.

[5] T. Kunitake, Y. Okahata, J. Am. Chem. Soc. 99 (1977) 3860.

[6] K. Ariga (Ed.), Organized Organic Thin Films: Fundamentals and Applications, Wiley-VCH, Berlin, 2012.

[7] A. Heppeler, S. Froidevaux, H.R. Mäcke, E. Jermann, M. Behe, P. Powell, M. Hennig, Chem. Eur. J. 5 (1999) 1974.

[8] X.Y. Liang, J.A. Parkinson, M. Weishaupl, R.O. Gould, S.J. Paisey, H.S. Park, H.T.M. Hunter, C.A. Blindauer, S. Parsons, P.J. Sadler, J. Am. Chem. Soc. 124 (2002) 9105.

[9] N.K. Mal, M. Fujiwara, Y. Tanaka, Nature 421 (2003) 350.

[10] C.-Y. Lai, B.G. Trewryn, D.M. Jeftinija, K. Jeftinija, S. Xu, S. Jeftinija, V.S.-Y. Lin, J. Am. Chem. Soc. 125 (2003) 4451.

[11] R. Casasús, E. Aznar, M.D. Marcos, R. Martínez-Máñez, F. Sancenón, P. Amorós, Angew. Chem. Int. Ed. 45 (2006) 6661.

[12] R. Hernandez, H.-R. Tseng, J.W. Wong, J.F. Stoddart, J.I. Zink, J. Am. Chem. Soc. 126 (2004) 3370.

[13] K. Ariga, Y. Yamauchi, G. Rydzek, Q. Ji, Y. Yonamine, K.C.-W. Wu, J.P. Hill, Chem. Lett. 43 (2014) 36.

[14] Q. Ji, M. Miyahara, J.P. Hill, S. Acharya, A. Vinu, S.B. Yoon, J.-S. Yu, K. Sakamoto, K. Ariga, J. Am. Chem. Soc. 130 (2008) 2376.

[15] D.G. Shchukin, A.A. Patel, G.B. Sukhorukov, Y.M. Lvov, J. Am. Chem. Soc. 126 (2004) 3374.

[16] K.N.A. Kumar, S.B. Ray, V. Nagaraja, A.M. Raichur, Mater. Sci. Eng. C 29 (2009) 2508.

[17] J. Liu, Y. Zhang, C. Wang, R. Xu, Z. Chen, N. Gu, J. Phys. Chem. C 114 (2010) 7673.

[18] A. Agarwal, Y. Lvov, R. Sawant, V. Torchilin, J. Control. Release 128 (2008) 255.

[19] Y. Lvov, A. Agarwal, R. Sawant, V. Torchilin, Pharma Focus Asia 7 (2008) 36.

[20] Z. Zheng, X. Zhang, D. Carbo, C. Clark, C.-A. Nathan, Y. Lvov, Langmuir 26 (2010) 7679.

[21] H. Izawa, K. Kawakami, M. Sumita, Y. Tateyama, J.P. Hill, K. Ariga, J. Mater. Chem. B 1 (2013) 2155.

[22] K. Ariga, T. Mori, S. Ishihara, K. Kawakami, J.P. Hill, Chem. Mater. 26 (2014) 519.

[23] K. Ariga, Y. Terasaka, D. Sakai, H. Tsuji, J. Kikuchi, J. Am. Chem. Soc. 122 (2000) 7835.

[24] T. Michinobu, S. Shinoda, T. Nakanishi, J.P. Hill, K. Fujii, T.N. Player, H. Tsukube, K. Ariga, J. Am. Chem. Soc. 128 (2006) 14478.

[25] T. Mori, K. Okamoto, H. Endo, J.P. Hill, S. Shinoda, M. Matsukura, H. Tsukube, Y. Suzuki, Y. Kanekiyo, K. Ariga, J. Am. Chem. Soc. 132 (2010) 12868.

[26] K. Ariga, T. Mori, J.P. Hill, Adv. Mater. 24 (2012) 158.

[27] K. Ariga, Y. Yamauchi, T. Mori, J.P. Hill, Adv. Mater. 25 (2013) 6477.

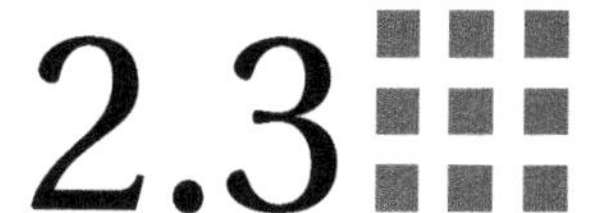

2.3 Injectable Hydrogels

Yuichi Ohya

DEPARTMENT OF CHEMISTRY AND MATERIALS ENGINEERING, FACULTY OF CHEMISTRY, MATERIALS AND BIOENGINEERING, KANSAI UNIVERSITY, SUITA, OSAKA, JAPAN; ORGANIZATION FOR RESEARCH AND DEVELOPMENT OF INNOVATIVE SCIENCE AND TECHNOLOGY (ORDIST), KANSAI UNIVERSITY, SUITA, OSAKA, JAPAN

CHAPTER OUTLINE

2.3.1 Introduction

Since physical properties of hydrogels are similar to those of the human body, various hydrogels have been studied over the past two decades as implantable biomaterials exhibiting good compatibility with soft tissue. During this time, *in situ* gel-forming polymer systems have attracted much attention in biomedical fields [1–7]. Such a polymer aqueous solution can be injected into the body by a simple syringe injection, and undergo gelation at the injected site in the body. Therefore, such a polymer is called an injectable polymer (IP). Especially, IPs that can be biodegraded and metabolized in the body are expected to be applied as implantable biomaterials because there is no need for them to be removed from the body after their usefulness has passed, which means that the possibility of toxicity may be low or negligible. For example, an aqueous solution of IP containing water-soluble drugs can be injected at a desired site and form a hydrogel. The hydrogel formed can act as a depot releasing the drug in a sustained manner, and provide a minimally invasive drug delivery system (DDS). IPs are also thought to be useful for tissue engineering and regenerative medicine. An IP solution containing living cells (such as patients' cells or stem cells) and/or growth factors can also be injected into the defective cite in the body. Then, the hydrogel formed can act as a scaffold for regeneration of the tissue. In addition, many applications such as antiadhesive materials after surgical operation, biodegradable glues, vascular embolization agents, and three-dimensional cell culture media can also be used as biodegradable IPs.

Gels can be categorized into chemical (covalent) gels and physical (noncovalent) gels. Polymer systems exhibiting sol–gel transition can also be categorized into these two gelation systems. One of the typical examples for chemical gelation systems is driven by polymerization reaction. In the polymerization system, polymer-carrying multiple polymerizable groups (typically, vinyl, acryl, or methacryl) can be polymerized with or without a comonomer using certain triggers such as photoirradiation [8,9]. Another type of chemical gelation system is that gelation can occur via chemical reaction between multifunctional reactive polymers forming covalent bonds [10,11]. In these chemical gelation systems, the gelation reactions are basically irreversible. On the other hand, in physical gelation systems, the most popular ones are temperature-responsive systems [6,12–14]. Gelation systems responsive for pH [14], or both pH and temperature [15,16], are also reported. Gelation processes in most of the external stimuli-responsive systems are basically reversible.

Generally, a chemical gelation system can provide a hydrogel exhibiting relatively high mechanical strength. However, the gelation time is usually difficult to control. On the contrary, upon injection stimuli-responsive systems show rapid gelation in response to external stimuli such as body temperature. But the mechanical strength of the hydrogel is relatively low. The gelation is basically reversible and the hydrogel formed may be return to the sol state under highly wet conditions because a noncovalent system is basically in the equilibrium state.

Polymers used in injectable systems can be categorized into biodegradable polymers and nonbiodegradable polymers. In the polymerization system described above, the polymerizable groups are limited to C=C groups, and the segments produced by the polymerization are not biodegradable. Some amphiphilic block copolymers are well known to exhibit temperature-responsive sol–gel transition, so-called thermogelling polymers. The triblock copolymer of poly(ethylene glycol) (PEG) and poly(propyrene glycol) (PPG) (PEG–PPG–PEG, called Pluronic) is a typical example [5]. Although Pluronic is a polyether and not biodegradable, amphiphilic block copolymers of PEG and aliphatic polyesters or polypeptides are also known to exhibit temperature-responsive sol–gel transition [13]. They are composed of biodegradable aliphatic polyesters or polypeptides and relatively low-molecular-weight PEG. As the hydrophobic segments can be degraded in the body and the degradation products and low-molecular-weight PEG can be excreted from the body, they are suitable for biomedical use.

In this chapter, biodegradable IP systems that can form hydrogels after injection into the body are introduced. Especially, recent progress in biodegradable copolymer systems exhibiting temperature-responsive sol–gel transition (thermogelling polymer) is mainly introduced from the viewpoint of polymer nanoarchitectonics.

2.3.2 Chemical Gel (Covalent Network) Systems

2.3.2.1 *In Situ* Polymerization Systems

Some *in situ* polymerization systems have been reported as covalent IP systems [8,9,17]. In these systems, linear or branched polymers, having multiple polymerizable functional

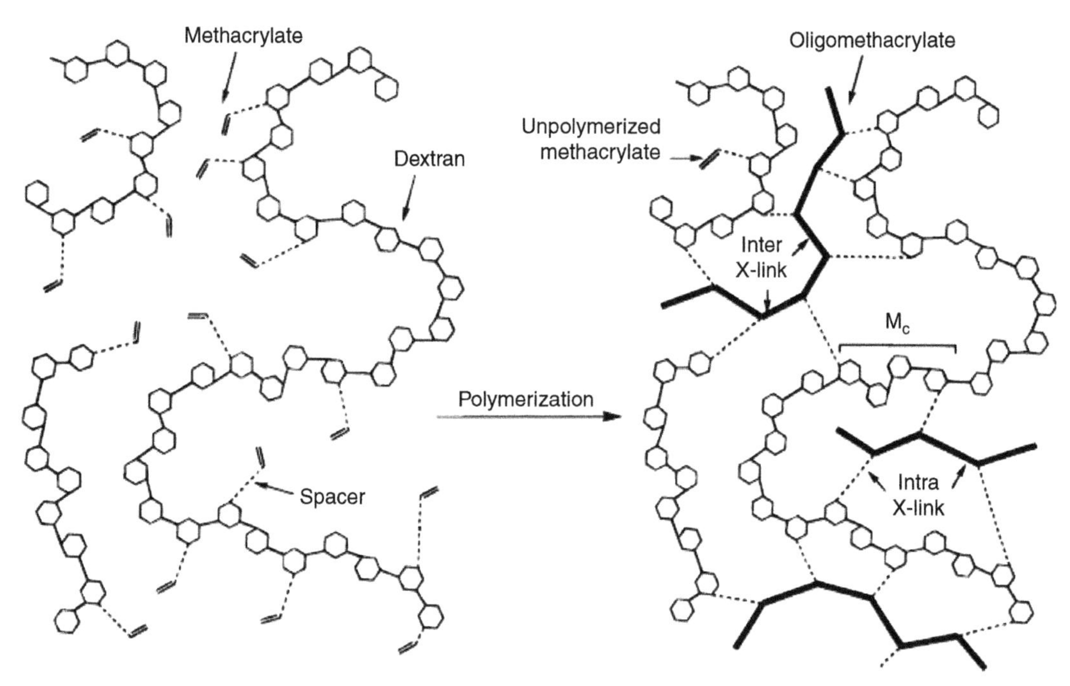

FIGURE 2.3.1 An example of polymerization systems: dextran carrying polymerizable methacrylate groups via biodegradable linkers can be polymerized to form biodegradable hydrogels. *Reprinted with permission from Ref. [17].*

groups (typically, vinyl, acryl, methacryl) at their termini or side chains, are used to form hydrogels (Fig. 2.3.1). Some triggers are used for initiation of the polymerization reactions, typically radical species produced by photoirradiation or redox reaction. In these cases, even if biodegradable prepolymers (macromonomers) were used, the newly produced segments by *in situ* polymerization must be nonbiodegradable. Therefore, these nonbiodegradable segments are desired to be water-soluble low-molecular-weight compounds. In addition, in the photoinitiating system, the biocompatibility of photoinitiators and the timing of photoirradiation are important and difficult problems.

2.3.2.2 Two-Polymer Solutions Mixing Systems

Two-polymer solutions mixing systems have also been reported as covalent IP systems. In these systems, a multifunctional polymer (linear, branched, or graft) is mixed with another bi- or multifunctional polymer carrying functional groups, which can act with functional groups on the first polymer to form a covalently cross-linked network (Fig. 2.3.2). Various combinations of the reactive functional groups forming covalent bonding spontaneously, such as activated esters (succinimide, *p*-nitrophenol, etc.) + primary amine for amide bonds, aldehyde + amine for Schiff base bond, and click chemistries (alkyne + azide, en + thiol, and Diels–Alder reaction) were reported [18–22]. Generally, two solutions containing each polymer would be mixed upon injection by a two-solution-mixing syringe to form a hydrogel. The gelation time in this system is usually difficult to control and an important key point

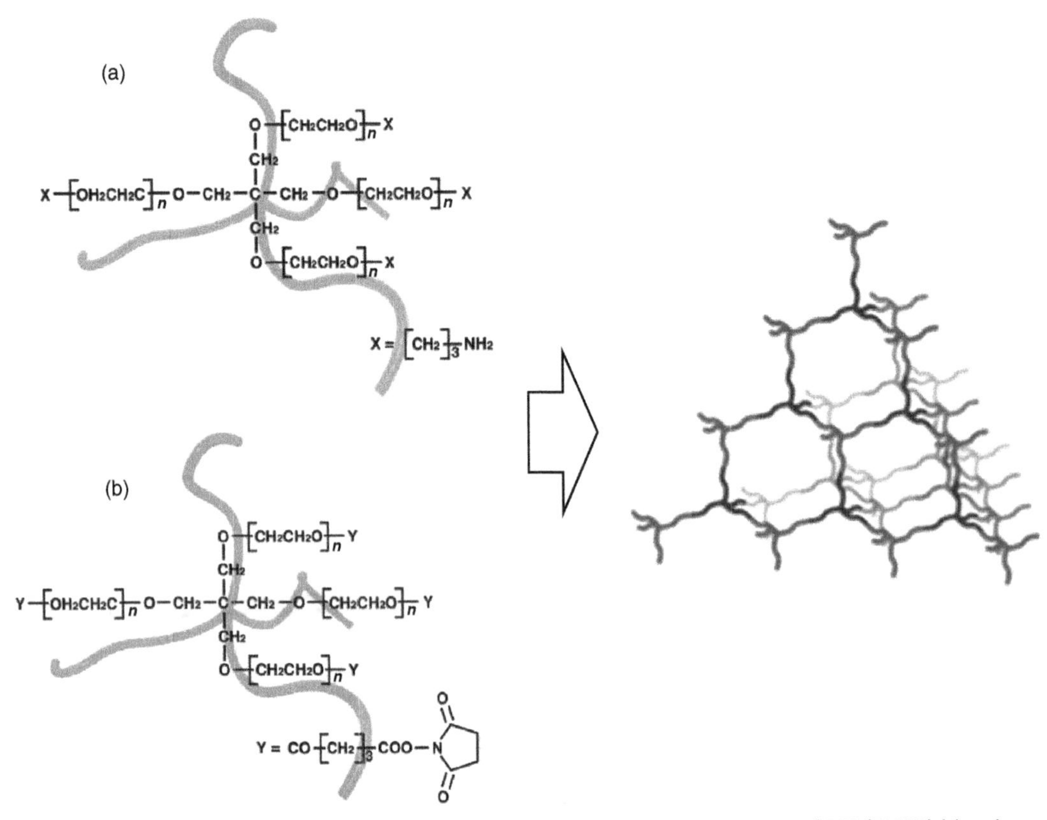

FIGURE 2.3.2 An example of a two-polymer solutions mixing system. Tetraamine-terminated PEG (TAPEG) (a) and tetra-*N*-hydroxysuccinimide glutarate-teminated PEG (TNPEG) (b) were mixed in solution to form tetra-PEG gel. *Reprinted with permission from Ref. [24].*

for the application. Slow reaction rate takes a long time for gelation to occur resulting in a flow from the injected site. On the other hand, too rapid reaction may lead to gelation in the syringe making it difficult to inject. As a recent example, Sakai et al. reported a tetra-PEG gel system produced by mixing two kinds of 4-arms PEG with a defined length of PEG arms in a tetrahedral symmetrical structure, where each tetra-PEG possessed activated ester groups or primary amine groups at their termini [11,23,24]. The obtained hydrogel (tetra-PEG gel) showed higher mechanical strength than usual hydrogels.

2.3.2.3 Enzymatic Reaction Systems

Covalent IP systems using enzymatic reactions are also reported [22,25–33]. Park et al. reported enzymatic gelation systems using gelatin and horseradish peroxidase (HRP) for biomedical use [25]. An enzyme-mediated cross-linking reaction using HRP and hydrogen peroxide provides an alternative method for the *in situ* formation of the hydrogels (Fig. 2.3.3). The HRP-mediated cross-linking reaction has several advantages, including

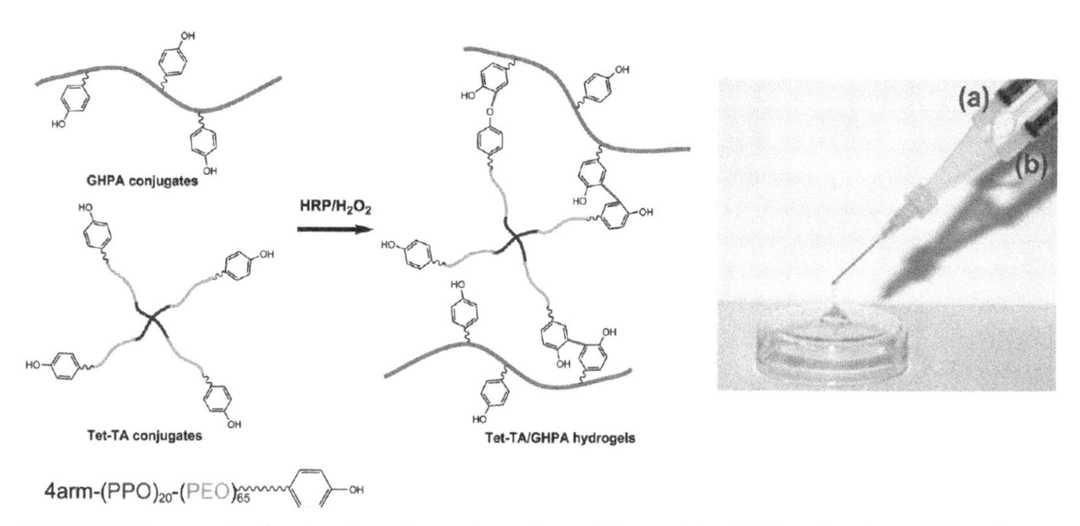

FIGURE 2.3.3 An example of enzymatic reaction systems. Horseradish peroxidase (HRP)-mediated cross-linking of tyramine conjugated 4arm-PPO-PEO (Tet–TA) and gelatin–hydroxyphenyl propionic acid (GHPA) conjugates, and the photograph of hydrogel formation using a dual syringe. *Reprinted with permission from Ref. [25].*

tunable reaction rate, mild reaction conditions, and good biocompatibility. The enzyme-mediated formable hydrogels are easy to handle and capable of loading with cells or bioactive molecules homogeneously because the viscosity of precursor polymer solutions is relatively low. They reported that the *in situ* cross-linkable gelatin hydrogels showed good tissue compatibility as well as a sufficiently long-term stability *in vivo* [23].

2.3.3 Physical Gel (Noncovalent Network) Systems

2.3.3.1 Temperature-Responsive Systems

2.3.3.1.1 Amphiphilic Block Copolymers

As mentioned previously, some biodegradable amphiphilic block copolymers showed sol–gel or gel–sol transition in response to temperature changes. PEG has often been used as hydrophilic segments of such thermogelling copolymer systems due to its biocompatibility and temperature-dependent dehydration behavior. Aliphatic polyesters such as poly(L-lactide) (PLLA), poly(D-lactide) (PDLA), poly(DL-lactide-*co*-glycolide) (PLGA), poly(ε-caprolactone) (PCL), and their copolymers have been used as hydrophobic segments based on their biodegradability and relatively good biocompatibility [34–40]. Biodegradable thermogelling copolymers containing amino acids as building blocks of the hydrophobic segments have also been developed [41–44].

In 1997, Jeong and Kim et al. reported biodegradable IP systems using a triblock copolymer of PEG and PLLA, PEG-*b*-PLLA-*b*-PEG [32]. After this achievement, many block copolymers with combinations of PEGs and aliphatic polyesters were reported [45–47] with various molecular architectures. Linear block, star-shaped block, and graft topologies

Table 2.3.1 Various Types of Thermogelling Biodegradable Polymers

Structure	Polymer	Remarks	References
Diblock	PEG-*b*-PLLA	Gel-to-sol transition	[47–49]
	PEG-*b*-L-PA	Enzymatic degradation	[42,43]
	PEG-*b*-PAF	Enzymatic degradation, low CGC	[45]
Triblock	PEG-*b*-PLGA-*b*-PEG	High CGC, low modulus	[52–54]
	PLGA-*b*-PEG-*b*-PLGA	High CGC, low modulus	[56,57]
	End-capped PLGA-*b*-PEG-*b*-PLGA	Low CGC, low modulus	[38,58]
	PLLA-*b*-PEG-*b*-PLLA/PDLA-*b*-PEG-*b*-PDLA	SC, thermo-stable	[35]
	PEG-*b*-PLLA-*b*-PEG/PEG-*b*-PDLA-*b*-PEG	SC, high modulus, gel-to-sol transition	[88]
	PDP-*b*-PEG-*b*-PDP	Reactive groups on main chain, tunable transition temperature	[41]
	OSM-PCLA-*b*-PEG-*b*-PCLA-*b*-OSM	pH/temperature responsive	[15,16]
Multiblock	(PEG-PLLA)$_n$	Controllable T_{gel}, low modulus	[46]
Graft	PLGA-*g*-PEG,	High CGC, low modulus	[63–65]
	PDG-DL-LA-*g*-PEG	High MW, slow gel degradation	[66,71,80]
Star shaped	PEG-*b*-(PLLA)$_8$/PEG-*b*-(PDLA)$_8$	SC, high modulus	[89,90]
	8-Arms PEG-*b*-PLLA-cholesterol	High MW, high modulus, low CGC, thermostable	[84]
	8-Arms PEG-*b*-PLLA-*b*-PEG/8-arms PEG-*b*-PDLA-*b*-PEG	SC, high MW, high modulus, irreversible sol–gel transition	[91]

have been reported as biodegradable thermogelling copolymer systems as summarized in Table 2.3.1. These copolymers exhibit various properties based on their molecular architectures and nature of the components. Among them, amphiphilic copolymers having linear block architectures were reported first and are still major among the biodegradable IP systems because of the simplicity of the synthetic procedure, etc. Typical examples of thermogelling block copolymers are shown in Fig. 2.3.4.

The mechanism of temperature-responsive sol–gel transition of the thermogelling copolymer aqueous solutions is explained as follows: these copolymers are dissolved as micelles in aqueous solution, dehydration of PEG chains occurs upon increase in temperature, and consequent perturbation and aggregation of the micelles lead to network formation of hydrogel [50,51]. The lengths of hydrophilic and hydrophobic segments strongly affect the phase transition behavior. When the hydrophobic polyester segment is too long, the copolymer is insoluble in aqueous solution. On the other hand, when the hydrophilic PEG block is too long, sol–gel transition temperature (T_{gel}) is increased and becomes higher than body temperature, or the sol–gel transition itself disappears. These phenomena indicate that hydrophobic/hydrophilic balance of the block copolymers is critical to their temperature-responsive phase transition behavior. The gelation properties including T_{gel} and critical gelation concentration (CGC) can roughly be modulated by several factors such as lengths of hydrophobic and hydrophilic segments, hydrophobic/hydrophilic segment ratios, crystallinity of the hydrophobic segments, and total molecular weights. These factors are also important for utility as drug delivery depots because the entrapment and release profiles of drugs and degradation properties can be affected by these factors, too.

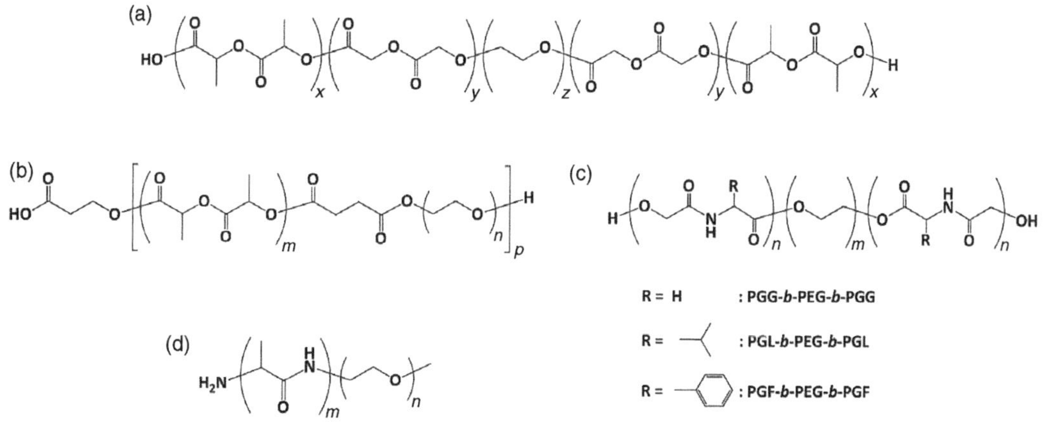

FIGURE 2.3.4 Chemical structures of linear-type biodegradable block polymers exhibiting temperature-responsive sol-to-gel transition in aqueous solutions. (a) PLGA-*b*-PEG-*b*-PLGA triblock copolymer, (b) PEG/PLLA multiblock copolymer, (c) PDP-*b*-PEG-*b*-PDP triblock copolymers, (d) PEG-*b*-PA diblock copolymer.

A triblock copolymer of PLGA and PEG, PLGA-*b*-PEG-*b*-PLGA, was reported in 1999, and has been extensively investigated as one of the representative examples of biodegradable thermogelling polymers [52–55]. This polymer solution usually shows sol–gel transition between 20°C and 37°C, and is utilized as an injectable DDS for both hydrophobic and hydrophilic drugs such as paclitaxel and insulin [56,57]. However, low mechanical strength and relatively high CGC value are often cited as problems of the PLGA-*b*-PEG-*b*-PLGA triblock and other similar linear block copolymer systems. The storage moduli of typical linear block-type thermogelling biodegradable polymers in the gel state are usually less than 100 Pa. To achieve good compatibility with natural tissues (normally storage modulus = 10 kPa–10 MPa) and to avoid flowing from the injected site in a human body under daily motion, higher mechanical strength is desired. End-capping approaches were reported for PLGA-*b*-PEG-*b*-PLGA copolymers to improve the mechanical strength and lower the CGC by tuning a hydrophobic/hydrophilic balance of the copolymer [41,58]. The storage modulus of the hydrogel was somewhat improved and the CGC was significantly decreased by introduction of diacetate or dipropionate end groups at the termini. Other approaches to improve mechanical strength by changing polymer architectures are described in the following sections.

Other problems with biodegradable thermogelling copolymer systems are solidification and solubility. Most thermogelling polymers reported previously are sticky paste in dry state at room temperature, and it usually takes a very long time (more than several hours) to be dissolved in aqueous solution. These characteristics of the copolymers are inconvenient for the preparation of the IP formulation in a clinical setting, and have been obstacles for clinical application of the thermogelling polymers. On this issue, Jeong and Deng reported that the amphiphilic block copolymer composed of PEG and PCL displayed solid (powder) form at dry state as well as thermogelling properties [59–61]. However, these systems still had problems in solubilization in aqueous solution. To dissolve

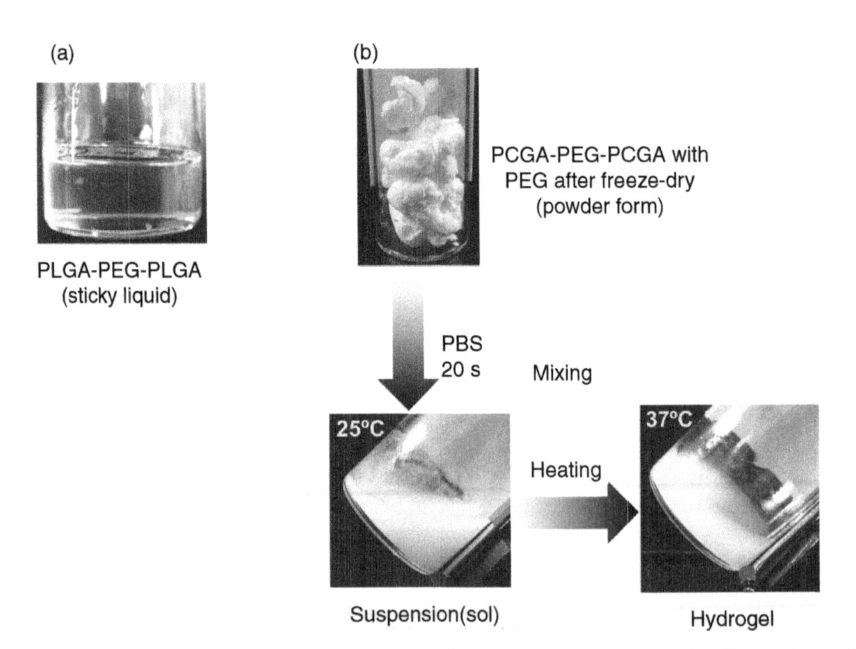

FIGURE 2.3.5 Photographs of (a) PLGA–PEG–PLGA (sticky liquid) and (b) PCGA–PEG–PCGA (solid, powder) and suspension of PCGA–PEG–PCGA containing PEG as an additive. *Reprinted with permission from Ref. [62].*

these copolymers, heating above the melting temperature of the copolymers was needed. In addition, the copolymer aqueous solution is likely to undergo spontaneously gelation after a certain period even at room temperature because of the relatively high-crystal-forming tendency of the hydrophobic segments. Recently, we developed a very quick and convenient preparative method for IP formulation [62]. We used a triblock polymer composed of poly(ε-caprolactone-*co*-glycolic acid) (PCGA) and PEG, PCGA-*b*-PEG-*b*-PCGA, and investigated the effects of various additives on the dispersion time and gelation behavior of the copolymers in phosphate buffered saline (PBS). As a result, we found the PEGs had appropriate molecular weights (3000–5000 Da) as additives were effective for quick preparation of IP suspension. It was possible to prepare a suspension from the freeze-dried mixture of PCGA-*b*-PEG-*b*-PCGA and PEG by the addition of PBS, and the obtained suspension exhibited temperature-responsive sol–gel transition at between room temperature and body temperature (Fig. 2.3.5). Although the obtained suspension was not a transparent solution, the sol–gel transition behavior was not so different from the clear solution obtained by the heating/cooling process. The formulation developed should be very convenient for use in a clinical setting.

2.3.3.1.2 Multiblock Copolymer Systems

One of the possible solutions to overcome low mechanical properties of thermogelling copolymer systems must be enlargement of their total molecular weights. But elongation of each segment (hydrophobic and hydrophilic) with keeping their hydrophobic/hydrophilic

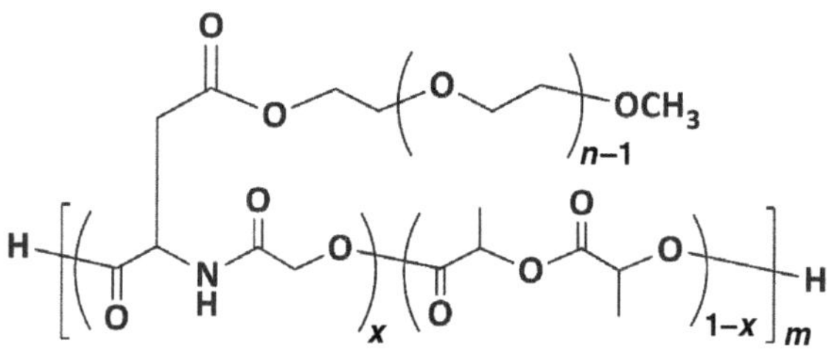

FIGURE 2.3.6 The chemical structure of P(DG-DL-LA)-*g*-PEG.

ratio was not successful because the dehydration temperature of PEG strongly depends on its length and the longer PEG chain lead disappearance of sol–gel transition properties. One solution for consistency of short PEG chains and larger molecular weight is a multiblock architecture. By employing multiblock architecture, enlargement of molecular weight was achieved by keeping the sol–gel transition properties of the resultant copolymers. Jeong et al. have reported multiblock copolymers having alternating PEG and PLLA segments $(PEG–PLLA)_n$ exhibiting temperature-responsive sol–gel transition at relatively lower polymer concentrations [46]. The mechanical strength was relatively high compared with triblock copolymer systems (modulus = 250 Pa at 37°C, 25 wt%).

2.3.3.1.3 Graft Copolymer Systems

Another possible solution for enlargement of molecular weight without elongation of each PEG block may be by employing graft architectures. Jeong et al. also reported the synthesis of a graft copolymer, PLGA-g-PEG [63–65]. However, the storage modulus of the hydrogel of PLGA-g-PEG graft copolymer (25 wt%) was ca. 100 Pa at 37°C 22 wt%, and was not high enough.

We also synthesized graft copolymers composed of PEG side chains and a polylactide copolymer main chain [66]. Polydepsipeptide is a category of copolymers consisting of α-amino acids and α-hydroxyl acids. We have reported the synthesis of biodegradable copolymers of depsipeptide and lactide, poly(depsipeptide-*co*-lactide), with reactive side-chain groups such as COOH, NH_2, OH, and SH, by ring-opening polymerization of cyclodepsipeptides (morphorin-2,5-dione derivative) consisting of the corresponding amino acids and glycolic acid [67–70]. Using the functionality of the side-chain group of these copolymers, various chemical modifications can be installed to provide functional biodegradable materials. We synthesized an amphiphilic graft copolymer of poly(depsipeptide-*co*-DL-lactide) with PEG, poly[(glycolic acid-*alt*-L-aspartic acid)-*co*-DL-lactide]-*g*-PEG [P(GD-DL-LA)-*g*-PEG] (Fig. 2.3.6), by the coupling reaction of carboxylic acid groups of P(GD-DL-LA) with monomethoxy-PEG (MeO-PEG) [66]. The obtained P(GD-DL-LA)-*g*-PEG showed temperature-responsive sol–gel transition. Then, we investigated the relationship between sol–gel transition behavior (T_{gel} and storage moduli) and molecular structure (PEG length and number of PEG chains per molecules) using graft copolymers having a wide variety of molecular structures [71]. The molecular weights of these graft copolymers were about 30,000 Da. T_{gel} of the P(DG-DL-LA)-*g*-PEG (20 wt%) controlled from 20°C to 60°C by varying PEG length and degree of introduction of PEG without a decrease in mechanical strength of the gels. The P(DG-DL-LA)-*g*-PEG gel formed showed significant higher storage modulus (ca. 700 Pa) at 37°C compared with the gels obtained from linear triblock copolymer systems using PEG and PLGA. The gel obtained from 20 wt% polymer solution was eroded gradually in PBS at 37°C for 60 days. These results suggest that graft approaches can overcome molecular weight constraint on designing biodegradable thermogelling polymers with controllable T_{gel} and mechanical strength.

2.3.3.1.4 Graft Copolymer Drug Conjugate

Biodegradable thermogelling systems have been widely investigated as a candidate for sustained drug releasing systems. Several factors must be considered for the release rates of drugs from hydrogels, such as hydrophilic or hydrophobic characters of drugs, molecular weights of drugs, degradation rates of hydrogels, and diffusion constants of drugs in hydrogels [72–74]. The release rates of low-molecular-weight hydrophilic drugs are generally faster than hydrophobic and/or high-molecular-weight drugs because the apparent pore sizes of the hydrogel networks are much larger than the size of low-molecular-weight drugs and the diffusion constants of such water-soluble molecules are relatively high. Thus, it is not easy to achieve sustained release of water-soluble low-molecular-weight drugs. In an ideal system, the release of drugs from IP hydrogels would be controlled independently by the hydrophilicity/hydrophobicity and molecular weights of the drugs.

A macromolecular prodrug is a category of prodrug systems used in DDS, where low-molecular-weight drugs are covalently attached to water-soluble polymers [75]. Our group previously reported various macromolecular prodrug systems of antitumor drugs using water-soluble biodegradable polymers as carriers [76,77]. Especially, covalent attachments of anticancer drugs to biocompatible water-soluble polymers were effective to deliver the drugs to tumor sites and give better *in vivo* antitumor activity. The phenomena are considered to be due to the enhancement permeability and retention effects [78,79] and the reduction of the side effects of the drugs by avoiding the distribution to unfavorable sites in the body. Usually the drugs are inactive and nontoxic while they remain attached to the backbone polymers, but they become active (toxic) by conversion to the parent drugs upon hydrolytic release from the backbone polymer. Therefore, these release and activation mechanisms of macromolecular prodrug systems can provide similar effects as a sustained release of drugs. The release rates of drugs from a backbone polymer can be controlled by the hydrolysis rate of the covalent bonds between the drugs and the backbone polymer, the attachment manner (type of chemical bonds), and the structure of spacer groups (hydrophilic/hydrophobic).

Using the amphiphilic graft copolymer system of P(DG-DL-LA)-*g*-PEG mentioned above, the unreacted residual carboxylic acid groups can be used for further functionalization of the thermogelling polymer system, in this case for drug immobilization. We proposed a macromolecular prodrug type of IP system exhibiting sustained release of water-soluble low-molecular-weight drugs [80]. Water-soluble antibiotic levofloxacin (LEV) was chosen

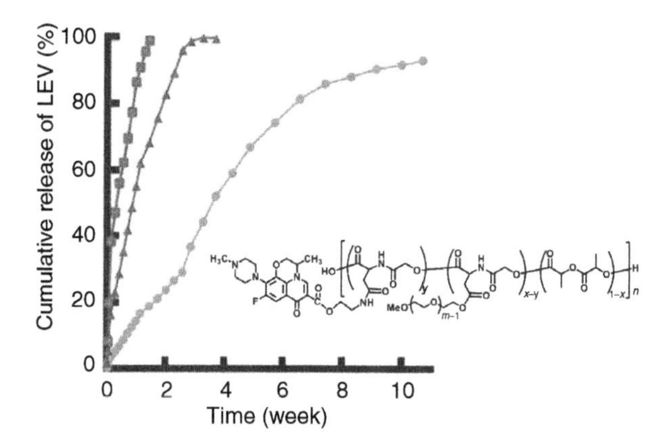

FIGURE 2.3.7 (a) Time course *in vitro* release of levofloxacin (LEV) derivatives from the hydrogels. (●) P(GD-DL-LA)-*g*-PEG/LEV conjugate gel, (▴) P(GD-DL-LA)-*g*-PEG gel entrapping LEV, and (■) PLGA-*b*-PEG-*b*-PLGA gel entrapping LEV. *Reprinted with permission from Ref. [80].*

as a model of a relatively hydrophilic low-molecular-weight drug. The LEV was attached to P(GD-DL-LA)-*g*-PEG to give a P(GD-DL-LA)-*g*-PEG/LEV conjugate. The aqueous solution of the conjugate showed temperature-responsive sol-to-gel transition behavior and the hydrogel showed much sustained release of LEV for 10 weeks in aqueous solution (Fig. 2.3.7).

2.3.3.1.5 Branched Copolymer Systems

As described earlier, amphiphilic multiblock copolymer systems and amphiphilic graft copolymer systems exhibited improved mechanical strength of gel state to some extent. We have developed some IP systems based on star-shaped block copolymers with branched architectures. The branched architecture was expected to accelerate efficient physical cross-link formation in the gel state. We have synthesized star-shaped diblock copolymers of PEG and PLLA, 8-arms PEG-*b*-PLLA as biocompatible materials [81–83]. Although some of the star-shaped diblock copolymers showed temperature responsiveness, the transition phenomena were not gel formation, but soluble–insoluble transition. Then, we introduced hydrophobic cholesterol groups to the termini of 8-arms PEG-*b*-PLLA to give 8-arms PEG-*b*-PLLA-cholesterol conjugates (Fig. 2.3.8) [84]. An aqueous solution of the conjugate having cholesterol end groups at 2–3 residues of total 8 termini exhibited temperature-responsive instantaneous gelation above 5 wt% in a polymer concentration below 37°C upon heating (Fig. 2.3.8). In contrast, aqueous solutions of virgin 8-arms PEG-*b*-PLLA without cholesterol moieties did not form gels at any concentrations and temperatures. The 8-arms PEG-*b*-PLLA-cholesterol conjugate system showed significantly higher mechanical strength (storage modulus = ca. 5000 Pa) compared with previously reported biodegradable thermogelling polymer systems. We then investigated the potential utility of the conjugate as an injectable scaffold for cell implantation and growth. L929 fibroblast cells encapsulated in the gel were viable and proliferated three dimensionally in the gel

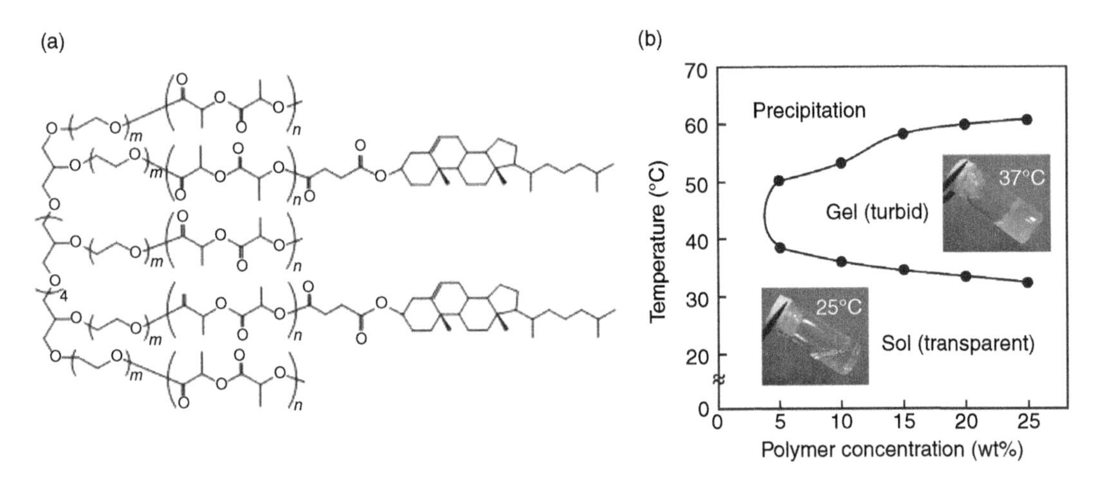

FIGURE 2.3.8 (a) The chemical structure of 8-arms PEG–PLLA-cholesterol. (b) Phase diagram of 8-arms PEG–PLLA-cholesterol solution, and the photographs of the solution in sol state and gel state. *Reprinted with permission from Ref. [84].*

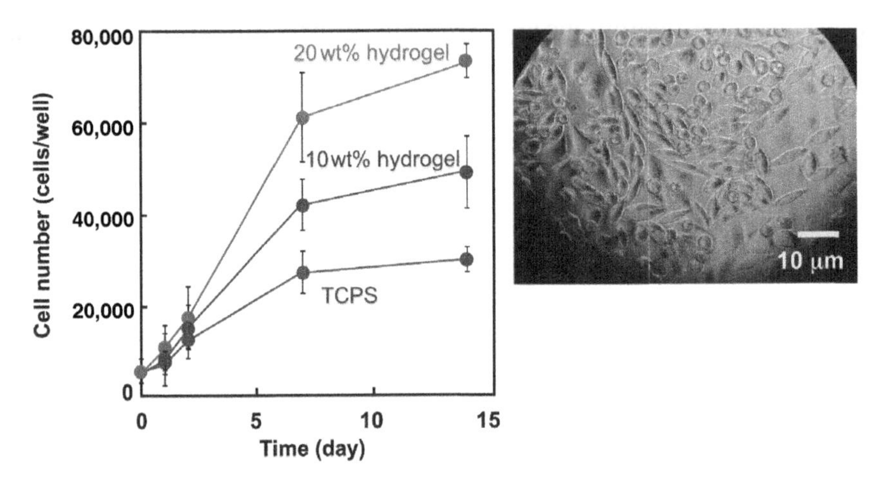

FIGURE 2.3.9 The growth of L929 cells proliferated inside the 10 and 20 wt% 8-arms PEG–PLLA-cholesterol hydrogel and the optical microscope image of the cross-section of the gel after 7 days. *Reprinted with permission from Ref. [84].*

for 2 weeks (Fig. 2.3.9). The gel prepared from 10 wt% conjugate solution eroded gradually in PBS at 37°C over a month, after which time the gel was completely dissociated. These results indicate that the 8-arms PEG-*b*-PLLA-cholesterol conjugate is a good candidate as an injectable cellular scaffold for tissue regeneration.

2.3.3.2 Stereocomplex Formation System

Polylactides (PLAs) have two enantiomeric forms, PLLA and PDLA. It is well known that a 1:1 mixture of PLLA and PDLA can form stable stereocomplex (SC) crystals, which have

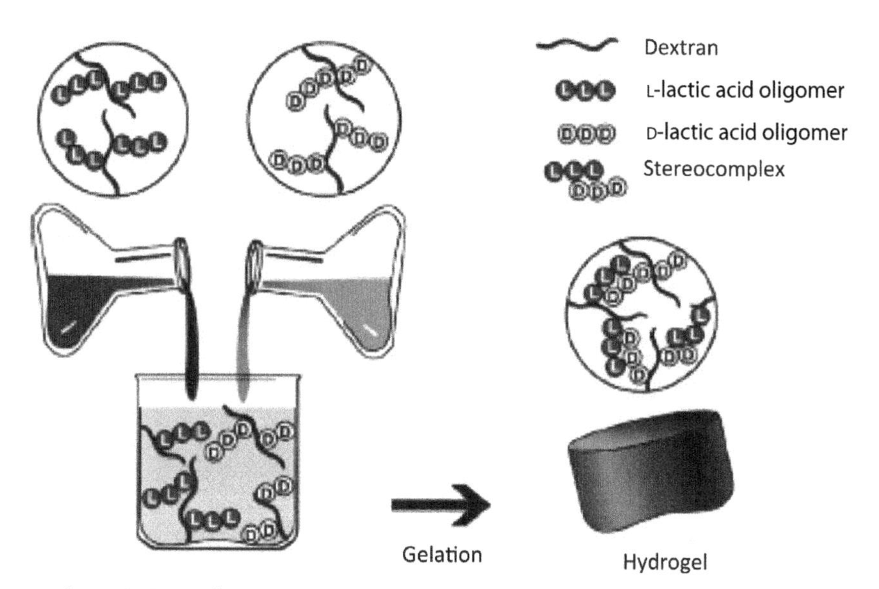

FIGURE 2.3.10 Schematic picture illustrating the formation of stereocomplex hydrogels from polymers containing either L- or D-lactic acid. *Reprinted with permission from Ref. [87].*

a higher T_m and higher mechanical strength than either of the homopolymer crystals [85]. The SC formation was also used as a noncovalent driving force for gel formation in IP systems. Hennink et al. reported a two-solution mixing gel formation system using dextran with PLLA graft chains (Dex-g-PLLA) and enantiomeric Dex-g-PDLA (Fig. 2.3.10). The solution of Dex-*g*-PLLA and the solution Dex-*g*-PDLA prepared separately were mixed together to form stable hydrogel [86,87].

Kimura et al. reported a combination system of temperature-responsive system and SC formation [35]. They prepared a mixture of aqueous solutions of PLLA-*b*-PEG-*b*-PLLA and PDLA-*b*-PEG-*b*-PDLA copolymers separately. Just after the mixing of each polymer aqueous solution, the solution was in sol state, but underwent gel state as temperature increased. Each solution of L- or D-isomer of the triblock copolymer did not show such temperature-responsive sol–gel transition behavior. These results suggest that an increase in temperature triggered perturbation of the polymer micelle through dehydration of PEG, which formed the shell layer of the micelle, and led to intermicellar aggregation by SC formation of PLLA and PDLA segments. The SC copolymer gels exhibited higher mechanical strength (modulus = 900 Pa at 37°C, 10 wt%) compared with that of simple triblock systems of PEG and aliphatic polyesters. They also reported reverse-type temperature-responsive gel-to-sol transition phenomenon using the PEG-*b*-PLLA-*b*-PEG and PEG-*b*-PDLA-*b*-PEG system [88].

Feijen et al. have reported the thermogelling system using SC formation of star-shaped diblock copolymers, PEG-*b*-$(PLLA)_8$ and PEG-*b*-$(PDLA)_8$ [89,90]. They have investigated the effects of arm number of the branched architecture on their temperature-responsive gelation by comparing the PEG-*b*-$(PLLA)_8$/PEG-*b*-$(PDLA)_8$ system with the

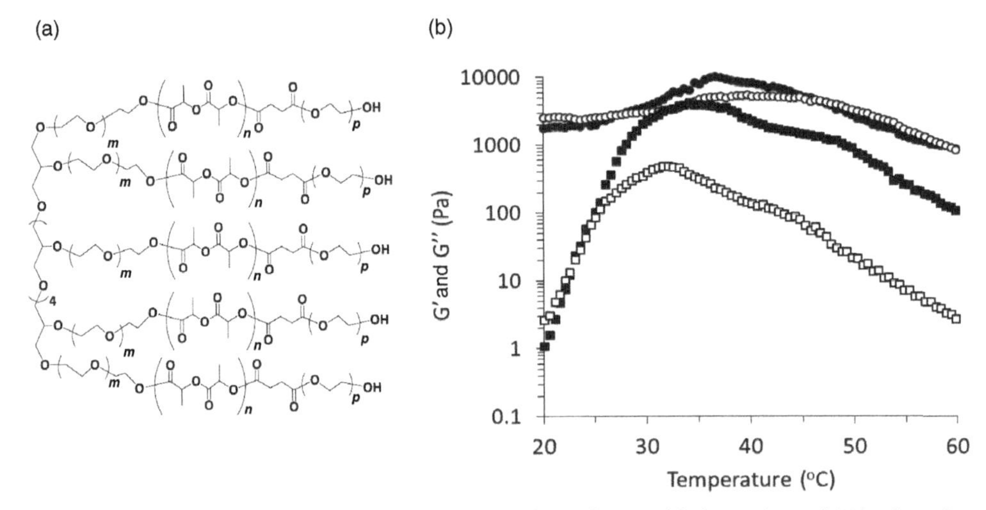

FIGURE 2.3.11 (a) Chemical structure of star-shaped 8-arms PEG-*b*-PLA-*b*-PEG triblock copolymer. (b) Rheological studies of aqueous solutions of a 1:1 mixture of 8-arms PEG-*b*-PLLA-*b*-PEG and 8-arms PEG-*b*-PDLA-*b*-PEG copolymers. *G*′ (solid symbols) and *G*′′ (open symbols) as a function of temperature for 10 wt% (square) and 15 wt% (circle) in PBS. *Reprinted with permission from Ref. [91].*

PLLA-*b*-PEG-*b*-PLLA/PDLA-*b*-PEG-*b*-PDLA system. Rheological studies revealed that star-shaped the PEG-*b*-$(PLLA)_8$/PEG-*b*-$(PDLA)_8$ mixture system showed a significantly higher storage modulus in the gel state (850–7000 Pa at 10 wt% depending on time after mixing) than the linear-type mixture system because of the higher cross-linking density of the former. These studies demonstrated, in addition to the block length of aliphatic polyester and PEG segments, that polymer architecture has a great influence on the temperature-responsive sol–gel transition behavior and the physical properties of the hydrogel formed.

We have also reported a thermogelling system using SC formation of star-shaped triblock copolymers consisting of 8-arms PEG and PLLA or PDLA, a mixture of 8-arms PEG-*b*-PLLA-*b*-PEG, and 8-arms PEG-*b*-PDLA-*b*-PEG (Fig. 2.3.11) [91]. An aqueous solution of a 1:1 mixture of these copolymers was in sol state at room temperature, but instantaneously formed gel in response to increasing temperature. The resulting gel exhibited a significantly higher storage modulus (ca. 10 kPa) at 37°C based on their branched structure, high molecular weight, and SC formation (Fig. 2.3.11). Interestingly, once formed above T_{gel}, the gel was stable even after cooling below the T_{gel} because of the stability of SC crystals formed in the physical cross-linking domains of the gel. The gel formed showed gradual hydrolytic degradation over 2 weeks. Sustained release of model protein drug (bovine serum albumin) was also observed. These characteristics render this polymer mixture system suitable for use in injectable biomedical materials such as a drug delivery depot or a biodegradable scaffold for tissue engineering.

2.3.4 Conclusions and Future Trends

Biodegradable IP systems, especially temperature-responsive sol–gel transition (thermogelling) systems were introduced. Mechanical strength of the hydrogel in thermogelling systems can be improved by employing multiblock, graft, and branched polymer architectures, and/or SC formation of polylactides. The handling conveniences (solidification and easy dissolving) were also improved by the polymer structures and the choice of appropriate additives. These improvements of biodegradable thermogelling IP systems provide high potential utility in clinical situations not only for noninvasive DDS exhibiting sustained release of drugs but also biodegradable scaffolds in tissue engineering, antiadhesive membranes on surgical operation, reversible cell stock devices, etc.

References

[1] B. Jeong, S.W. Kim, Y.H. Bae, Adv. Drug Deliv. Rev. 54 (2002) 37.
[2] B. Jeong, Y.K. Choi, Y.H. Bae, G. Zentner, S.W. Kim, J. Control. Release 65 (1999) 109.
[3] A. Hatefi, B. Amsden, J. Control. Release 80 (2002) 9.
[4] S.V. van Tomme, G. Storm, W.E. Hennink, Int. J. Pharm. 355 (2008) 1.
[5] L. Yu, J. Ding, Chem. Soc. Rev. 37 (2008) 1473.
[6] K. Nagahama, A. Takahashi, Y. Ohya, React. Funct. Polym. 73 (2013) 979.
[7] Y. Ohya, A. Takahashi, K. Nagahama, Adv. Polym. Sci. 247 (2012) 65.
[8] K.T. Nguyen, J.L. West, Biomaterials 23 (2002) 4307.
[9] L.J. Suggs, A.G. Mikos, Cell Transplant 8 (1999) 293.
[10] B. Balakrishnan, A A Jayakrishnan, Biomaterials 26 (2005) 3941.
[11] X. Li, Y. Tsutsui, T. Matsunaga, M. Shibayama, U. Chung, T. Sakai, Macromolecules 44 (2011) 3567.
[12] H.J. Moon, D.Y. Ko, M.H. Park, M.K. Joo, B. Jeong, Chem. Soc. Rev. 41 (2012) 4860.
[13] M.H. Park, M.K. Joo, B.G. Choi, B. Jeong, Acc. Chem. Res. 45 (2012) 424.
[14] C. He, S.W. Kim, D.S. Lee, Control. Release 127 (2008) 189.
[15] W.S. Shim, J.S. Yoo, Y.H. Bae, D.S. Lee, Biomacromolecules 6 (2005) 2930.
[16] W.S. Shim, S.W. Kim, D.S. Lee, Biomacromolecules 7 (2006) 1935.
[17] W.N.E. van Dijk-Wolthuis, J.A.M. Hoogeboom, M.J. van Steenbergen, S.K.Y. Tsang, W.E. Hennink, Macromolecules 30 (1997) 4639.
[18] H.P. Tan, C.R. Chu, K.A. Payne, K.G. Marra, Biomaterials 30 (2009) 2499.
[19] E.A. Phelps, N.O. Enemchukwu, V.F. Fiore, J.C. Sy, N. Murthy, T.A. Sulchek, Adv. Mater. 24 (2012) 64.
[20] B.D. Fairbanks, M.P. Schwartz, A.E. Halevi, C.R. Nuttelman, C.N. Bowman, K.S. Anseth, Adv. Mater. 21 (2009) 5005.
[21] C.A. DeForest, B.D. Polizzotti, K.S. Anseth, Nat. Mater. 8 (2009) 59.
[22] F. Yu, X.D. Cao, Y.L. Li, L. Zeng, B. Yuan, X.F. Chen, Polym. Chem. 5 (2014) 1082.
[23] H. Kamata, Y. Akagi, Y.K. Kariya, U. Chung, T. Sakai, Science 343 (2014) 873.
[24] T. Sakai, T. Matsunaga, Y. Yamamoto, C. Ito, R. Yoshida, S. Suzuki, N. Sasaki, M. Shibayama, U. Chung, Macromolecules 41 (2008) 5379.

[25] K.M. Park, Y. Lee, J.Y. Son, D.H. Oh, J.S. Lee, K.D. Park, Biomacromolecules 13 (2012) 604.

[26] R. Jin, C. Hiemstra, Z. Zhong, J. Feijen, Biomaterials 28 (2007) 2791.

[27] M. Kurisawa, J.E. Chung, Y.Y. Yang, S.J. Gao, H. Uyama, Chem. Commun. 34 (2005) 4312.

[28] S. Sakai, K.J. Kawakami, Biomed. Mater. Res. A 85A (2008) 345.

[29] S. Sakai, Y. Ogushi, K. Kawakami, Acta Biomater. 5 (2009) 554.

[30] S. Sakai, K. Hirose, K. Taguchi, Y. Ogushi, K. Kawakami, Biomaterials 30 (2009) 3371.

[31] L.S. Wang, J. Boulaire, P.P.Y. Chan, J.E. Chung, M. Kurisawa, Biomaterials 31 (2010) 8608.

[32] L.S. Wang, J.E. Chung, P.P.Y. Chan, M. Kurisawa, Biomaterials 31 (2009) 1148.

[33] S. Sakai, T. Matsuyama, K. Hirose, K. Kawakami, Biomacromolecules 11 (2010) 1370.

[34] B. Jeong, Y.H. Bae, D.S. Lee, S.W. Kim, Nature 388 (1997) 860.

[35] T. Fujiwara, T. Mukose, T. Yamaoka, H. Yamane, S. Sakurai, K. Kimura, Macromol. Biosci. 1 (2001) 204.

[36] B. Jeong, Y.H. Bae, S.W. Kim, Macromolecules 32 (1999) 7064.

[37] M.J. Hwang, J.M. Suh, Y.H. Bae, S.W. Kim, B. Jeong, Biomacromolecules 6 (2005) 885.

[38] L. Yu, H. Zhang, J. Ding, Angew. Chem. Int. Ed. 45 (2006) 2232.

[39] X.J. Loh, Y.X. Tan, Z. Li, L.S. Teo, S.H. Goh, J. Li, Biomaterials 29 (2008) 2164.

[40] X.J. Loh, K.B.C. Song, J. Li, Biomaterials 29 (2008) 3185.

[41] Y. Ohya, H. Yamamoto, K. Nagahama, T. Ouchi, J. Polym. Sci. A 47 (2009) 3892.

[42] Y.Y. Choi, M.K. Joo, Y.S. Sohn, B. Jeong, Soft Matter 4 (2008) 2383.

[43] H.J. Oh, M.K. Joo, Y.S. Sohn, B. Jeong, Macromolecules 41 (2008) 8204.

[44] Y.Y. Choi, J.H. Jang, M.H. Park, B.G. Choi, B. Chi, B. Jeong, J. Mater. Chem. 20 (2010) 3416.

[45] Y. Jeong, M.K. Joo, K.H. Bahk, Y.Y. Choi, H.T. Kim, W.K. Kim, H.J. Lee, Y.S. Sohn, B. Jeong, J. Control. Release 137 (2009) 25.

[46] J. Lee, Y.H. Bae, Y.S. Sohn, B. Jeong, Biomacromolecules 7 (2006) 1729.

[47] B. Jeong, D.S. Lee, J.I. Shon, Y.H. Bae, S.W. Kim, J. Polym. Sci. A 37 (1999) 751.

[48] S.W. Choi, S.Y. Choi, B. Jeong, S.W. Kim, D.S. Lee, J. Polym. Sci. A 37 (1999) 2207.

[49] M.S. Kim, K.S. Seo, G. Khang, S.H. Cho, H.B. Lee, J. Polym. Sci. A 42 (2004) 5784.

[50] M.S. Kim, H. Hyun, Y.H. Cho, K.S. Seo, W.Y. Jang, S.K. Kim, G. Khang, H.B. Lee, Polym. Bull. (Berlin) 55 (2005) 149.

[51] D.S. Lee, M.S. Shim, S.W. Kim, H. Lee, I. Park, T. Chang, Macromol. Rapid Commun. 22 (2001) 587.

[52] B. Jeong, Y.H. Bae, S.W. Kim, Coll. Surf. B 16 (1999) 185.

[53] K.W. Kwon, M.J. Park, Y.H. Bae, H.D. Kim, K. Char, Polymer 43 (2002) 3353.

[54] M.J. Park, K. Char, Langmuir 20 (2004) 2456.

[55] D.S. Lee, M.S. Shim, S.W. Kim, H. Lee, I. Park, T. Chang, Macromol. Rapid Commun. 22 (2001) 587.

[56] G.M. Zentner, R. Rathi, C. Shih, J.C. McRea, M.H. Seo, H. Oh, B.G. Rhee, J. Mestecky, Z. Moldoveanu, M. Morgan, S. Weitman, J. Control. Release 72 (2001) 203.

[57] C.A. Bagley, M.J. Bookland, J. Neurosurg. 104 (2006) A653.

[58] L. Yu, G.T. Chang, H. Zhang, J.D. Ding, J. Polym. Sci. A 45 (2007) 1122.

[59] S.J. Bae, J.M. Suh, Y.S. Sohn, Y.H. Bae, S.W. Kim, B. Jeong, Macromolecules 38 (2005) 5260.

[60] Z. Jiang, Y. You, X. Deng, J. Hao, Polymer 48 (2007) 4786.

[61] L. Yu, W. Sheng, D. Yang, J. Ding, Macromol. Res. 21 (2013) 207.

[62] Y. Yoshida, A. Takahashi, A. Kuzuya, Y. Ohya, Polym. J. 46 (2014) 632.
[63] B. Jeong, L.Q. Wang, A. Gutowska, Chem. Commun. 16 (2001) 1516.
[64] B. Jeong, M.R. Kibbey, J.C. Birnbaum, Y.Y. Won, A. Gutowska, Macromolecules 33 (2000) 8317.
[65] S.J. Lee, B.R. Han, S.Y. Park, D.K. Han, S.C. Kim, J. Polym. Sci. A 44 (2006) 888.
[66] K. Nagahama, Y. Imai, T. Nakayama, J. Ohmura, T. Ouchi, Y. Ohya, Polymer 50 (2009) 3547.
[67] T. Ouchi, T. Nozaki, A. Ishikawa, I. Fujimoto, Y. Ohya, J. Polym. Sci. A 35 (1997) 377.
[68] Y. Ohya, H. Matsunami, E. Yamabe, T. Ouchi, J. Biomed. Mater. Res. 65A (2003) 79.
[69] F. Tasaka, Y. Ohya, T. Ouchi, Macromolecules 34 (2001) 5494.
[70] T. Ouchi, H. Seike, T. Nozaki, Y. Ohya, J. Polym. Sci. A 36 (1998) 1283.
[71] A. Takahashi, M. Umezaki, Y. Yosida, A. Kuzuya, Y. Ohya, J. Biomat. Sci. Polym. Ed. 25 (2014) 444.
[72] B. Jeong, Y.H. Bae, S.W. Kim, J. Control. Release 63 (2000) 155.
[73] M. Qiao, D. Chen, X. Ma, Y. Liu, Int. J. Pharm. 294 (2005) 103.
[74] D.P. Huynh, W.S. Shim, J.H. Kim, D.S. Lee, Polymer 47 (2006) 7918.
[75] T. Ouchi, Y. Ohya, Prog. Polym. Sci. 20 (1995) 211.
[76] Y. Ohya, H. Oue, K. Nagatomi, T. Ouchi, Biomacromolecules 2 (2001) 927.
[77] T. Ouchi, M. Tada, M. Matsumoto, Y. Ohya, K. Hasegawa, Y. Arai, K. Kadowaki, S. Akao, T. Matsumoto, S. Suzuki, M. Suzuki, J. Bioact. Compat. Polym. 13 (1998) 257.
[78] Y. Matsumura, H. Maeda, Cancer Res. 46 (1986) 6387.
[79] H. Maeda, Y. Matsumura, Crit. Rev. Ther. Drug Carrier Syst. 6 (1989) 1939.
[80] A. Takahashi, M. Umezaki, Y. Yosida, A. Kuzuya, Y. Ohya, Polym. Adv. Technol. 25 (2014) 1226.
[81] K. Nagahama, Y. Ohya, T. Ouchi, Macromol. Biosci. 6 (2006) 412.
[82] K. Nagahama, Y. Ohya, T. Ouchi, Polym. J. 38 (2006) 852.
[83] K. Nagahama, Y. Nishimura, Y. Ohya, T. Ouchi, Polymer 48 (2007) 2649.
[84] K. Nagahama, T. Ouchi, Y. Ohya, Adv. Funct. Mater. 18 (2008) 1220.
[85] H. Tsuji, Y. Ikada, Macromolecules 26 (1993) 6918.
[86] S.J. de Jong, S.C. De Smedt, M.W.C. Wahls, J. Demeester, J.J. Kettenes-van den Bosch, W.E. Hennink, Macromolecules 33 (2000) 3680.
[87] C.F. van Nostrum, T.F.J. Veldhuis, G.W. Bos, W.E. Hennink, Macromolecules 37 (2004) 2113.
[88] T. Mukose, T. Fujiwara, J. Nakano, I. Taniguchi, M. Miyamoto, Y. Kimura, I. Teraoka, C.W. Lee, Macromol. Biosci. 4 (2004) 361.
[89] C. Hiemstra, Z. Zhong, P.J. Dijkstra, J. Feijen, Macromol. Symp. 224 (2005) 119.
[90] C. Hiemstra, Z. Zhong, L. Li, P.J. Dijkstra, J. Feijen, Biomacromolecules 7 (2006) 2790.
[91] K. Nagahama, K. Fujiura, S. Enami, T. Ouchi, Y. Ohya, J. Polym. Sci. A 46 (2008) 6317.

2.4 Nature-Inspired Polymers

Yohei Kotsuchibashi*, Ravin Narain**

*INTERNATIONAL CENTER FOR YOUNG SCIENTISTS (ICYS) AND INTERNATIONAL CENTER FOR MATERIALS NANOARCHITECTONICS (MANA), NATIONAL INSTITUTE FOR MATERIALS SCIENCE (NIMS), TSUKUBA, JAPAN; **DEPARTMENT OF CHEMICAL AND MATERIALS ENGINEERING, UNIVERSITY OF ALBERTA, EDMONTON, AB, CANADA

CHAPTER OUTLINE

2.4.1 Introduction

With considerable and advanced developments in nanotechnological tools and techniques, it has become remarkably easy and fascinating to study materials at the micro- and nanoscale. For example, the lotus leaf shows super-hydrophobicity known as the "lotus effect" because of their waxy and hierarchical nano/microstructure surface, which explains its self-cleaning properties [1,2]. Miyauchi et al. prepared a silver ragwort leaf-like super-hydrophobic polystyrene fiber, having a contact angle beyond 150°, by electrospinning [3]. Inspired by the inner surface structure of the *Nepenthes* pitcher plants, Wong et al. created a slippery surface that can eliminate water, oil, and several mixed solutions [4]. Cai et al. were inspired by the rough skin of the *N. septentrionalis* for anisotropic oleophobicity under water [5]. The artificial fish skin was fabricated on a poly(dimethylsiloxane) layer that was also treated with soft lithography and oxygen-plasma treatment. The oil droplets on the artificial fish skin tend to roll off along a head-to-tail (HT) direction, but tend to pin in the opposite direction (TH direction). These oil-sliding angles were 22.5 ± 7.3° (HT direction) and 38.7 ± 3.7° (TH direction), respectively. We have efficiently prepared the nanoscale roughness on substrates for water repelling using a mixture of the size different silica nanoparticles (SiNPs) (average diameters: 20 and 128 nm) coated with the pH-responsive polymers [6–8]. The roughness was constructed on glass surface, polymeric nanofibers, and on paper via simple coating methods such as dip, cast, and spray coating. Moreover, the polymer-coated SiNPs could

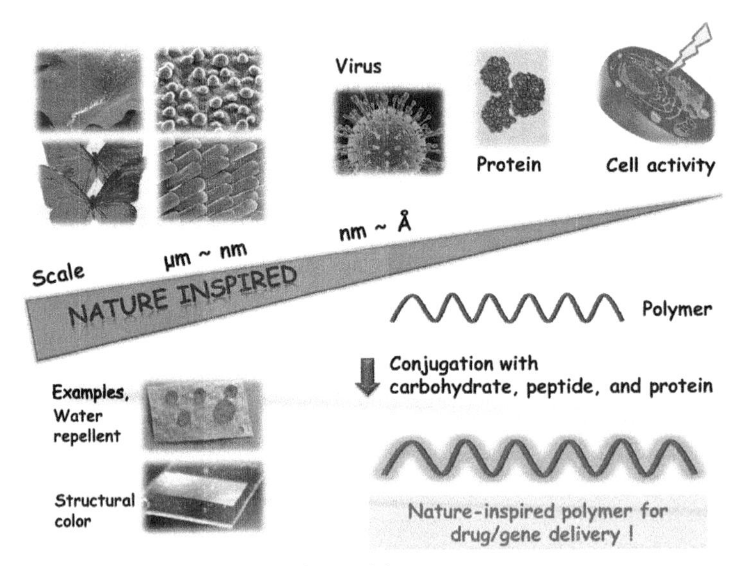

FIGURE 2.4.1 Nature-inspired polymers for drug and gene delivery system.

easily be removed from the substrates by washing with an acidic solution including lemon water due to the pH-responsive nature of the polymers.

The big question is: "What type of structures/phenomena of living things can we mimic using synthetic materials, particularly for drug and gene delivery applications?" Recently, with the rapid development in nanotechnology, it is possible to trace the work of an organelle in the cytoplasm of a living cell including its signal transduction. These observational techniques have been combined with smart polymers for understanding the local information on the living cell (Fig. 2.4.1). A temperature-responsive polymer with fluorescent units was used as a monitor of local temperature in living cells with the difference in fluorescence intensity depending on the organelles [9]. Chang et al. have prepared pH-responsive fluorescent hybrid nanoparticles for real-time cell labeling and endocytosis tracking [10]. The hybrid nanoparticles were composed of amphiphilic block copolymers, a silica-rich shell, rapid CPPs (HIV-1 TAT), and an encapsulated pH-responsive fluorophore. The fluorescent signal on the cell organelles of the human breast cancer cells (MCF-7) was tracked using confocal laser scanning microscopy and a flow cytometry analysis. The signal increased in acidic lysosomes with an increase of the incubation time (1, 4, and 8 h). Hayashi et al. achieved the selective labeling and profiling of glycoproteins on living cells using semisynthetic lectin-4-dimethylaminopyridine conjugates [11]. In addition, by a combination of immunoprecipitation with mass spectrometry fingerprinting techniques, some low-abundant glycoproteins including epidermal growth factor receptor and neuropilin-1 were identified from glycoproteins expressed on HeLa cells. These artificial nature-inspired polymers are expected to fit the cell cycle and cell activity, which makes them not only excellent drug/gene carriers but also a compass for understanding biological mechanisms.

2.4.2 Carbohydrate-Inspired Polymers

Carbohydrates (including glycoproteins) play important roles in biological processes such as cell–cell interactions, cell growth regulation, differentiation, adhesion, cancer cell metastasis, cellular trafficking, immunities, and inflammation [12–16]. Natural polymers consisting of carbohydrates (such as cellulose, starch, chitin, etc.) are abundant materials and have been actively used as biomaterials [17–19]. These natural polymers possess some unique biological properties and can avoid the stimulation of chronic inflammation, immunological reactions, and toxicity. However, it is still difficult to engineer these materials, and strict polymeric design is necessary in the biomedical field in order to avoid any unexpected side effects.

Synthetic glycopolymers have therefore received much attention due to the myriad of possibilities that can be achieved by the combination of controlled living radical polymerization (CLRP) and click chemistry [20–25]. However, when the glycomonomers are synthesized, the synthesis usually requires protection and deprotection group chemistries, which make the process tedious and economically not viable. We have directly synthesized (meth)acrylate and (meth)acrylamide types of glycomonomers without using protecting group chemistry [26–29]. Moreover, these monomers can be easily copolymerized with typical (meth)acrylate and (meth)acrylamide monomers. In recent years, several types of glycopolymers including linear polymers, branched polymers, cyclic polymers, and conjugated particles were prepared [12]. These biocompatible glycomonomers have been copolymerized with cationic monomers and the copolymers have been used to form conjugated nanoparticles with nucleic acids for gene delivery. In addition, glycopolymers are well known to interact with specific proteins and cells [15,16]. The carbohydrateprotein interaction is very important for the various types of biological systems (Fig. 2.4.2) [30]. For example, glycoproteins are proteins with one or more carbohydrate chains with fixed order such as sialic acid(Sia)-galactose(Gal)-*N*-acetylglucosamine and the terminal Sia group can be removed with the degradation of the protein, which leads to exposure of the Gal resulting in it becoming the new terminal group. The glycoprotein that exposes the Gal group is known as an asialoglycoprotein. The hepatocyte can recognize the asialoglycoprotein through the asialoglycoprotein receptor (ASGP-R), which is C type lectin and is overexpressed on these cells. Degraded glycoproteins from the blood flow are removed by the liver via the initial interactions with ASGP receptors.

Galactose-based DNA conjugated nanoparticles prepared by our group are efficiently uptaken in HepG2 cells by exploiting the interaction between galactose residues and ASGP-R. Random or block copolymers consisting of cationic 3-aminopropyl methacrylamide (APMA) or 2-aminoethyl methacrylamide (AEMA) and a glycomonomer of GAPMA have been prepared with a range of molecular weights and compositions by reversible addition fragmentation chain transfer polymerization [31]. These glyco-copolymers were used to form polyplexes with deoxyribonucleic acid (DNA) via an electrostatic interaction for a nonviral gene delivery system. Interestingly, the polyplexes consisting of random glycopolymers were found to have lower cellular toxicity and higher gene expression, both in

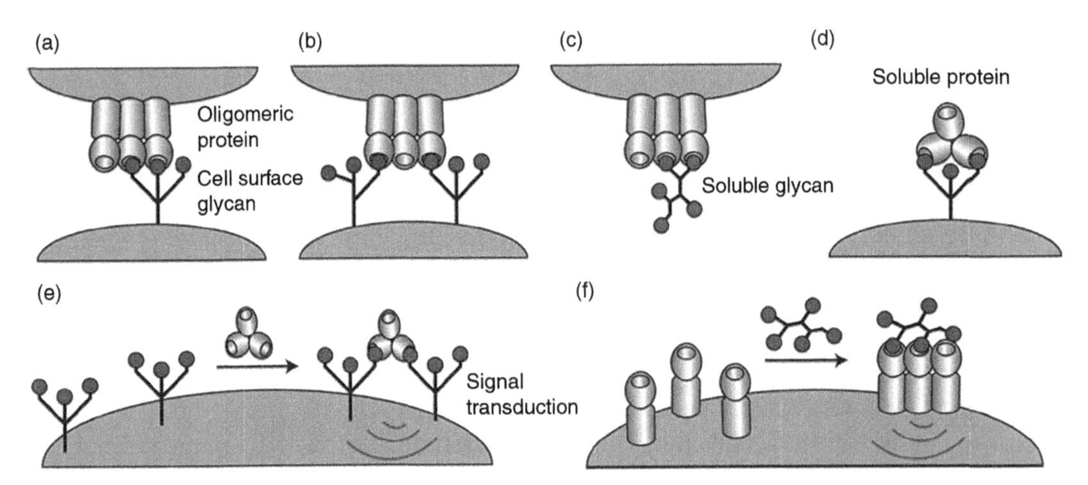

FIGURE 2.4.2 Interaction between carbohydrate-binding proteins and glycans through a variety of mechanisms. An oligomeric protein can interact with an individual cell-surface glycan (a) or with multiple difference cell-surface glycans simultaneously (b). Oligomeric proteins can also interact with soluble glycans or soluble oligomeric lectins can engage cell-surface glycans (c and d). Soluble proteins can cluster cell-surface glycoproteins to mediate signal transduction (e). Likewise, soluble glycans can cluster cell-surface receptors to mediate signal transduction (f) [30].

the presence and absence of serum, as compared to block copolymer-based polyplexes. The polyplexes prepared from block copolymers showed weak interactions with serum proteins, resulting in low cellular uptake and gene expression in HepG2 and HeLa cells. Moreover, the transfection efficiency of the DNA was strongly dependent on the structures consisting of galactose-based polymers such as statistical copolymers, block copolymers, and hyperbranched copolymers. Among them, the polyplexes consisting of hyperbranched copolymers showed high gene expression with low toxicity [14,32]. The ASGP-R may recognize the different glycopolymer structures in the polyplexes. Chen et al. prepared doxorubicin (DOX)-loaded nanoparticles consisting of poly(ε-caprolactone)-*g*-SS-lactobionic acid (PCL-*g*-SS-LBA) for a target drug delivery system (DDS) [33]. There were two kinds of nanoparticles (NPs) with or without S–S cross-linking, that is, SS–NPs and non-SS–NPs, respectively. The diameter of the SS–NPs was around 80 nm and the DOX loading capacity was 12.0 wt%. After 24 h in a reducing environment, 80.3% of DOX was released from the nanoparticles due to the dissociation of the S–S bond. On the other hand, in a nonreducing environment, the release was reduced to <21%. As the target cells, HepG2 cells (ASGP-R overexpression) and MCF-7 cells (ASGP-R negative) were selected. Both SS–NPs and non-SS–NPs showed low toxicity in HepG2 and MCF-7 (MTT assay: cell viabilities >95%, up to a tested concentration of 1.0 mg/mL). The half maximum inhibitory concentration (IC_{50}) of DOX-loaded SS–NPs in HepG2 was 0.1 μg DOX equiv./mL, which was 56 times lower than non-SS–NPs (free DOX, 0.24 μg). The high cell toxicity of the DOX-loaded SS–NPs was due to the rapid drug release after uptake under the intracellular reduction condition. Also, the IC50 of SS–NPs for the MCF-7 cells (ASGP-R negative) was 0.58 μg DOX equiv./mL.

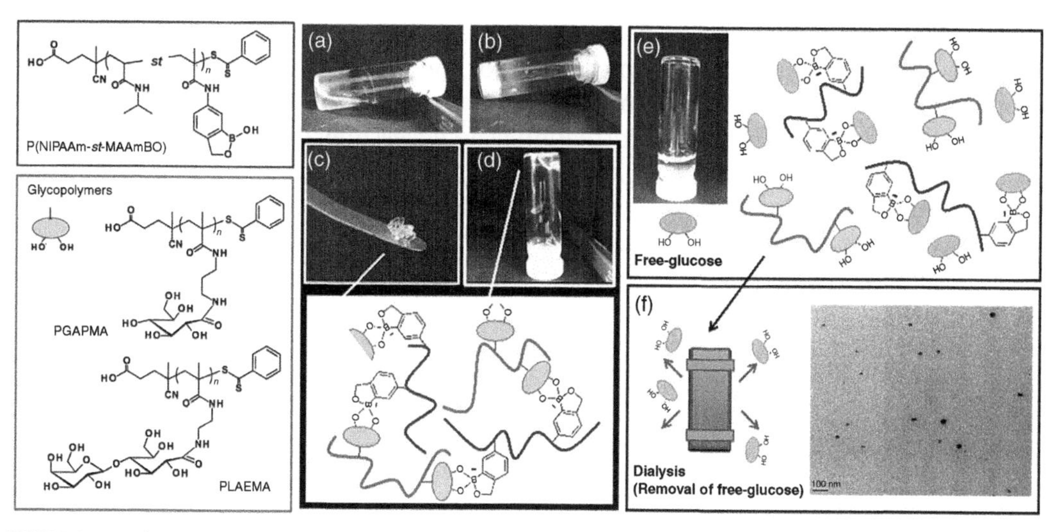

FIGURE 2.4.3 P ($NIPAAm_{90}$-*st*-$MAAmBO_{12}$) in pH 7.4 phosphate buffered saline (400 μL 10 wt%) at (a) 4 and (b) 30°C. Gel formation between P ($NIPAAm_{90}$-*st*-$MAAmBO_{12}$) (400 μL, 10 wt%) and (c) $PGAPMA_{30}$ (200 μL, 20 wt%) or (d) $PLAEMA_{21}$ (200 μL, 20 wt%) in pH 13 at 4°C. (e) Highlight gel formation by adding excess free glucose solution (600 μL, 10 wt%) into P($NIPAAm_{90}$-*st*-$MAAmBO_{12}$)-$PGAPMA_{30}$ gel sample in pH 13 at 4°C. (f) Transmission electron microscope image of nanogel consisting of P($NIPAAm_{90}$-*st*-$MAAmBO_{12}$) and $PGAPMA_{30}$ by dialysis in a large amount of pH 12 solution at 4°C [34].

It was found that glycopolymers could form a gel structure by simple mixing with the boroxole-based copolymers due to the reversible boronic-*cis*-diol interaction [34,35] (Fig. 2.4.3). Boronic acids and their esters have been applied to a wide range of fields such as catalysis for stereo-controlled synthesis, diagnosis, and medical treatment for human immunodeficiency virus (HIV), obesity, diabetes, and cancer [36]. For example, the reversible interaction between phenylboronic acid (PBA) and glucose was particularly used as a trigger for insulin release in the designed polymeric structure, that is, copolymers, particles, and gels [37–42]. Recently, Hall et al. reported the benzoxaborole group, which has a higher affinity than PBA toward saccharides in a buffer solution at a pH of 7.4 [43]. The K_a (M^{-1}) values were 28 ± 4 (glucose) and 43 ± 5 (*N*-acetylneuraminic acid [Neu5Ac]) in the benzoxaborole, respectively, which were higher than the K_a values with PBA (5 ± 1: glucose, 13 ± 1: Neu5Ac) [44]. The boroxole monomer of 5-methacrylamido-1,2-benzoxaborole (MAAmBO) was copolymerized with a typical temperature-responsive polymer, poly(*N*-isopropylacrylamide) (poly[NIPAAm]) (copolymers: poly[NIPAAm-*co*-MAAmBO]). The poly(NIPAAm-*co*-MAAmBO)s were mixed with glycopolymers of PGAPMA and poly(2-lactobionamidoethyl methacrylamide) (poly[LAEMA]) and the gel formation was observed in both glycopolymers [34]. This gelation system is promising for the incorporation/conjugation of various materials for several applications including DDS. Combination of this glycopolymer–boroxole gel system with photoinduced proton transfer chemistry (photoacid generators [PAGs]) can be used for local and remote controllable gel disintegration and drug release [35]. The PAGs can rapidly release the proton by UV irradiation and show local pH change in the solution/gel [45–48]. The pH decrease will lead to breakage of the glycopolymer–boroxole interaction for the pKa (7~8) of the boroxole group. In our system, one of the PAG samples, *o*-nitrobenzaldehyde (*o*-NBA), was loaded into glycopolymer–boroxole gel. The gel formation was successfully disintegrated upon UV irradiation with the local pH decrease in the gel resulting in release of the loaded drug and subsequently in the collapse of the glycopolymer–boroxole interaction.

Glycopolymers are also able to act as a drug for their specific interaction with biomolecules, resulting in control of the immune system, antibacterium, and virus neutralization. Tanaka et al. prepared the glycopolymers bearing sialyloligosaccharide, which could interact with both human and avian influenza virus [49]. The hemagglutinin is one of the spike proteins of the influenza virus that can recognize the sialic acid on the host cell during the infection process. Therefore, the glycopolymers are expected to neutralize the influenza virus due to the interaction of the virus with the sialyloligosaccharide. Among the acrylamide types of glycopolymers, the *N*-glycan-based glycopolymer showed the strongest interaction with both human and avian influenza virus. By the hemagglutination inhibition test, the minimum concentrations of the *N*-glycan-based glycopolymer for human and avian influenza virus were 4.9×10^{-7} and 6.3×10^{-5} g/mL, respectively. These values were lower than control fetuin (human influenza virus: 7.8×10^{-5} g/mL, avian influenza virus: 5.0×10^{-3} g/mL), which suggested strong interaction of the glycopolymer with both influenza viruses. This strong interaction was caused by the glyco-cluster effect [50] and the biantenna structure of the *N*-linked oligosaccharide; these glycopolymers are applied not only in virus neutralization but also in sensitive virus diagnosis. Zhang et al. reported linear glycopolymers with precise control of the numbers/orders of the monomer units [51]. The glycopolymers were composed of 12~27 units of sugar residues (having mannose and glucose groups) that were polymerized through six steps by the CLRP. These short chains of glycopolymers were expected to prevent interactions between dendritic cell-specific intercellular (DC-SIGN) and gp120 protein on HIV virus. In fact, the glycopolymers were found to show strong interactions with DC-SIGN with increasing mannose content and the bond orders of sugar units can also affect these interactions. Therefore, these glycopolymers can be useful in various types of anti-infection systems. The same group also tried drug delivery of anti-HIV drug using the β-cyclodextrin (CD)-based glycoconjugates of different structures (CD-based glyco-clusters and CD-based star glycopolymers) [52] (Fig. 2.4.4). These CD-based glycoconjugates can interact with human transmembrane lectin DC-SIGN and prevent the interaction with HIV envelope protein gp120. The IC50 (measured by surface plasmon resonance) of a CD-based glycoconjugate of β-CD-$[(Man)9.6]_{16}$ was ~30 nM, which was slightly higher than the control of the envelope protein gp120 (~11 nM). This result suggests that the CD-based glycoconjugate can be satisfyingly used as an inhibitor for interaction between HIV and DG-SIGN. As an anti-HIV drug, saquinavir, which is an important class of archetypal HIV protease inhibitors, was selected [53]. The saquinavir was efficiently encapsulated into a star block copolymer β-CD-$[(DEGEEA)_{10}$-*b*-$(Man)5]_{16}$ due to the hydrophobic DEGEEA segment, and the calculated drug loading amount in each CD-based glycoconjugate was four saquinavir mesylate molecules on average.

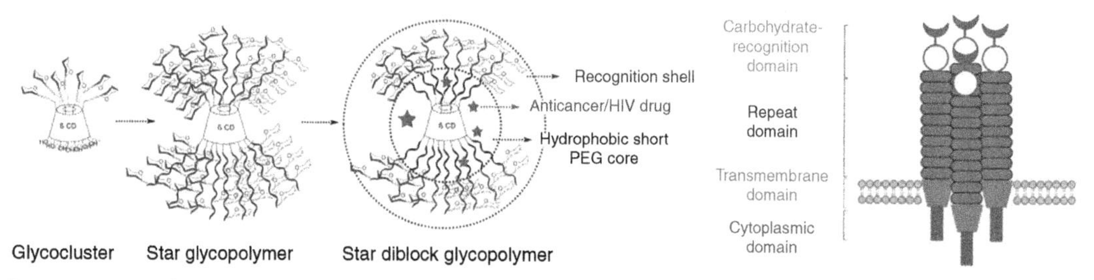

FIGURE 2.4.4 Synthesis route from glycocluster to star diblock glycopolymer and schematic structure of human DC-SIGN lectin [52].

2.4.3 Peptide/Protein-Inspired Polymers

Peptides play an important role in several physiological activities such as neurotransmitter, neurotrophic factor, growth factor, and cytokine. Among them, cell-targeting and CPP have the potential for efficient drug delivery. These cell-targeting peptides are summarized in Table 2.4.1 [54–56]. The advantage of nanoparticles with cell-targeting peptides is their switchable surface properties. The peptides on the nanoparticle can be customized based on the target cell line and tissue [57].

CPP are mainly divided into two types: (1) amphipathic helical peptides such as transportin and model amphipathic peptide having lysine as a main contributor to the positive charge, and (2) arginine-rich peptides such as transactivating transcriptional activator (TAT) and homeodomain of antennapedia (Antp) [54]. The HIV-1 TAT peptide is composed of six arginine units and two lysine units in the sequence and is known to show high permeability to the cell membrane, which has been combined with several materials for effective delivery into the cytoplasm [58,59]. Mao et al. prepared a fluorescein isothiocyanate (FITC)-SiNPs-TAT peptide (around 200 nm), and estimated their ability for

Table 2.4.1 Some of the Peptides Evidenced to Target-Specific Tissues or Cell Types [56]

Peptide Sequence	Length	Targeted Tissue	Cellular Target
TSPLNIHNGQKL	12	Human head and neck solid tumors	Unknown
CGKRK	5	Tumor neovasculature	Heparan sulfate
CGNKRTRGC	7*	Breast carcinoma	Unknown
SMSIARL	7	Prostate vasculature	Unknown
FQHPSFI	7	Hepatocellular carcinoma cell line	Unknown
RGD	3	Integrin receptor	$\alpha V\beta 3$
NGR	3	Tumor neovasculature	Amino peptidase N
VHSPNKK	7	Endothelial VCAM-1 expressing cells	VCAM-1
RRPYIL	6	Adenocarcinoma cells	Neurotensin receptor
EDYELMDLLAYL	12	Various carcinomas	Unknown
LTVSPWY	7	Breast carcinoma	erbB2
ATWLPPR	7	Tumor neovasculature	VEGF receptor

*Excluding the cysteine residues used for peptide cyclization.

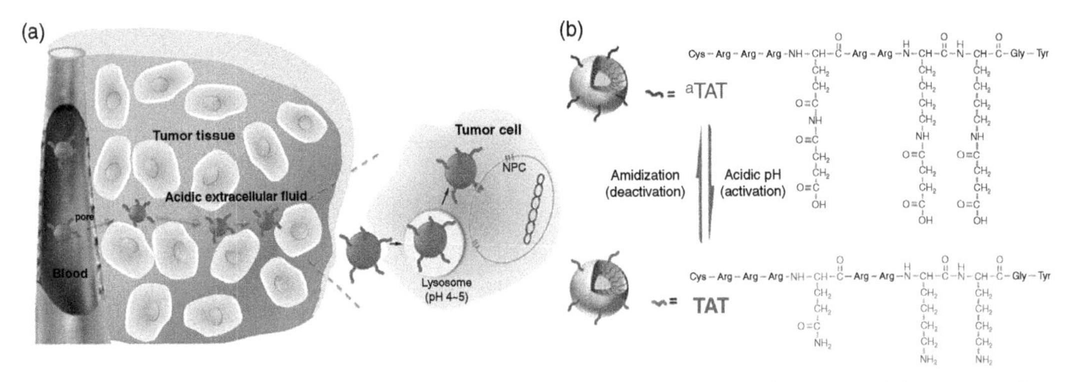

FIGURE 2.4.5 (a) Illustration of the use of TAT as an example of a CPP to demonstrate the concept of deactivation of a CPP in the blood compartment and its activation in the tumor interstitium or cells for *in vivo* tumor-targeted drug delivery. (b) Amidization of TAT's primary amines to succinyl amides and their acid-triggered hydrolysis [65].

permeability and targeting to the nucleus at differential modified TAT peptide amounts [60]. These FITC-SiNPs-Tat peptides were incubated with HepG2 cells. After incubation for 8 h, the fluorescence intensity of the FITC-SiNPs-TAT peptide was 4.5 times higher than that of the FITC-SiNPs-NH_2. Moreover, the FITC-SiNPs-TAT peptides were observed to transfer into the nucleus after 24 h. Wu et al. prepared mesoporous organosilica nanoparticles (MOSiNPs) with large pore size for efficient nuclear-targeted gene delivery [61]. The mesoporous silica nanoparticles (MSiNPs) are known as an excellent drug carrier [62–64]. For gene delivery, however, the gene is adsorbed on the silica surface due to the relatively small pore size (<3 nm). The prepared MOSiNPs had the large-pore size (N_2 adsorption: 6.2 nm, and transmission electron microscope 8–13 nm) and the diameter was 51 nm. The surface of the MOSiNPs was modified with cationic polyethyleneimine (PEI) and TAT peptide for gene delivery (MOSiNPs-PEI-TAT). The loading amount of a plasmid DNA into the MOSiNPs-PEI-TAT was 66.67 μg/mg that was twice higher than that of the control MSiNPs-PEI-TAT (33.3 μg/mg). These SiNPs were incubated with HeLa cells and the intracellular silicon amount was observed. In the MOSiNPs-PEI-TAT, the intranuclear silicon amount was 18~21 times higher than MOSiNPs-PEI. Interestingly, no remarkable difference was observed between MOSiNPs-PEI-TAT and MOSiNPs-PEI in the total intracellular silicon amount (1.7~2.4 times). In addition, the MOSiNPs-PEI-TAT showed high transfection efficiency (35.5%) as compared with MOSiNPs-PEI (13.5%) and MSiNPs-PEI-TAT (4.97%). Thus, TAT peptide possesses the cell penetration ability. There is the possibility, however, to induce a nonspecific interaction due to the lysine-based positive charge. Jin et al. protected the TAT peptide on the PEG-PCL micelle to prevent the nonspecific interaction as an efficient nuclear DDS (Fig. 2.4.5) [65]. The lysine residues' amines of the TAT peptide were converted to succinyl amides (^{a}TAT). The protected ^{a}TAT is expected to convert TAT in acidic tumor interstitium or internalized into cell endo/lysosomes. In fact, at pH 5, almost all of the ^{a}TAT peptide was converted to the original TAT peptide after 24 h. The ^{a}TAT-PEG-PCL micelle encapsulates drugs and the diameters were 75 (DOX: drug loading 13.6wt%) and 92 nm (a near-IR fluorescence dye, DiR: drug loading 14.3wt%), respectively. The aTAT-PEG-PCL micelle was incubated in SKOV-3 ovarian cancer cells, and after 24 h, the micelle had accumulated around the nucleus. On the other hand, there was no accumulation at the nucleus in the case of the PEG-PCL micelle. The clearance of the aTAT-PEG-PCL was prolonged *in vivo* with reduced nonspecific interactions and enhanced blood compatibility. The calculated tumor-inhibition rates were 47% (aTAT-PEG-PCL micelle/DOX), 29% (PEG-PCL micelle/DOX), and 18% (TAT-PEG-PCL micelle/DOX), respectively, which suggested that aTAT-PEG-PCL micelle/DOX has enhanced cancer therapeutic efficacy. Moreover, the cancer tissue cells treated with the aTAT-PEG-PCL micelle/DOX were observed to induce apoptosis.

Synthetic poly(amino acid)s (polypeptides) are biodegradable and biocompatible polymers that have similar structures to natural proteins [66]. These polypeptides have been used for drug and gene delivery [67,68]. Unlike typical synthetic polymers, polypeptide possesses a secondary structure (α-helix and β-sheet) due to the cooperative hydrogen bonding, which leads to their specific self-assembled structures [69,70]. For example, some polypeptides (including comb-like polymers with polypeptide) can form a fiber structure due to the supramolecular self-assembly. These fiber structures can occur *in vivo* due to the aggregation/precipitation of the denatured proteins, and in many cases, they can lead to serious diseases such as neurodegenerative disease including Alzheimer's and Parkinson's diseases. The cause of the neurodegenerative disease is a result of the misfolding of proteins, and subsequent aggregation of the denatured proteins (amyloid fiber) whose accumulation causes toxicity to nerve cells [71,72]. Many natural proteins are also known to convert amyloid fibers (width: 8–30 nm and lengths: several micrometers) at high concentration under destabilizing conditions and with Young's moduli ranges from 0.2 GPa to 20 GPa [73–76]. With these unique properties, amyloid fibers have recently been used as biomaterials for tissue engineering, drug delivery, protein films, and for retroviral gene transfer enhancers [77–83]. Moreover, the "on/off" switchable peptide-based fibers have been reported for controlled cell toxicity. In these cases, therefore, the peptide-based fiber itself acts as a drug. Shi et al. reported that an induced necrotic cell death triggered by the aggregation of molecules due to the ligand–receptor interaction [84]. Self-aggregating materials in aqueous conditions usually have hydrophobic properties. Therefore, organic solvents are often required for their dissolution and the aggregates are formed once the mixed solvent is added to water followed by evaporation. In addition, it is difficult to control the size of aggregates. The size of aggregated particles usually increases with time, and finally precipitates out of solution. To overcome the problems, they selected a ligand–receptor interaction between vancomycin and D-Ala-D-Ala, which works as a trigger for the controlled aggregation. D-Ala-D-Ala is a peptidoglycan that is one of the essentials of cell wall bacteria. The vancomycin can specifically interact with the D-Ala-D-Ala, which leads to antimicrobial activity. In addition, the binding of cancomycine and D-Ala-D-Ala is known to promote self-assembled nanofiber aggregation [85,86]. The D-Ala-D-Ala and aromatic groups containing small peptides were synthesized for controlling the fiber aggregation through the interaction with vancomycin. The fiber aggregation of the

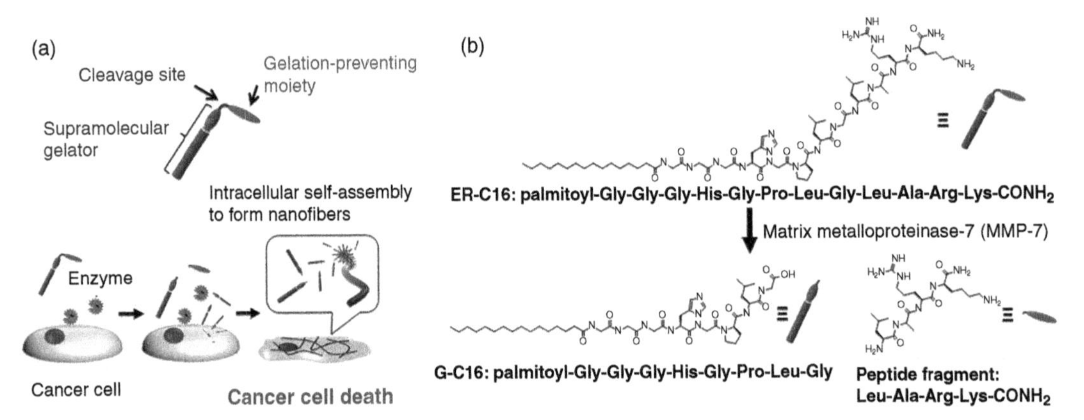

FIGURE 2.4.6 (a) Cancer cell death induced by molecular self-assembly of an enzyme-responsive supramolecular gelator and (b) molecular structures of *N*-palmitoyl-Gly-Gly-Gly-His-Gly-Pro-Leu-Gly-Leu-Ala-Arg-Lys-$CONH_2$ (ER-C16), *N*-palmitoyl-Gly-Gly-Gly-His-Gly-Pro-Leu-Gly (G-C16), and Leu-Ala-Arg-Lys-$CONH_2$ (peptide fragment) [87].

D-Ala-D-Ala/aromatic group containing small peptides and vancomycin caused cell necrosis by the inhibition of cell growth (concentration: 0.2 mg/mL). On the other hand, as a control, no cell toxicity was observed in the small peptides with L-Ala-L-Ala and small peptides without aromatic groups. Both ligand–receptor and aromatic–aromatic interactions play a key role in the fiber aggregation process, resulting in the induction of necrotic cell death. Tanaka et al. prepared an enzyme-responsive supramolecular gelator for an induced cancer cell death (Fig. 2.4.6) [87]. The supramolecular gelator is a peptide–lipid precursor that is composed of palmitoyl-Gly-Gly-Gly-His-Gly-Pro-Leu-Gly-Leu-Ala-Arg-Lys-CONH2 (ER-C16). The alkyl chain of the Fly-Gly-Gly-His part has both hydrogen bonding donor and acceptor. Moreover, the terminal cationic peptide Arg-Lys prevents precursor aggregation due to the electrostatic repulsion. When the peptide–lipid precursor ER-C16 is exposed to a cancer-related enzyme of matrix metalloproteinase-7 (MMP-7), the Gly-Leu part is cleaved and the generated palmitoyl-Gly-Gly-Gly-His-Gly-Pro-Leu-Gly (G-C16) forms intercellular self-assembled nanofibers. The peptide–lipid precursor ER-C16 is an aqueous solution at 0.2 wt% (50 mM tris-HCl containing 150 mM NaCl, 2 mM CaCl2, pH 7.4). On the other hand, nanofibers were observed by adding 2 μg/mL of MMP-7 in ER-C16 solution after 2 h. Under this condition, over 50% of ER-C16 is converted to G-C16 by MMP-7, which is formed into nanofibers. As a result of the cell toxicity test, HeLa cells and normal human dermal microvascular endothelial (MvE) cells were selected. For the HeLa cells, cell viability was down to 35% by the peptide–lipid precursor ER-C16 (0.01 wt%). On the other hand, the ER-C16 displayed no cell toxicity with MvE cells. The specific HeLa cell toxicity was explained by the formation of MMP-7 in HeLa cells. The MMP-7 became a trigger for transformation from ER-C16 to assemble G-C16 (nanofibers) in the cell, and the prepared nanofibers led to cell death. In fact, the intracellular MMP-7 in HeLa cells was six times higher than MvE cells. The treated HeLa cells with ER-C16 were lysed by ultrasonication and the cell lysate showed a gelation that was composed of nanofibers.

Protein therapeutics has received a lot of attention because cellular functions are in large part carried out by proteins [88]. However, therapeutic proteins are often decomposed *in vivo* and are immediately excreted from blood circulation. To solve this problem and to add more function, proteins have been conjugated with synthetic polymers. For example, proteins conjugated with poly(ethylene glycol) (PEG) (known as PEGylation) can have extended circulation time [89,90]. Stayton et al. reported an "on/off" switch of the protein function by combining the temperature-responsive polymer [91]. Cummings et al. polymerized a dual temperature-responsive polymer, poly(sulfobetaine methacrylamide [SBMAm])-*b*-poly(NIPAAm) from a protein chymotrypsin (CT) [92]. The poly(SBMAm)-*b*-poly(NIPAAm) on the CT could control the access of the CT substrate due to the structures depending on the temperature. Also, the activity of modified CT was kept around 70% after incubation for 75 min in pH 1 with pepsin. These high stabilities on the modified CT were explained by the hydration/dehydration of poly(SBMAm)-*b*-poly(NIPAAm) resulting in the restriction of the access to CT molecules. Recently, the conjugation of proteins with polymers has been achieved under bioinert conditions such as body temperature, buffer solution, and toxic-free material [93]. Hu et al. prepared a cyclized protein–polymer conjugate for enhanced thermal stability and cancer accumulation [94]. The cyclization of protein was achieved by sortase-mediated protein ligation, which is known as one of the effective synthesis methods for the cyclized protein with improved thermal stability [95,96]. Green fluorescence protein (GFP) was selected as a model protein and was cyclized to combine its N- and C-termini (*c*-GFP). Biocompatible oligo(ethylene glycol) methyl ether methacrylate (OEGMA) was synthesized from the *c*-GFP and linear (*l*)-GFP (*c*-GFP-POEGMA and *l*-GFP-POEGMA). These conjugated proteins were heated to 90°C for 5 min, and the fluorescence recovery of *c*-GFP-POEGMA was 31%, which was 310-fold and ninefold higher than that of *l*-GFP-POEGMA and *l*-GFP, respectively. This high thermal stability was due to the cyclized protein structure. In addition, enhanced accumulation of the cyclized protein in cancer was also observed. After 48 h postinjection, *c*-GFP-POEGMA was found to remain in cancer tissue and the fluorescence intensity was over sixfold higher than that of *l*-GFP-POEGMA. Lu et al. prepared an antibody–polymer conjugate for siRNA delivery [97] (Fig. 2.4.7). Anti-HER2 antibodies including the S202-pAcF Fab were combined with the cationic polymers (S202-Fab-polymer). A conjugated S202-Fab-polymer/FITC-siRNA was incubated with $HER2^+$-positive SKBR-3 cells and HER2-HeLa cells, and the fluorescence was only observed in the $HER2^+$-positive SKBR-3 cells. Moreover, for the selective gene knockdown, the S202-Fab-polymer was conjugated with a GAPDH-specific siRNA, and the conjugates showed 88% knockdown of the targeted GAPDA mRNA.

2.4.4 Conclusion and Future Trends

This chapter introduced the nature-inspired polymers with the ability to mimic cell activity for advanced drug and gene delivery. These polymers have been combined with biomolecules such as carbohydrates, peptides, and proteins, which played the prominent roles not only of excellent drug carriers but also of drug molecules themselves. For further

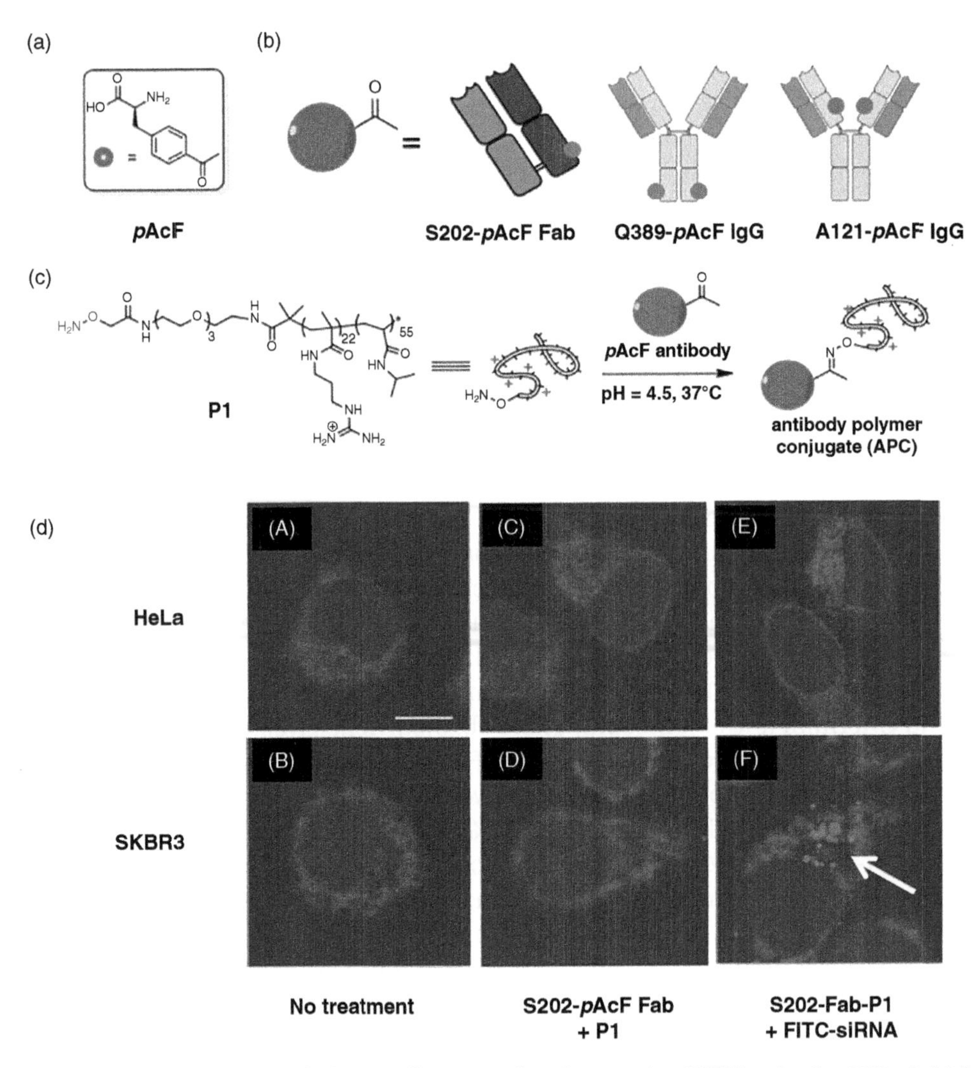

FIGURE 2.4.7 (a) Structure of *p*AcF. (b) Schematic illustration of *p*AcF mutated anti-HER2 antibodies, S202-*p*AcF Fab, Q389-*p*AcF IgG, and A121-*p*AcF IgG. (c) Synthetic scheme for the antibody–polymer conjugates. (d) Confocal microscopy of internalization of siRNA mediated by S202-Fab-P1. HeLa (A, C, E) and SKBR-3 (B, D, F) cells were treated with buffer (A, B), 200 nM S202-pAcF Fab + 200 nM P1 + 50 nM siRNA-FITC (C, D), or 200 nM S202-Fab-P1 + 50 nM siRNA-FITC (E, F) for 4 h. Cells were then stained with Hoechst 33342 (blue) and ER-Tracker (red) and imaged with a Leica 710 confocal microscope. Bar = 10 μm [97].

development of the nature-inspired polymers, greater structure control is indispensable, and the preparation methods such as CLRP and click chemistry will play a key role in overcoming this challenge. Recently, by these preparation methods, the linear polymer structures have been controlled on a monomer unit scale. Moreover, the multiblock copolymers (over 10 blocks) have been synthesized [98–100]. However, their molecular weights are relatively small (<10,000 g/mol), and the short polymer chain is not enough to form the folding structures like natural proteins. Understandably, it is very difficult to mimic these complex protein structures via conventional polymers. In the near future, polymers with remarkable structures and properties will be designed and fabricated to mimic more closely the natural macromolecules. Therefore, nature-inspired polymers combined with advanced preparation techniques will open a new platform for drug/gene delivery systems.

References

[1] W. Barthlott, C. Neinhuis, Planta 202 (1997) 1.

[2] L. Feng, S. Li, Y. Li, H. Li, L. Zhang, J. Zhai, Y. Song, B. Liu, L. Jiang, D. Zhu, Adv. Mater. 14 (2002) 1857.

[3] Y. Miyauchi, B. Ding, S. Shiratori, Nanotechnology 17 (2006) 5151.

[4] T.-S. Wong, S.H. Kang, S.K.Y. Tang, E.J. Smythe, B.D. Hatton, A. Grinthal, J. Aizenberg, Nature 477 (2011) 443.

[5] Y. Cai, L. Lin, Z. Xue, M. Liu, S. Wang, L. Jiang, Adv. Funct. Mater. 24 (2014) 809.

[6] Y. Kotsuchibashi, A. Faghihnejad, H. Zeng, R. Narain, Polym. Chem. 4 (2013) 1038.

[7] Y. Kotsuchibashi, Y. Wang, Y.-J. Kim, M. Ebara, T. Aoyagi, R. Narain, ACS Appl. Mater. Interfaces 5 (2013) 10004.

[8] Y. Kotsuchibashi, M. Ebara, T. Aoyagi, R. Narain, Polym. Chem. 3 (2012) 2545.

[9] K. Okabe, N. Inada, C. Gota, Y. Harada, T. Funatsu, S. Uchiyama, Nat. Commun. 3 (2012) 705.

[10] S. Chang, X. Wu, Y. Li, D. Niu, Y. Gao, Z. Ma, J. Gu, W. Zhao, W. Zhu, H. Tian, J. Shi, Biomaterials 34 (2013) 10182.

[11] T. Hayashi, Y. Sun, T. Tamura, K. Kuwata, Z. Song, Y. Takaoka, I. Hamachi, J. Am. Chem. Soc. 135 (2013) 12252.

[12] R. Narain, Engineered Carbohydrate-Based Materials for Biomedical Applications, John Wiley & Sons, Inc, New York, NY, (2011).

[13] M. Ahmed, R. Narain, Biomaterials 32 (2011) 5279.

[14] M. Ahmed, R. Narain, Biomaterials 33 (2012) 3990.

[15] A. Maruyama, T. Ishihara, J.-S. Kim, S.W. Kim, T. Akaike, Bioconjug. Chem. 8 (1997) 735.

[16] U. Hasegawa, S.-M. Nomura, S.C. Kaul, T. Hirano, K. Akiyoshi, Biochem. Biophys. Res. Commun. 331 (2005) 917.

[17] J.F. Mano, G.A. Silva, H.S. Azevedo, P.B. Malafaya, R.A. Sousa, S.S. Silva, L.F. Boesel, J.M. Oliveira, T.C. Santos, A.P. Marques, N.M. Neves, R.L. Reis, J. R. Soc. Interface 4 (2007) 999.

[18] L.I.F. Moura, A.M.A. Dias, E. Carvalho, H.C. de Sousa, Acta Biomater. 9 (2013) 7093–7114.

[19] G. Siqueira, J. Bras, A. Dufresne, Polymers 2 (2010) 728.

[20] M.K. Georges, R.P.N. Veregin, P.M. Kazmaier, G.K. Hamer, Macromolecules 26 (1993) 2987.

[21] M. Kato, M. Kamigaito, M. Sawamoto, T. Higashimura, Macromolecules 28 (1995) 1721.

[22] J.-S. Wang, K. Matyjaszewski, Macromolecules 28 (1995) 7572.

[23] J. Chiefari, Y.K. Chong, F. Ercole, J. Krstina, J. Jeffery, T.P.T. Le, R.T.A. Mayadunne, G.F. Meijs, C.L. Moad, G. Moad, E. Rizzardo, S.H. Thang, Macromolecules 31 (1998) 5559.

[24] Y.K. Chong, T.P.T. Le, G. Moad, E. Rizzardo, S.H. Thang, Macromolecules 32 (1999) 2071.

[25] H.C. Kolb, M.G. Finn, K.B. Sharpless, Angew. Chem. Int. Ed. 40 (2001) 2004.

[26] R. Narain, S.P. Armes, Chem. Commun. 23 (2002) 2776.

[27] R. Narain, S.P. Armes, Macromolecules 36 (2003) 4675.

[28] Z. Deng, M. Ahmed, R. Narain, J. Polym. Sci. A 47 (2009) 614.

[29] M. Ahmed, M. Jawanda, K. Ishihara, R. Narain, Biomaterials 33 (2012) 7858.

[30] L.L. Kiessling, J.C. Grima, Chem. Soc. Rev. 42 (2013) 4476.

[31] M. Ahmed, R. Narain, Biomaterials 32 (2011) 5279.

[32] M. Ahmed, P. Wattanaarsakit, R. Narain, Eur. Polym. J. 49 (2013) 3010.

[33] W. Chen, Y. Zou, F. Meng, R. Cheng, C. Deng, J. Feijen, Z. Zhong, Biomacromolecules 15 (2014) 900.

[34] Y. Kotsuchibashi, R.V.C. Agustin, J.-Y. Lu, D.G. Hall, R. Narain, ACS Macro. Lett. 2 (2013) 260.

[35] Y. Kotsuchibashi, M. Ebara, T. Sato, Y. Wang, R. Rajender, D.G. Hall, R. Narain, T. Aoyagi, J. Phys. Chem. B 119 (2015) 2323.

[36] D.G. Hall, Boronic Acids: Preparation and Applications in Organic Synthesis, Medicine and Materials, second ed., Wiley-VCH, Weinheim, Germany, (2011).

[37] J. Böeseken, Adv. Carbohydr. Chem. 4 (1949) 189.

[38] A. Matsumoto, K. Yamamoto, R. Yoshida, K. Kataoka, T. Aoyagi, Y. Miyahara, Chem. Commun. 46 (2010) 2203.

[39] K. Kataoka, H. Miyazaki, M. Bunya, T. Okano, Y. Sakurai, J. Am. Chem. Soc. 120 (1998) 12694.

[40] A. Matsumoto, S. Ikeda, A. Harada, K. Kataoka, Biomacromolecules 4 (2003) 1410.

[41] Y. Qin, G. Cheng, A. Sundararaman, F. Jäkle, J. Am. Chem. Soc. 124 (2002) 12672.

[42] D. Roy, J.N. Cambre, B.S. Sumerlin, Chem. Commun. 30 (2009) 2106.

[43] M. Dowlut, D.G. Hall, J. Am. Chem. Soc. 128 (2006) 4226.

[44] G.A. Ellis, M.J. Palte, R.T. Raines, J. Am. Chem. Soc. 134 (2012) 3631.

[45] M. Irie, J. Am. Chem. Soc. 105 (1983) 2078.

[46] J. Choi, N. Hirota, M. Terazima, J. Phys. Chem. A 105 (2001) 12.

[47] S. Abbruzzetti, M. Carcelli, D. Rogolino, C. Viappiani, Photochem. Photobiol. Sci. 2 (2003) 796.

[48] M.V. George, J.C. Scaiano, J. Phys. Chem. 84 (1980) 492.

[49] T. Tanaka, H. Ishitani, Y. Miura, K. Oishi, T. Takahashi, T. Suzuki, S. Shoda, Y. Kimura, ACS Macro. Lett. 3 (2014) 1074.

[50] Y.C. Lee, R.T. Lee, Acc. Chem. Res. 28 (1995) 321.

[51] Q. Zhang, J. Collins, A. Anastasaki, R. Wallis, D.A. Mitchell, C.R. Becer, D.M. Haddleton, Angew. Chem. Int. Ed. 52 (2013) 4435.

[52] Q. Zhang, L. Su, J. Collins, G. Chen, R. Wallis, D.A. Mitchell, D.M. Haddleton, C.R. Becer, J. Am. Chem. Soc. 136 (2014) 4325.

[53] C.M. Buchanan, N.L. Buchanan, K.J. Edgar, J.L. Little, M.G. Ramsey, K.M. Ruble, V.J. Wacher, M.F. Wempe, Biomacromolecules 9 (2007) 305.

[54] B. Gupta, T.S. Levchenko, V.P. Torchilin, Adv. Drug Deliver. Rev. 57 (2005) 637.

[55] U. Hersel, C. Dahmen, H. Kessler, Biomaterials 24 (2003) 4385.

[56] E. Vivès, J. Schmidt, A. Pèlegrin, Biochim. Biophys. Acta 1786 (2008) 126.

[57] Y. Zhong, F. Meng, C. Deng, Z. Zhong, Biomacromolecules 15 (2014) 1955.

[58] A.G. Tkachenko, H. Xie, D. Coleman, W. Glomm, J. Ryan, M.F. Anderson, S. Franzen, D.L. Feldheim, J. Am. Chem. Soc. 125 (2003) 4700.

[59] V.A. Sethuraman, Y.H. Bae, J. Control. Release 118 (2007) 216.

[60] Z. Mao, L. Wan, L. Hu, L. Ma, C. Gao, Colloids Surf. B 75 (2010) 432.

[61] M. Wu, Q. Meng, Y. Chen, Y. Du, L. Zhang, Y. Li, L. Zhang, J. Shi, Adv. Mater. 27 (2015) 215.

[62] I.I. Slowing, J.L. Vivero-Escoto, C.W. Wu, V.S. Lin, Adv. Drug Delivery Rev. 60 (2008) 1278.

[63] Q.J. He, J.M. Zhang, J.L. Shi, Z.Y. Zhu, L.X. Zhang, W.B. Bu, L.M. Guo, Y. Chen, Biomaterials 31 (2010) 1085.

[64] Q.J. He, J.L. Shi, J. Mater. Chem. 21 (2011) 5845.

[65] E. Jin, B. Zhang, X. Sun, Z. Zhou, X. Ma, Q. Sun, J. Tang, Y. Shen, E.V. Kirk, W.J. Murdoch, M. Radosz, J. Am. Chem. Soc. 135 (2013) 933.

[66] T.J. Deming, Prog. Polym. Sci. 32 (2007) 858.

[67] N. Nishiyama, K. Kataoka, Pharmacol. Therapeut. 3 (2006) 630.

[68] I.W. Hamley, Soft Matter 7 (2011) 4122.

[69] A. Carlsen, S. Lecommandoux, Curr. Opin. Colloid Interface Sci. 14 (2009) 329.

[70] H. Schlaad, Adv. Polym. Sci. 202 (2006) 53.

[71] R.W. Carrell, D.A. Lomas, Lancet 350 (1997) 134.

[72] C.M. Dobson, Nature 426 (2003) 884.

[73] L. Goldschmidt, P.K. Teng, R. Riek, D. Eisenberg, Proc. Natl. Acad. Sci. USA 107 (2010) 3487.

[74] C.M. Dobson, Nature 426 (2003) 884.

[75] J. Adamcik, J.-M. Jung, J. Flakowski, P. De Los Rios, G. Dietler, R. Mezzenga, Nat. Nanotechnol. 5 (2010) 423.

[76] D. Li, E.M. Jones, M.R. Sawaya, H. Furukawa, F. Luo, M. Ivanova, S.A. Sievers, W. Wang, O.M. Yaghi, C. Liu, D.S. Eisenberg, J. Am. Chem. Soc. 136 (2014) 18044.

[77] T.C. Holmes, S. de Lacalle, X. Su, G. Liu, A. Rich, S. Zhang, Proc. Natl. Acad. Sci. USA 97 (2000) 6728.

[78] S.L. Gras, A.K. Tickler, A.M. Squires, G.L. Devlin, M.A. Horton, C.M. Dobson, C.E. MacPhee, Biomaterials 29 (2008) 1553.

[79] S.K. Maji, D. Schubert, C. Rivier, S. Lee, J.E. Rivier, R. Riek, PLoS Biol. 6 (2008) e17.

[80] G. Bhak, S. Lee, J.W. Park, S. Cho, S.R. Paik, Biomaterials 31 (2010) 5986.

[81] S. Koutsopoulos, L.D. Unsworth, Y. Nagai, S. Zhang, Proc. Natl. Acad. Sci. USA 106 (2009) 4623.

[82] T.P. Knowles, T.W. Oppenheim, A.K. Buell, D.Y. Chirgadze, M.E. Welland, Nat. Nanotechnol. 5 (2010) 204.

[83] M. Yolamanova, C. Meier, A.K. Shaytan, V. Vas, C.W. Bertoncini, F. Arnold, O. Zirafi, S.M. Usmani, J.A. Muller, D. Sauter, C. Goffinet, D. Palesch, P. Walther, N.R. Roan, H. Geiger, O. Lunov, T. Simmet, J. Bohne, H. Schrezenmeier, K. Schwarz, L. Standker, W.G. Forssmann, X. Salvatella, P.G. Khalatur, A.R. Khokhlov, T.P. Knowles, T. Weil, F. Kirchhoff, J. Munch, Nat. Nanotechnol. 8 (2013) 130.

[84] J. Shi, X. Du, Y. Huang, J. Zhou, D. Yuan, D. Wu, Y. Zhang, R. Haburcak, I.R. Epstein, B. Xu, J. Am. Chem. Soc. 137 (2015) 26.

[85] Y. Zhang, Z. Yang, F. Yuan, H. Gu, P. Gao, B. Xu, J. Am. Chem. Soc. 126 (2004) 15028.

[86] M.-C. Lo, H. Men, A. Branstrom, J. Helm, N. Yao, R. Goldman, S. Walker, J. Am. Chem. Soc. 122 (2000) 3540.

[87] A. Tanaka, Y. Fukuoka, Y. Morimoto, T. Honjo, D. Koda, M. Goto, T. Maruyama, J. Am. Chem. Soc. 137 (2015) 770.

[88] S.D. Putney, P.A. Burke, Nat. Biotechnol. 16 (1998) 153.

[89] R. Duncan, Nat. Rev. Drug Discov. 2 (2003) 347.

[90] A.S. Hoffman, P.S. Stayton, Prog. Polym. Sci. 32 (2007) 922.

[91] P.S. Stayton, T. Shimoboji, C. Long, A. Chilkoti, G. Chen, J.M. Harris, A.S. Hoffman, Nature 30 (1995) 472.

[92] C. Cummings, H. Murata, R. Koepsel, A.J. Russell, Biomacromolecules 15 (2014) 763.

[93] B.S. Sumerlin, ACS Macro. Lett. 1 (2012) 141.

[94] J. Hu, W. Zhao, Y. Gao, M. Sun, Y. Wei, H. Deng, W. Gao, Biomaterials 47 (2015) 13.

[95] H. Iwai, A. Pluckthun, FEBS Lett. 459 (1999) 166.

[96] J.M. Antos, M.W.L. Popp, R. Ernst, G.L. Chew, E. Spooner, H.L. Ploegh, J. Biol. Chem. 284 (2009) 16028.

[97] H. Lu, D. Wang, S. Kazane, T. Javahishvili, F. Tian, F. Song, A. Sellers, B. Barnett, P.G. Schultz, J. Am. Chem. Soc. 135 (2013) 13885.

[98] J.-F. Lutz, M. Ouchi, D.R. Liu, M. Sawamoto, Science 341 (2013) 1238149.

[99] J. Sun, R.N. Zuckermann, ACS Nano 7 (2013) 4715.

[100] F.S. Bates, M.A. Hillmyer, T.P. Lodge, C.M. Bates, K.T. Delaney, G.H. Fredrickson, Science 336 (2012) 434.

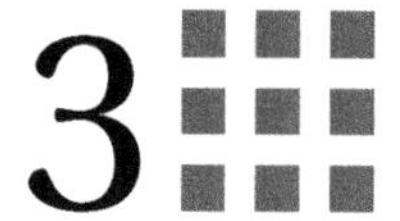

Regenerative Medicines

3.1

Preparation of Polymer Scaffolds by Ice Particulate Method for Tissue Engineering

Guoping Chen, Naoki Kawazoe

TISSUE REGENERATION MATERIALS UNIT, INTERNATIONAL CENTER FOR MATERIALS NANOARCHITECTONICS (MANA), NATIONAL INSTITUTE FOR MATERIALS SCIENCE (NIMS), TSUKUBA, JAPAN

CHAPTER OUTLINE

3.1.1 Introduction

Porous scaffolds of biodegradable polymers have been broadly used in tissue engineering because of their versatile properties of biodegradation, good biocompatibility, and easy formation into different porous structures [1]. They serve as temporary supports for cell adhesion and provide various signals for cell proliferation, cell differentiation, and secretion of extracellular matrix, thus guiding the formation of new tissues and organs [2,3]. Porous scaffolds should have pore structures that facilitate cell seeding and cell penetration into all the spaces in the scaffolds. In general, cells are easily allocated and distributed in the peripheral areas, resulting in partial tissue regeneration in the outermost peripheral layers of the scaffolds. Regeneration of functional tissues and organs requires smooth cell delivery and distribution throughout the whole scaffolds [4,5].

Many methods have been developed and used to prepared porous scaffolds of biodegradable polymers. They include particle leaching [6], freeze-drying [7], phase separation [8], gas foaming [9], electrospinning [10], fiber bonding [11], and rapid prototyping [12]. Although these methods have their respective advantages, there are many challenges.

Scaffolds prepared by the first five methods have the problem of partially closed surface pore structures that inhibit cell penetration into the inner body of the scaffolds and result in uneven cell distribution. Scaffolds prepared by the latter two methods have straight-through pore structures that present the problems of cell leakage and low cell loading in the scaffolds. To solve these problems, a method using preprepared ice particulates as a template or a porogen material has been established [13–16]. Ice particulates can not only provide their negative replica for pore formation but also initiate generation of new ice crystals during the freezing process. The pre-prepared ice particulates and the newly formed ice crystals can create open and well-interconnected pore structures. In other words, ice particulates can grow during the freezing process and thus serve as an active porogen material. Funnel-like porous scaffolds with open surface pores and interconnected inner body pores can be prepared by using ice particulates embossing on a substrate as a template. Porous scaffolds with high interconnectivity can be prepared by using free ice particulates as a porogen material. Funnel-like porous scaffolds of naturally derived biodegradable polymers such as collagen, gelatin, chitosan, hyaluronic acid (HA), and glycosaminoglycans (GAGs) have been prepared by using embossing ice particulates as a template [8–10]. Highly interconnected porous scaffolds of biodegradable synthetic polymers such as poly(L-lactic acid) (PLLA) and poly(DL-lactic-*co*-glycolic acid) (PLGA) and naturally derived polymers have be prepared by using free ice particulates as a porogen material ([16–18]). The porous scaffolds of biodegradable polymers have been used for tissue engineering of skin and cartilage. This chapter describes the details of the ice particulate method and some of the porous scaffolds of biodegradable polymers prepared by this method.

3.1.2 Preparation of Funnel-Like Polymer Porous Scaffolds

Open surface pore structure is important for cell penetration into the inner body of scaffolds during cell seeding. Cells stay and stack at the surface of scaffolds if their surface pores are not open, resulting in tissue regeneration predominantly on the scaffold surface. Open surface pores are required for homogeneous cell distribution and functional tissue engineering. Ice particulates embossing on a substrate have been used to prepare open pore structures in porous scaffolds of naturally derived biodegradable polymers such as collagen [13,19–21]. The preparation scheme of collagen porous scaffolds by this method is shown in Fig. 3.1.1. At first, water droplets are formed by spraying pure water onto a hydrophobic surface, for example, perfluoroalkoxy (PFA) film wrapped on a copper plate. The size of water droplets can be controlled by the number of spraying times. Embossing ice particulates are formed on the PFA film surface after the water droplets are frozen at –30°C. Embossing ice particulates having a diameter of 181 ± 43, 398 ± 113, and 719 ± 149 μm can be prepared by spraying pure water 10, 20, and 30 times, respectively. After preparation, the ice particulate templates are placed at a designated temperature for 1 h to allow the templates to reach a designated temperature to control the freezing temperature during the next step when the mixture suspension of ice particulates and aqueous collagen solution is frozen. To investigate the effect of freezing temperature on

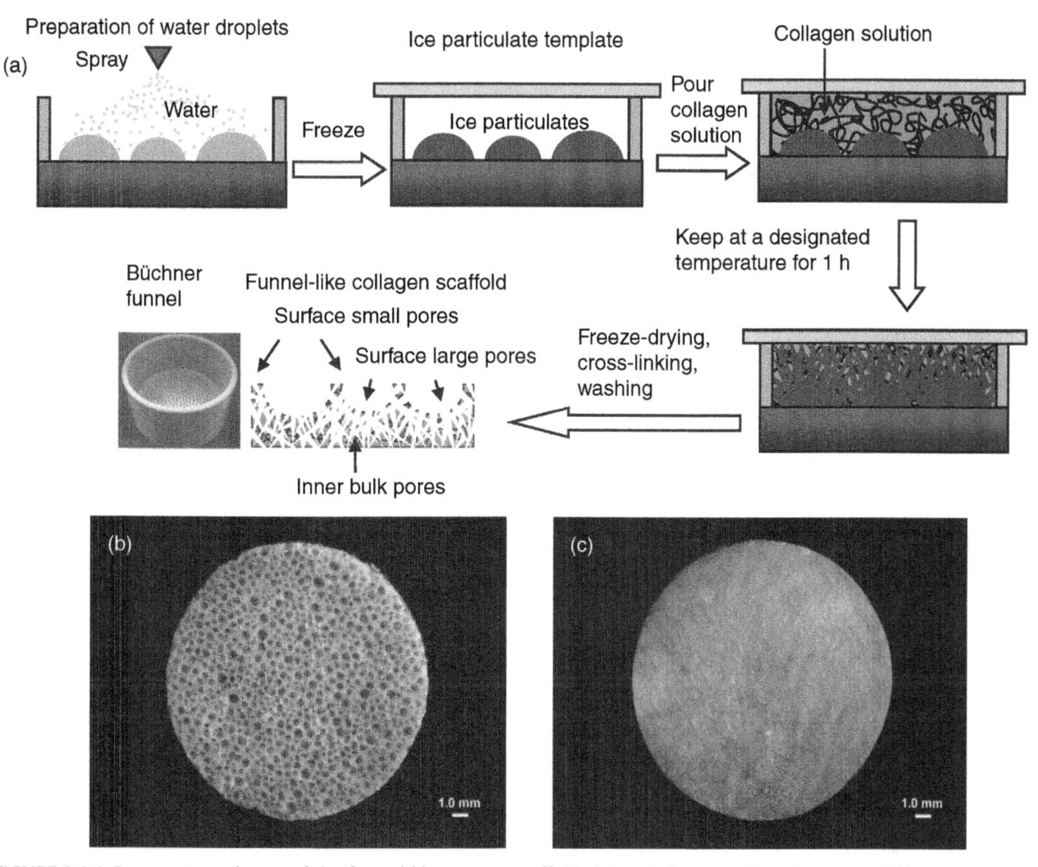

FIGURE 3.1.1 Preparation scheme of the funnel-like porous scaffolds (a) and photographs of the funnel-like collagen porous scaffold prepared with 398-mm diameter ice particulate template at −3°C (b) and control collagen porous scaffold prepared without ice particulates at −3°C (c). *Adapted from Ref. [13].*

the porous structure of the collagen porous scaffolds, four temperatures (−1, −3, −5, and −10°C) are chosen.

Subsequently, collagen aqueous solution is eluted onto the embossing ice particulates and is kept at the designated temperatures (−1, −3, −5, and −10°C) for 1 h to gradually freeze. During the freezing process, the ice particulates serve as nuclei to initiate the formation of new ice crystals starting from their semispherical surfaces. The collagen aqueous solution is kept at −1°C for 24 h to allow the temperature to reach −1°C before being eluted onto the ice particulates that are balanced to the four different temperatures (−1, −3, −5, and −10°C).

Finally, the frozen construct of ice particulates and aqueous collagen solution is freeze-dried. The ice particulate template and newly formed ice crystals are removed by freeze-drying. After freeze-drying, the dried scaffolds are cross-linked. After cross-linking, blocking of any nonreacted cross-linking agent, washing, and a second freeze-drying, collagen porous scaffolds with open surface pores are prepared. The embossing ice particulates define the surface porous structure and the newly formed ice crystals define the bulk porous structure of the funnel-like collagen sponges. The unique porous structure of the collagen scaffolds is somewhat like that of a Büchner funnel (insert in Fig. 3.1.1a). For this reason, the collagen porous scaffolds prepared with the embossing ice particulates template are referred as to funnel-like collagen scaffolds.

Figure 3.1.1b and c shows the collagen scaffolds prepared with and without use of the embossing ice particulates. The surface structures of the two types of collagen sponges are different. Large pores are visible and evenly distributed only on the surface of the funnel-like collagen porous scaffolds. The control collagen scaffolds prepared without ice particulates do not have large surface pores.

Observation by a scanning electron microscope (SEM) shows the detailed porous structures of collagen scaffolds. The funnel-like collagen scaffolds prepared with an ice particulates template having a diameter of 398 μm and a freezing temperature of –1, –3, –5, and –10°C are shown in Fig. 3.1.2. The template temperature is adjusted to be the same as that

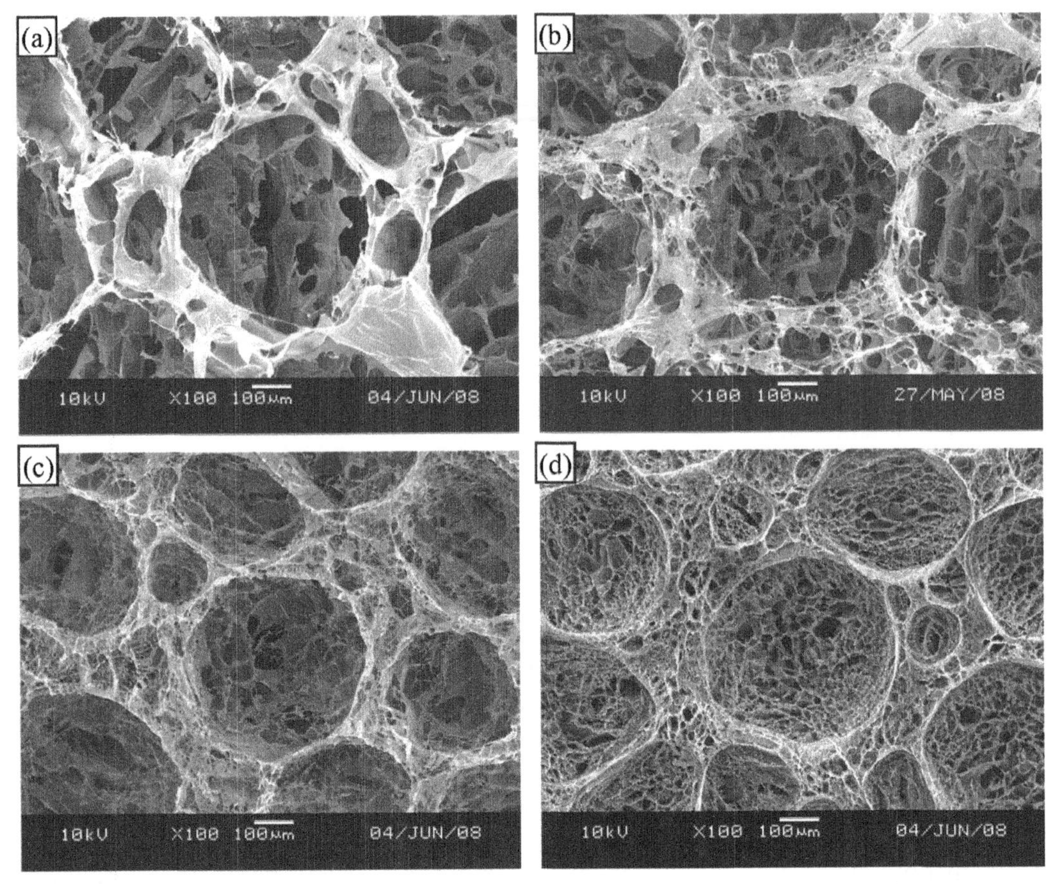

FIGURE 3.1.2 SEM photomicrographs of top surfaces of funnel-like collagen porous scaffolds prepared with ice particulates having a diameter of 398 mm at different temperatures: (a) –1°C, (b) –3°C, (c) –5°C, and (d) –10°C. *Adapted from Ref. [13].*

of the freezing temperature. The funnel-like collagen scaffolds have a hierarchical porous structure of two layers: a surface porous layer and a bulk porous layer. The surface porous layer consists of large open pores and some small pores. The mean diameters of the large surface pores are almost the same as those of the respective ice particulates used as templates. There is no significant difference among the pore sizes of the large surface pores since ice particulates with the same sizes and shapes are used to prepare these collagen sponges. However, the pore sizes of the inner body pores and the small surface pores decrease with a decrease of the ice particulates temperature (the same as freezing temperature). The inner body pores and small surface pores are dense and small when being prepared at a low temperature, and sparse and large when being prepared at a high temperature.

The funnel-like collagen sponge prepared with a template of 398-μm diameter embossing ice particulates at –3°C and the control collagen sponge prepared at –3°C without ice template are used for the culture of human dermal fibroblasts [13]. The cell seeding efficiencies of the funnel-like and control collagen sponges are 93.2 ± 1.0% and 92.1 ± 1.1%, respectively. Both collagen scaffolds show high cell seeding efficiency. The fibroblasts are observed both on the top surface and within the inner body pores of the funnel-like collagen scaffolds. The cells are distributed throughout the funnel-like collagen scaffolds. However, the fibroblasts are mostly distributed on the surface and few cells are observed in the inner body part of the control collagen scaffolds. The difference in cell distribution should be caused by the different porous structures of the scaffolds. The large surface open pores and high interconnectivity of the inner body pores of the funnel-like collagen scaffolds facilitate cell delivery and penetration into the body pores of the funnel-like collagen scaffolds. However, a low ratio of surface open pores and low interconnectivity in the control collagen scaffolds retard cell diffusion into the inner body pores of the control scaffolds.

Cell viability analysis after 2 weeks' culture shows many red-stained dead cells are detected in the control collagen scaffolds while few are detected in the funnel-like collagen scaffolds (Fig. 3.1.3a). The open surface pores and interconnected porous structure in the funnel-like collagen scaffolds improve cell delivery and distribution, and provide enough extra area for cell spreading and proliferation, thus avoiding overcell aggregation and overgrowth. However, in the case of the control collagen scaffolds, most of the cells are stacked up on the scaffold surface, resulting in the accumulation and overgrowth of the fibroblasts that may result in the death of some cells. Hematoxylin and eosin (HE) staining of the 2 weeks' cultured cells shows more cells are observed on the surface than in the inner body part of the control collagen scaffolds (Fig. 3.1.3b). In contrast, the fibroblasts are distributed homogeneously throughout the funnel-like collagen scaffolds. The funnel-like collagen scaffolds facilitate cell seeding and homogeneous cell distribution and promote dermal tissue formation.

The embossing ice particulate template method has also been used to prepare porous scaffolds of other naturally derived polymers such as chitosan, HA and GAGs [19–21]. The funnel-like porous scaffolds of chitosan and HA and collagen–GAG composite prepared by this method also show the hierarchical two-layer pore structures (Fig. 3.1.4). Depending on the type of naturally derived polymers, the cross-linking method is different. The

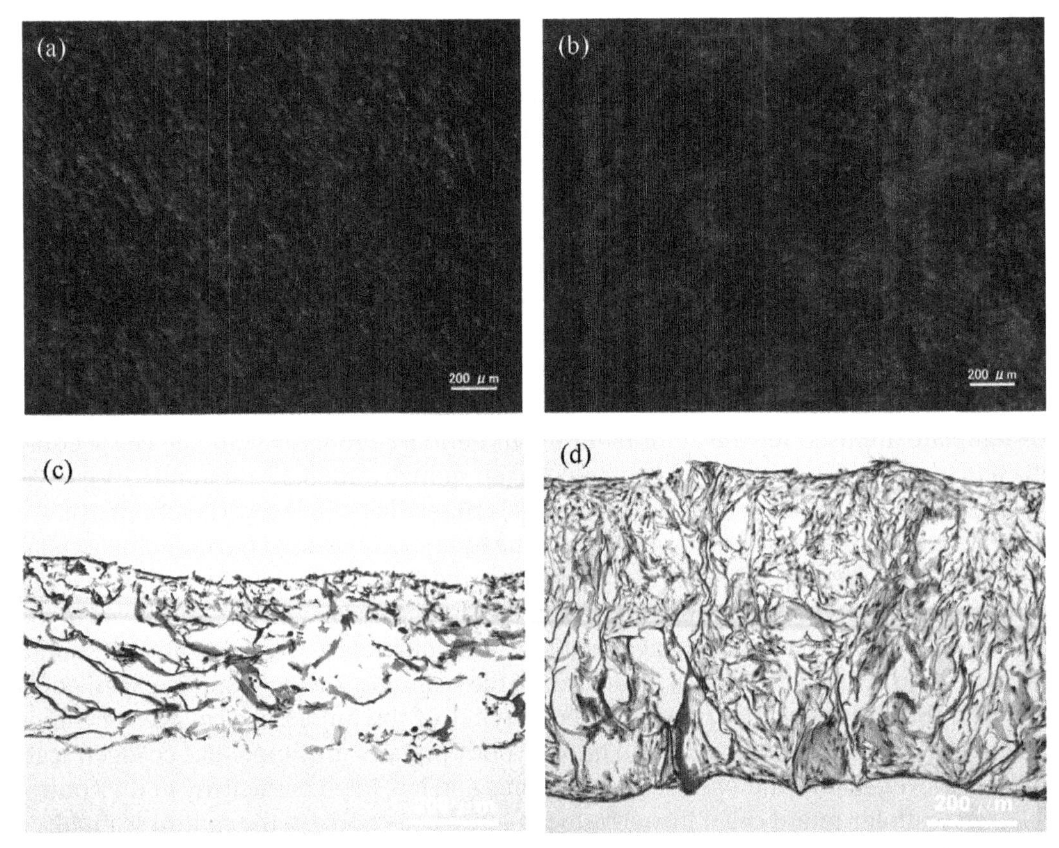

FIGURE 3.1.3 Live/dead staining (a, b) and HE staining (c, d) of fibroblasts after being cultured in the control collagen scaffold (a, c) and funnel-like collagen porous scaffold (b, d) for 2 weeks. *Adapted from Ref. [13].*

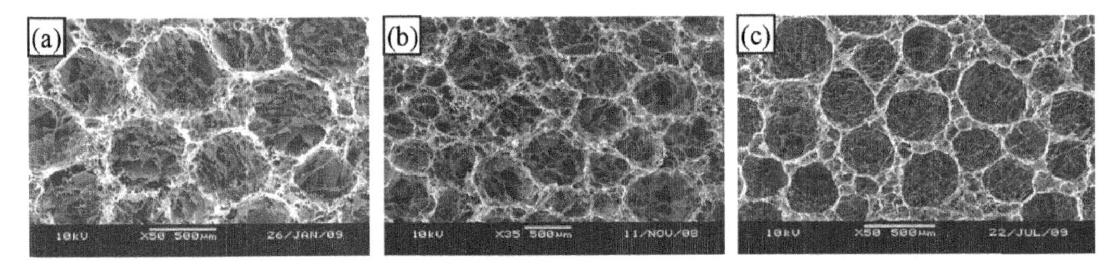

FIGURE 3.1.4 SEM photomicrographs of top surface of funnel-like porous scaffolds of chitosan (a), hyaluronic acid (b), and collagen–GAG composite (c) prepared by using templates embossed with ice particulates having a diameter of about 400 μm. The freezing temperature is −3°C. *Adapted from Refs [19–21], with permissions from John Wiley and Sons and Taylor & Francis.*

lyophilized HA sponges are cross-linked by water-soluble carbodiimide dissolved in an aqueous solution of ethanol at room temperature for 24 h [20].

3.1.3 Preparation of Micropatterned Polymer Porous Scaffolds

The embossing ice particulates method can be used to introduce micropatterned structures in three-dimensional porous scaffolds [14]. The micropatterned structures include micropatterned pore structures and micropatterns of bioactive substances such as growth factors.

Three-dimensional porous polymer scaffolds with micropatterned pores can be prepared by using micropatterned ice particulates or ice lines of pure water as a template. The ice particulate and ice line templates can be prepared by ejecting water droplets through a dispensing machine on a low-temperature copper plate that is wrapped with a PFA film. The low temperature of the copper plate is achieved by a circulation cooler that is set at –20°C. The micropatterns of the ice particulates and ice lines can be designed using a computer program. Apart from the fabrication of micropatterned ice particulates or ice lines templates, the other processes of manipulation are the same as those for preparation of funnel-like collagen porous scaffolds. The balance temperature and freezing temperature are set at –5°C. Figure 3.1.5 shows four types of micropatterned ice templates (three types of ice particulates and one type of ice line) and their respective micropatterned collagen scaffolds. The micropatterned pores are the negative replica of the micropatterned ice particulates or ice lines. The other pores and inner body pores are formed from the ice crystals that are generated during the freezing process.

The scaffolds shown in Fig. 3.1.5b, d, f, and h have one layer of micropatterned pores and lines on their top surfaces. The micropatterned pore layer can be laminated to construct collagen porous scaffolds with three-dimensionally micropatterned pores. Figure 3.1.5i and j shows the top surface and cross-section pore structures of collagen porous scaffolds with three-dimensionally micropatterned pores. To prepare the three-dimensionally micropatterned pore structures, the frozen collagen solution on the first layer of micropatterned ice particulates, as prepared above, is used to prepare the second layer of micropatterned ice particulates instead of the PFA film-wrapped copper plate. Collagen aqueous solution is eluded onto the second layer of micropatterned ice particulates and frozen, as described above. By repeating the procedure and later following it with the freeze-drying, cross-linking, and washing processes, a collagen porous scaffold with a three-layer laminated micropatterned structure is prepared (Fig. 3.1.5i and j). An SEM image of its top surface showed a pore structure similar to that of the collagen scaffold with one layer of micropatterned structure. The cross-section had the laminated pore structure. The micropatterned pores are hemispheric.

Three-dimensional porous polymer scaffolds with micropatterned bioactive substances can be prepared by using micropatterned ice particulates or ice lines of an aqueous

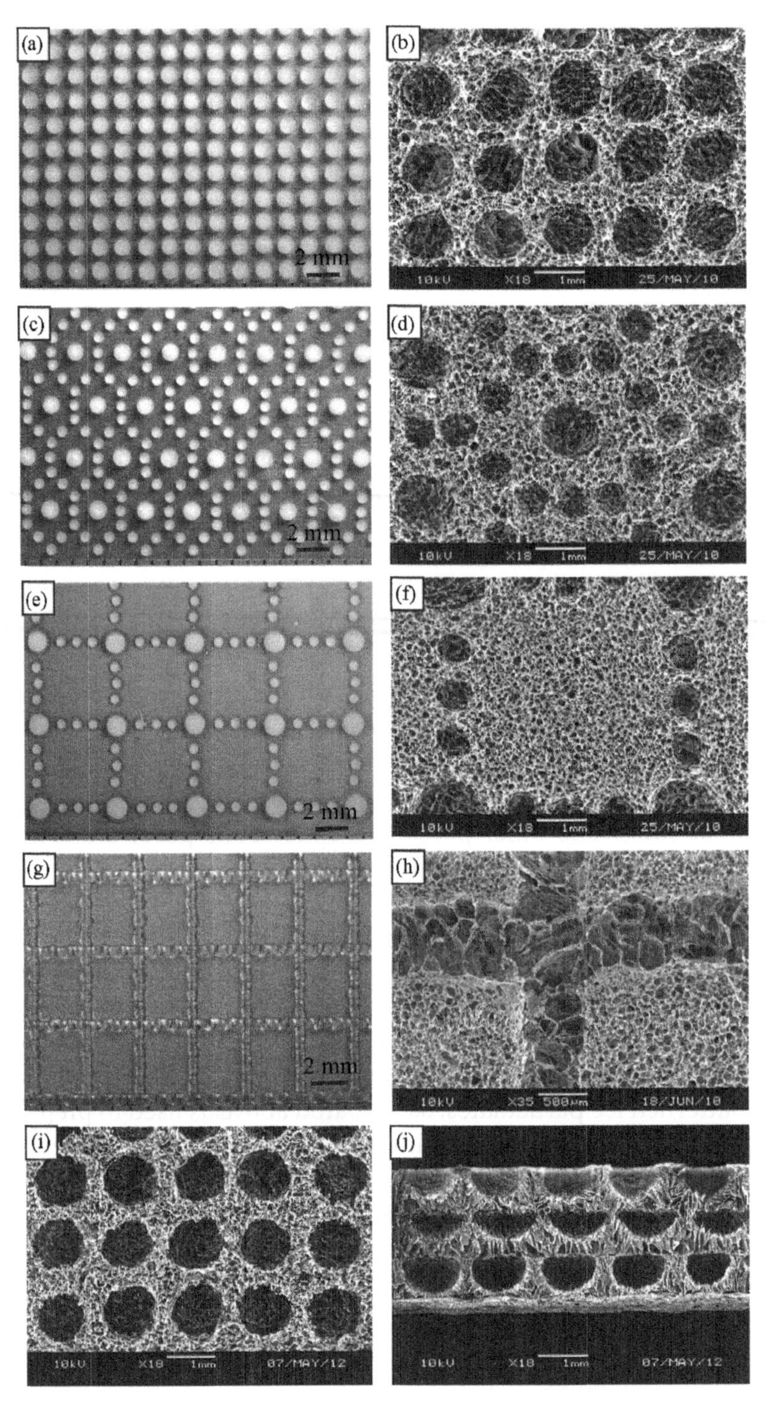

FIGURE 3.1.5 Photographs of four types of ice micropattern templates (a, c, e, and g), SEM photomicrographs of top surfaces of collagen porous scaffolds with one layer of micropatterned pores that are prepared with the respective ice micropattern templates (b, d, f, and h), and SEM photomicrographs of top surface (i) and cross-section (j) of a collagen scaffold with three-dimensionally micropatterned pores that are prepared with an ice micropattern template. *Adapted from Ref. [14], with permission from John Wiley and Sons.*

solution containing the bioactive substances as a template. For example, a collagen aqueous solution containing bioactive substances can be used to prepare the templates instead of generating the ice templates from pure water. Figure 3.1.6 shows collagen porous scaffolds micropatterned with three types of bioactive substances (vascular endothelial growth factor [VEGF], nerve growth factor [NGF], and fibronectin). VEGF, NGF, or fibronectin is mixed with a collagen aqueous solution. The mixture solution is ejected onto the low-temperature copper plates through a nozzle using a dispensing machine. Three different ice micropattern designs (square, diamond, and circle) composed of the collagen/bioactive substance solution are prepared. The diameter of the ice lines in the micropatterns of the bioactive substance can be adjusted by controlling the ejection pressure, the distance between the copper and nozzle and the nozzle caliber. The ice micropatterns of bioactive substances are used to prepare collagen porous scaffolds with micropatterned bioactive substances. Immunological staining of VEGF, NGF, and fibronectin shows that the three types of bioactive substances are micropatterned on the top surface of collagen porous scaffolds. The micropatterns can be designed by a program of the dispensing machine. Not only one single type of bioactive substance but also a few types of bioactive substances can be comicropatterned in collagen porous scaffolds. For comicropatterns of a few types of bioactive substances, the mixture solution of collagen aqueous solution and different bioactive substances should be subsequently ejected onto the –20°C copper plate to prepare their micropatterned ice particulates or ice lines. Bioactive substances can also be three dimensionally micropatterned in collagen porous scaffolds by repeating the above-mentioned micropatterning procedure. The laminating method is similar to that of collagen scaffolds with three-dimensionally micropatterned pores. A stripe micropattern of NGF is three dimensionally introduced in a collagen porous scaffold. Immunological staining demonstrates the three-dimensionally micropatterned NGF structure (Fig. 3.1.6m and n).

Micropattern structures of porous scaffolds are important to guide the regeneration of tissues and organs with complex structures. They can arrange cells into a predesigned location and guide the regeneration of complex networks, such as capillary and neuronal networks, in accordance with the micropatterns. To demonstrate the effect of micropatterned VEGF, the collagen porous scaffolds micropatterned with VEGF stripes are subcutaneously implanted into the dorsa of athymic nude mice [15]. After 6 weeks of implantation, the implants are harvested for examination of capillary blood vessel regeneration. More blood vessels are formed in the VEGF-micropatterned collagen porous scaffolds than in the control collagen scaffolds that are prepared without VEGF (Fig. 3.1.7). The blood vessel network formed in the VEGF-micropatterned collagen scaffolds follows the micropattern of the immobilized VEGF. In the control scaffolds, however, the blood vessel network is regenerated randomly. Staining with an antibody for von Willebrand factor (a marker of endothelial cells) shows that the blood vessel density in the VEGF-micropatterned lines is significantly higher than that in the regions without VEGF. These results demonstrate that the immobilized VEGF promotes blood vessel formation and that the blood vessel network is regenerated according to the micropattern of immobilized VEGF.

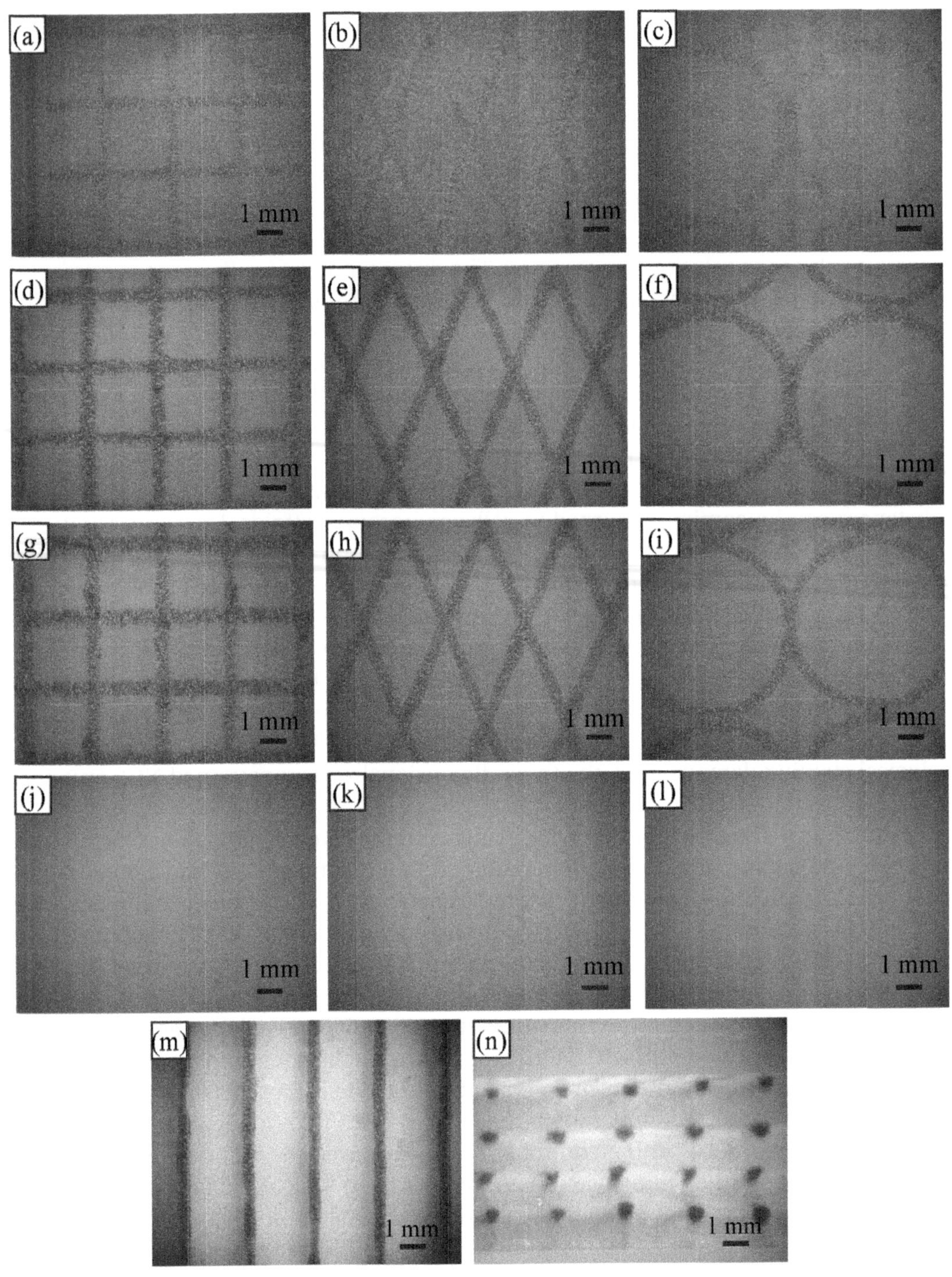

FIGURE 3.1.6 Immunological staining of collagen porous scaffolds with one layer of micropatterned VEGF (a–c), NGF (d–f), fibronectin (g–i), and pure collagen as control (j–l) in square- (a, d, g, and j), diamond- (b, e, h, and k), and circle-shaped (c, f, i, and l) micropatterns and a collagen porous scaffold with a three-dimensional micropattern of NGF (m: top surface, n: cross-section). *Adapted from Ref. [14], with permission from John Wiley and Sons.*

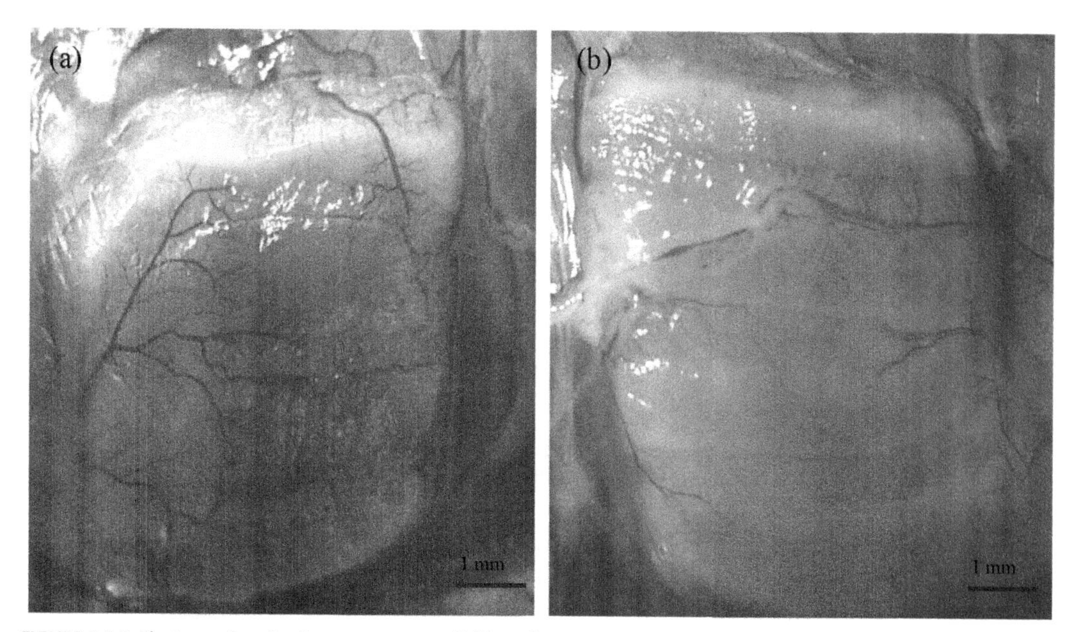

FIGURE 3.1.7 Photographs of collagen porous scaffolds with micropatterned lines of VEGF (a) and control collagen scaffold (b) after subcutaneous implantation in the back of nude mice for 6 weeks. *Adapted from Ref. [15], with permission from Taylor & Francis.*

3.1.4 Preparation of Porous Scaffolds of Biodegradable Synthetic Polymers

The embossing ice particulates can be used to control the surface pore structures and to create micropatterned structures in porous scaffolds of naturally derived biodegradable polymers. When free ice particulates that are not embossed on a substrate are used, the inner body pore structures of biodegradable polymers can be controlled. In this case, pre-prepared ice particulates are used as a porogen material. The ice particulates are mixed with precooled polymer solution. The mixture is subsequently frozen slowly and freeze-dried. This method has been used to prepare porous scaffolds of biodegradable synthetic polymers and biodegradable naturally derived polymers [16–18,22].

When the ice particulates method is used for preparation of porous scaffolds of biodegradable synthetic polymers, the synthetic polymers are dissolved in solvent and pre-cooled to a temperature below 0°C [22]. The pre-prepared ice particulates are added in the precooled polymer solutions and mixed to let the ice particulates distribute homogeneously in the polymer solution. The mixture suspension is subsequently frozen and freeze-dried. The porous scaffolds of PLLA and PLGA prepared by this method are shown in Fig. 3.1.8. PLLA or PLGA is dissolved in chloroform and the polymer solution is cooled to −20°C. Subsequently, pre-prepared ice particulates are added to the precooled PLLA or PLGA solution. The dispensing solution is homogeneously mixed and frozen in liquid nitrogen. Finally, the frozen constructs are freeze-dried for 48 h under the freezing of liquid

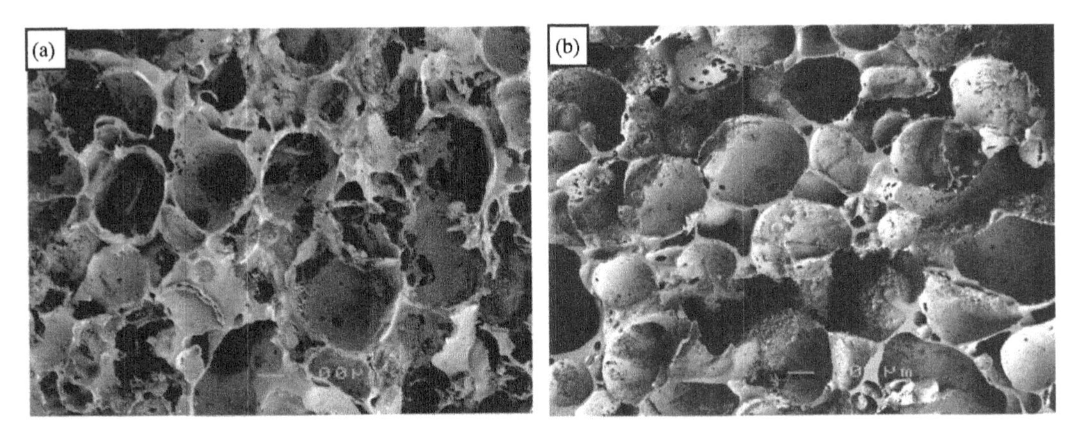

FIGURE 3.1.8 SEM photomicrographs of cross-sections of porous scaffolds of PLLA (a) and PLGA (b) prepared with a weight ratio of ice microparticulates of 90%. *Adapted from Ref. [22], with permission from Elsevier.*

nitrogen to remove the ice particulates and solvent and for another 48 h at room temperature to completely remove the solvent. The PLLA and PLGA scaffolds are highly porous with evenly distributed pore structures. The pore shapes are almost the same as those of the ice particulates. The scaffolds become further interconnected as the weight fraction of the ice microparticulates increases. The polymer concentration also has some effect on the pore wall structure. Low polymer concentration results in more porous pore wall structures.

3.1.5 Preparation of Porous Scaffolds of Biodegradable Naturally Derived Polymers

The free ice particulates method has been used to prepare porous scaffolds of naturally derived polymers such as collagen (Fig. 3.1.9) [16]. Free ice particulates with a diameter range from 355 μm to 425 μm are first prepared by spraying Milli Q water into liquid nitrogen using a sprayer and sieving the ice particulates with sieves having 335 and 425 μm mesh pores. Subsequently, the ice particulates are mixed with an aqueous solution of collagen that is prepared by dissolving collagen in a solution of ethanol and acetic acid. The solution of acetic acid and ethanol is used to dissolve collagen to decrease the freezing temperature of the collagen solution below –4°C. Before mixing, the ice particulates and collagen solution are kept in a low-temperature chamber (–4°C) for 6 h for temperature balance. The mixing process is conducted at –4°C. At –4°C, the ice particulates do not melt and the collagen aqueous solution does not freeze, which is beneficial for complete mixing of the two components to obtain an even distribution of ice particulates in the collagen aqueous solution. Finally, the mixture of ice particulates and collagen aqueous solution is frozen at –80°C and freeze-dried. The freeze-dried collagen porous scaffolds are cross-linked for 6 h with glutaraldehyde vapor, which is saturated with a 25% aqueous glutaraldehyde solution at 37°C in a closed box. After cross-linking, the scaffolds are immersed in

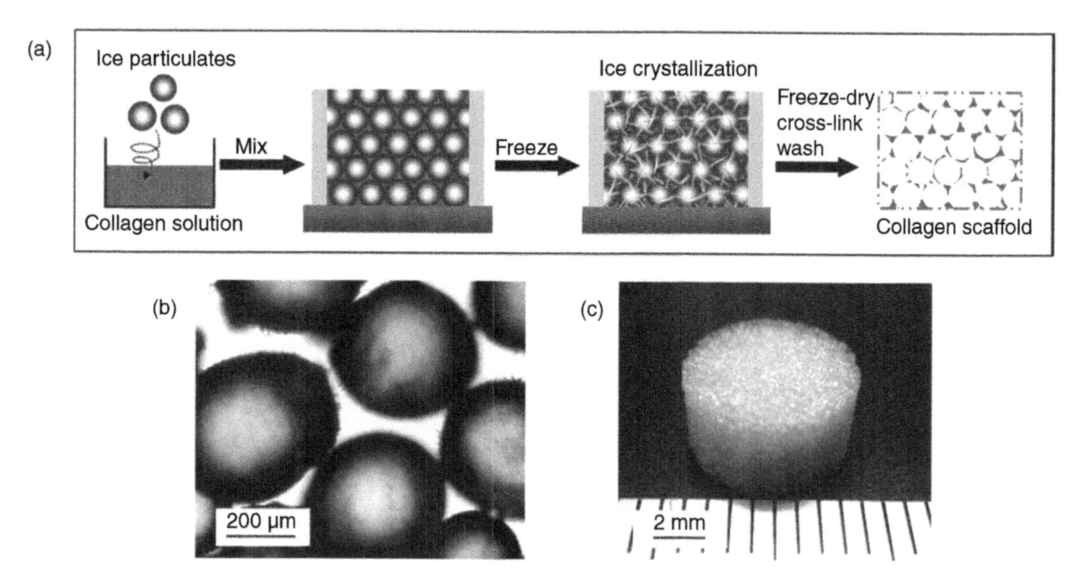

FIGURE 3.1.9 Preparation scheme of collagen porous scaffold by using free ice particulates as a porogen material (a), photomicrograph of ice particulates (b), and photograph of collagen porous scaffold prepared with the ice particulates (c). *Adapted from Ref. [16].*

a 0.1 M glycine aqueous solution to block any unreacted aldehyde groups. The scaffolds are completely washed with pure water and freeze-dried again to obtain the dried collagen scaffolds.

The collagen porous scaffolds prepared by this method have interconnected large pores and small pores (Fig. 3.1.10). The large pores are spherical and have the same size as that of the ice particulates. The small pores have a random morphology and different sizes. The small pores surround the large spherical pores. The large pores should be negative replicas of the pre-prepared free ice particulates, while the small ice particulates are from the ice crystals formed during the freezing process. The density of the large spherical pores is dependent on the ratio of ice particulates used to prepare the scaffolds. The large pore density increases when the ratio of ice particulates increases. The collagen porous scaffolds prepared with 50% ice particulates show the most homogeneous pore structure. When fewer ice particulates are used, the large spherical pores are sparsely distributed, meaning there is some distance between the large pores. When a high ratio of ice particulates is used, some collapsed large pores are observed. With a high ratio of ice particulates, the collagen aqueous solution filling the spaces between the spherical ice particulates decreases and the collagen matrix surrounding the large pores decreases. In addition, mixing of the ice particulates and the collagen aqueous solution becomes difficult when the ice particulate ratio is high. The collapsed large pores should be due to the less dense collagen matrix and incomplete mixing.

Collagen concentration also affects the pore structure. When 1, 2, and 3% (w/v) of collagen aqueous solution is used for preparation of the scaffolds, some collapsed large pores can be observed in the scaffolds prepared with 1 and 3% collagen aqueous solutions. The

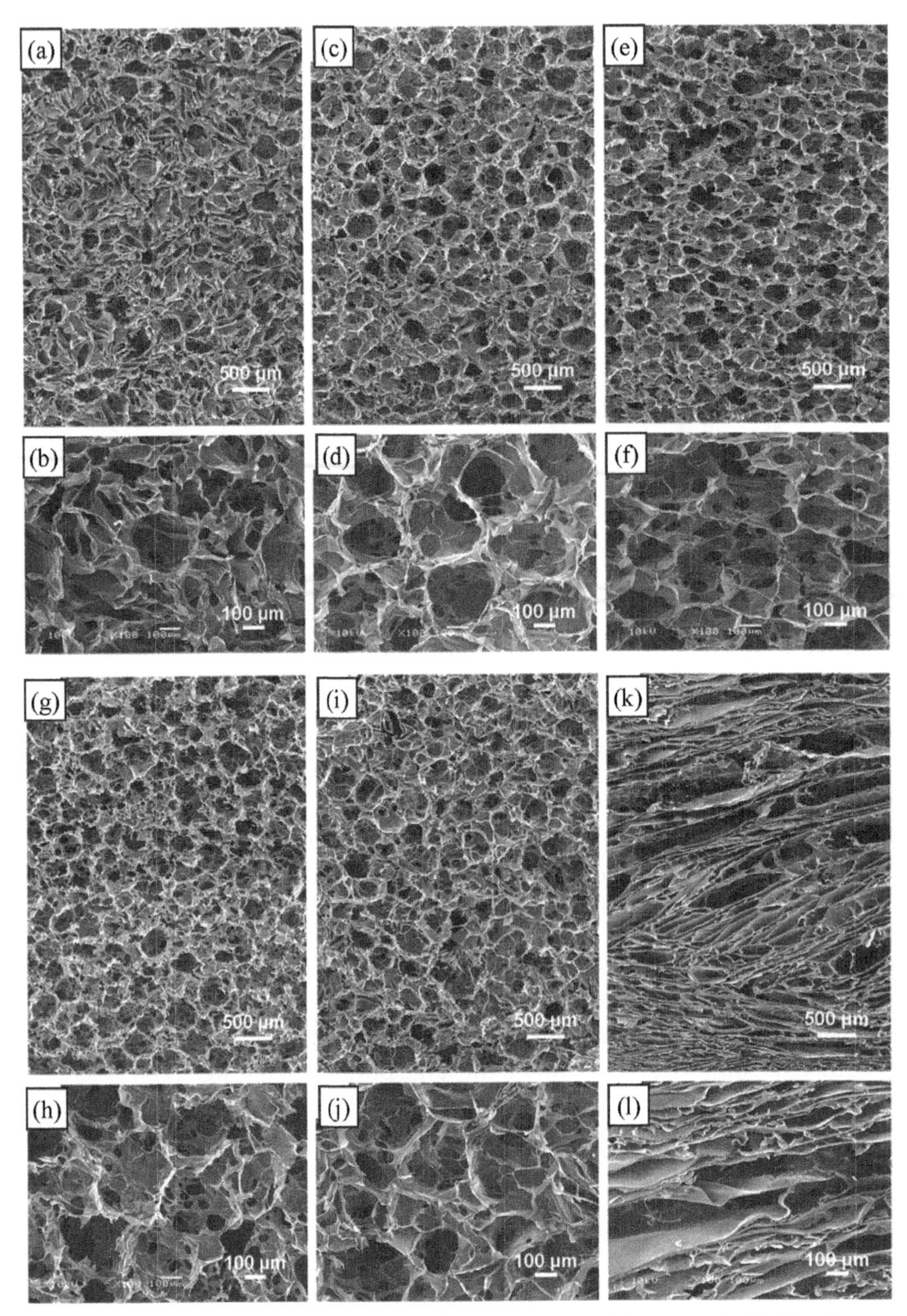

FIGURE 3.1.10 SEM photomicrographs of cross-sections of collagen porous scaffolds prepared with 2% collagen aqueous solution and ice particulates at a ratio of ice particulates/collagen solution of 25% (a, b), 50% (c, d), and 75% (e, f); collagen porous scaffolds prepared with a ratio of ice particulates/collagen solution of 50% and a collagen solution concentration of 1% (g, h) and 3% (i, j) and control collagen porous scaffolds prepared with 2% collagen aqueous solution without the use of ice particulates (k, l). *Adapted from Ref. [16].*

collapsed large pores in collagen scaffolds prepared with the 1% collagen aqueous solution may have occurred because the low concentration resulted in a less dense collagen matrix surrounding the large pores. The case involving the 3% collagen aqueous solution may be due to incomplete mixing because the 3% collagen solution is too viscous. The porous scaffolds prepared with the 2% collagen solution and an ice particulate/collagen solution ratio of 50% show the most homogeneous pore structure. The control scaffolds prepared without ice particulates have a heterogeneous lamellar pore structure.

Because the ice particulates can increase the interconnectivity among the pores of scaffolds, it can be used to make well-interconnected pore gradient scaffolds (Fig. 3.1.11) [17]. At first, an aqueous collagen solution as well as ice particulates are made. Two percent (w/v) aqueous collagen solution is prepared by dissolving freeze-dried porcine type I collagen in a mixture of ethanol and acetic acid. The ice particulates are prepared by spraying Milli Q water into liquid nitrogen using a sprayer. The ice particulates are sieved by sieves with mesh pores of 150, 250, 355, 425, and 500 μm to obtain ice particulates having diameters of 150–250, 250–355, 355–425, and 425–500 μm. The sieving process is conducted at −15°C in a low-temperature chamber. The sieved ice particulates are stored in closed glass

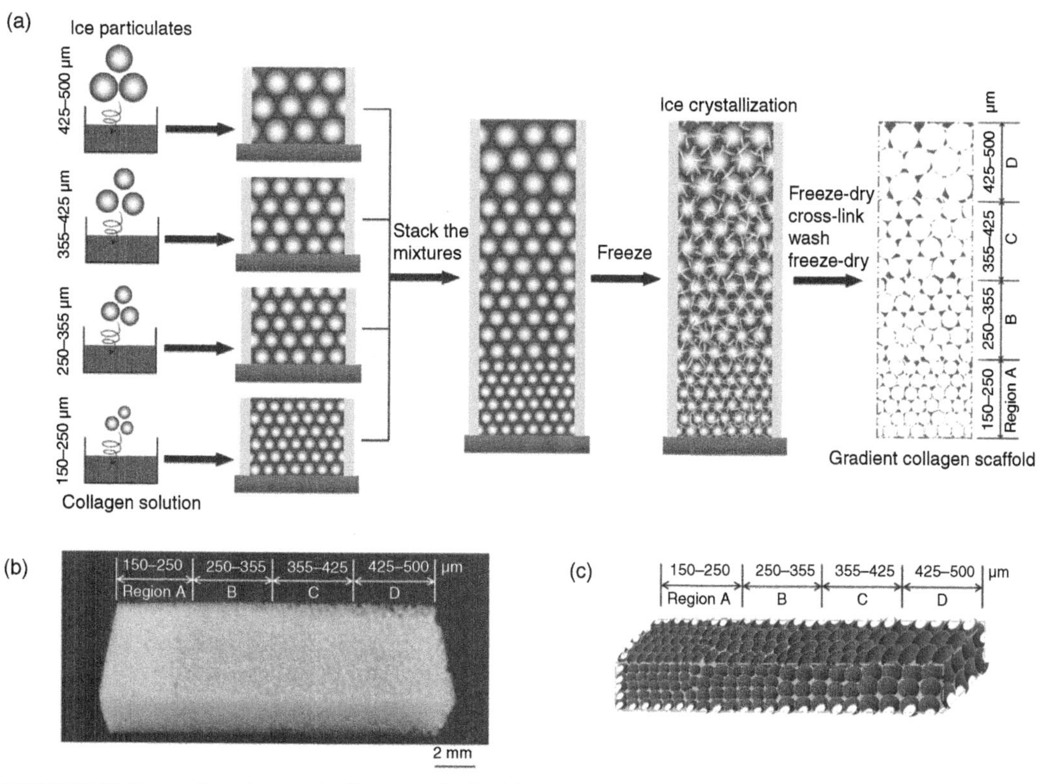

FIGURE 3.1.11 Preparation scheme of collagen scaffolds with a gradient pore structure by using ice particulates as a porogen material (a). Photograph (b) and an illustration of the pore structure (c) of the collagen gradient scaffolds. *Adapted from Ref. [17], with permission from Elsevier.*

bottles in a –80°C freezer until their use. Subsequently, the 2% (w/v) aqueous collagen solution is mixed with the sieved ice particulates. Before mixing, the collagen solution and the ice particulates are moved to a –4°C low-temperature chamber for 6 h to balance their temperatures. The four sets of ice particulates, each with different diameters, are separately added to four batches of precooled collagen aqueous solution in a 50:50 (v/w) ratio. The components are mixed thoroughly with a steel spoon. Each of the four mixtures of collagen solution and ice particulates is poured into a silicone frame that is then placed on a PFA film-wrapped copper plate and the mixture surface is flattened with a steel spatula. The four mixtures in their frames are stacked together with ice particulate sizes increasing from bottom to top (Fig. 3.1.11a). The top surface of the stacked mixtures is pressed to compact the four trays together and is then covered with a glass plate wrapped with polyvinylidene chloride film. Finally, the entire set is frozen at –80°C for 6 h and the frozen constructs are freeze-dried for 3 days. After cross-linking and afterward blocking the unreacted aldehyde groups as described above, collagen scaffolds with a gradient pore size are prepared.

The gross appearance of the gradient collagen scaffolds and their illustrated pore structure are shown in Fig. 3.1.11b and c. SEM observation shows interconnected spherical pores are formed. Four regions of different pore sizes are confirmed. The spherical large pores are compactly stacked. Many small pores are seen on the walls of the spherical large pores. The small pores connect the spherical large pores, making the scaffold well interconnected. The sizes of the large pores in the four regions, which are prepared with ice particulates having diameters of 150–250, 250–355, 355–425, and 425–500 μm, are 165 ± 33, 259 ± 41, 357 ± 35, and 431 ± 36 μm, respectively. The sizes of the large pores are in good agreement with the sizes of the prepared ice particulates.

The gradient collagen porous scaffolds are cut into cuboids (6 mm × 16 mm × 3 mm, $W \times L \times H$, where L represents the direction of the pore gradient), which covers the entire pore range. The gradient collagen porous scaffolds are seeded with bovine articular chondrocytes. Cellular nucleus staining shows that the chondrocytes distribute on the walls of all of the spherical pores. The distribution of cells on the pore walls is homogeneous for all four regions. However, the cells seem denser in the regions with smaller pore sizes. A smaller pore size makes the cell distribution look denser. The homogeneous cell distribution in all four regions should be due to the good interconnectivity of the entire scaffold. The interconnectivity among the spherical large pores in the gradient collagen scaffolds facilitates the smooth delivery of cells throughout the scaffolds, even to areas of smaller pores. The cell/scaffold constructs are subcutaneously implanted into nude mice for 8 weeks. The implants appear glisteningly white (Fig. 3.1.12). HE staining shows that the spatial cell and ECM distribution are uniform and that tissue formation is homogeneous in the gradient collagen scaffold (Fig. 3.1.12b). The chondrocytes show their typical round morphology in all four regions. Safranin O staining shows that GAG is abundant and mainly distributed around the central parts in the scaffolds (Fig. 3.1.12c). The region with the smallest pore size, 150–250 μm, shows the most compact and abundant GAG production by the chondrocytes. Based on the HE and Safranin O staining results, the degree of

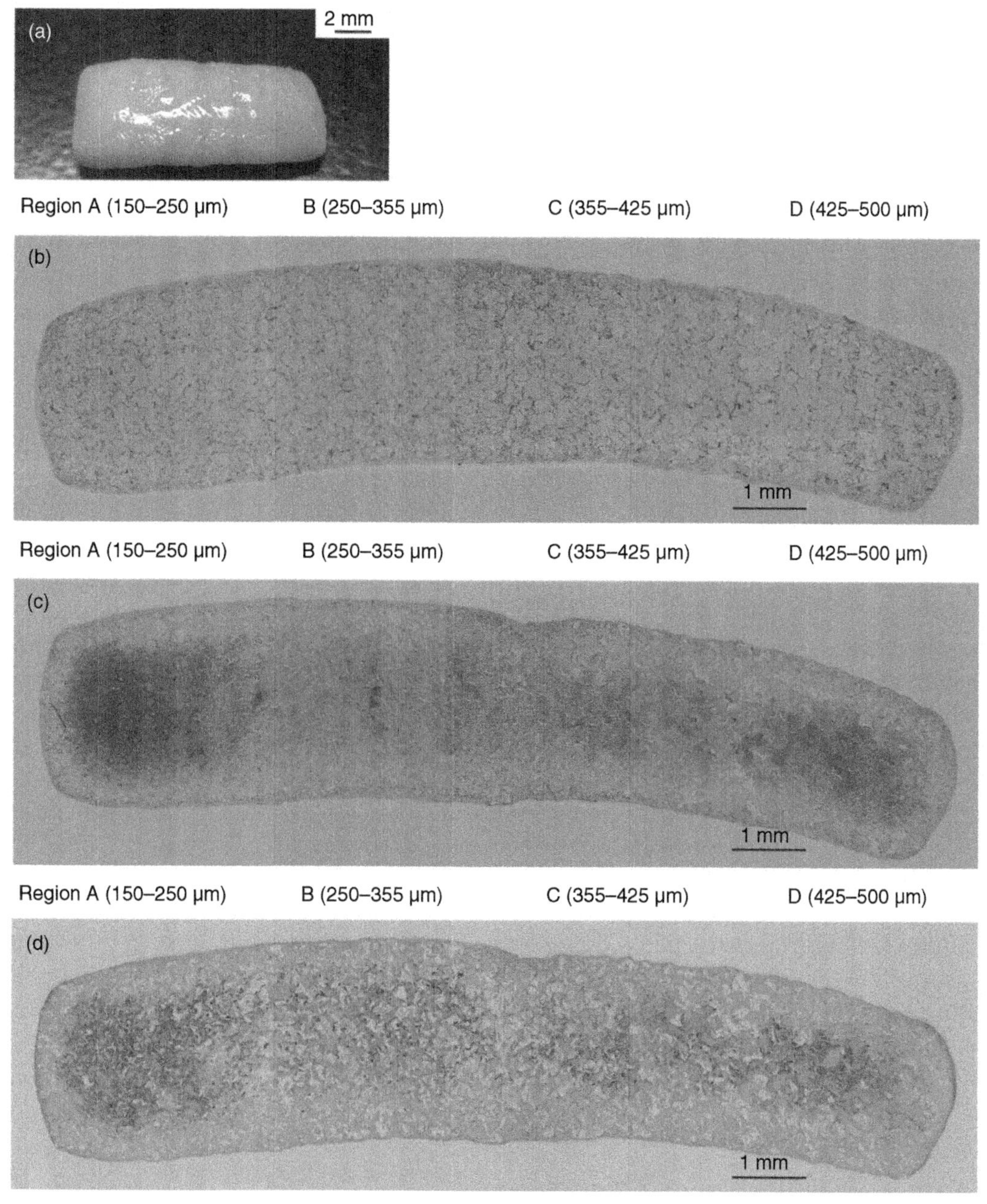

FIGURE 3.1.12 Gross appearance (a) and photomicrographs of HE staining (b), Safranin O/light green staining (c), and immunostaining of type II collagen (d) of chondrocytes/collagen gradient scaffold construct after 8 weeks of subcutaneous implantation. *Adapted from Ref. [17], with permission from Elsevier.*

cartilage regeneration in the four regions is determined to increase in the following order: region C ≈ region B < region D < region A. The smallest pore size, prepared with the 150–250 μm ice particulates, best promotes cartilaginous matrix formation. The promotion effect of cartilage regeneration in the four regions is in the following order: 250–355 μm region ≈ 355–425 μm region < 425–500 μm region < 150–250 μm region. Usually large pores are more easily accessible to cells than are small pores. However, interconnectivity is also a very important factor for cell delivery and spatial distribution. The good interconnectivity among the spherical large pores in the gradient collagen scaffolds facilitates the smooth delivery of cells throughout the scaffolds. Therefore, the cells can be smoothly delivered and homogeneously distributed not only in the larger pore region, but also in the smaller pore region. Although all four regions show similarly homogeneous cell distribution, the larger pores require more cells to fill the entire free space, while the smaller pores are more easily filled with cells. Filling the pores can increase the cell–cell interactions and provide a real three-dimensional microenvironment to promote chondrogenic differentiation and cartilage tissue formation. This may explain the best promotive effect of the 150–250 μm region on cartilaginous matrix formation.

3.1.6 Conclusions and Future Trends

The ice particulate method has the advantage of initiating the growth and formation of new ice crystals during the freezing process, thus creating unique pore structures in the scaffolds of biodegradable polymers. The surface large pores and inner body large pores are replicas of the pre-prepared ice particulates. Their size, density, and distribution can be controlled by the size, density, and location of the pre-prepared ice particulates. The small pores and interconnecting pores are replicas of ice crystals that are newly generated during the freezing process, which can be controlled by freezing temperature. Funnel-like porous scaffold, highly interconnected scaffolds, and micropatterned porous scaffolds can be prepared by using the ice particulate method. The unique pore structures of these scaffolds facilitate smooth cell seeding and homogeneous cell distribution in the whole spaces of the scaffolds. Cells have high viability and regenerate new tissues when being cultured in the scaffolds. The micropatterned scaffolds facilitate regeneration of capillary network. These scaffolds should be useful for tissue engineering.

References

[1] M.S. Shoichet, Macromolecules 43 (2010) 581–591.

[2] M.R. Badrossamay, K. Balachandran, A.K. Capulli, H.M. Golecki, A. Agarwal, J.A. Goss, H. Kim, K. Shin, K.K. Parker, Biomaterials 35 (2014) 3188–3197.

[3] F. Causa, P.A. Netti, L. Ambrosio, Biomaterials 28 (2007) 5093–5099.

[4] S.W. Choi, J.W. Xie, Y.N. Xia, Adv. Mater. 21 (2009) 2997–3001.

[5] D.J. Griffon, M.R. Sedighi, D.V. Schaeffer, J.A. Eurell, A.L. Johnson, Acta Biomater. 2 (2006) 313–320.

[6] A.G. Mikos, A.J. Thorsen, L.A. Czerwonka, Y. Bao, R. Langer, D.N. Winslow, J.P. Vacanti, Polymer 35 (1994) 1068–1077.

[7] H.F. Zhang, I. Hussain, M. Brust, M.F. Butler, S.P. Rannard, A.I. Cooper, Nat. Mater. 4 (2005) 787–793.

[8] F. Yang, R. Murugan, S. Ramakrishna, X. Wang, Y.X. Ma, S. Wang, Biomaterials 25 (2004) 1891–1900.

[9] L.D. Harris, B.S. Kim, D.J. Mooney, J. Biomed. Mater. Res. 42 (1998) 396–402.

[10] W. Meng, S.Y. Kim, J. Yuan, J.C. Kim, O.H. Kwon, N. Kawazoe, G.P. Chen, Y. Ito, I.K. Kang, J. Biomater. Sci. – Polym. Ed. 18 (2007) 81–94.

[11] A.G. Mikos, Y. Bao, L.G. Cima, D.E. Ingber, J.P. Vacanti, R. Langer, J. Biomed. Mater. Res. 27 (1993) 183–189.

[12] W. Sun, B. Starly, A. Darling, C. Gomez, Biotechnol. Appl. Biochem. 39 (2004) 49–58.

[13] Y.G. Ko, N. Kawazoe, T. Tateishi, G. Chen, J. Bioactive Comp. Polym. 25 (2010) 360–373.

[14] H.H. Oh, Y.G. Ko, H. Lu, N. Kawazoe, G. Chen, Adv. Mater. 24 (2012) 4311–4316.

[15] H.H. Oh, H. Lu, N. Kawazoe, G. Chen, J. Biomat. Sci. - Polym. Ed. 23 (2012) 2185–2195.

[16] Q. Zhang, H. Lu, N. Kawazoe, G. Chen, J. Bioactive Comp. Polym. 28 (2013) 426–438.

[17] Q. Zhang, H. Lu, N. Kawazoe, G. Chen, Mater. Lett. 107 (2013) 280–283.

[18] Q. Zhang, T. Nakamoto, S. Chen, N. Kawazoe, K. Lin, J. Chang, G. Chen, J. Nanosci. Nanotechnol. 14 (2014) 3221–3227.

[19] Y.G. Ko, N. Kawazoe, T. Tateishi, G. Chen, J. Biomed. Mater. Res. B 93B (2010) 341–350.

[20] Y.G. Ko, S. Grice, N. Kawazoe, T. Tateishi, G. Chen, Macromol. Biosci. 10 (2010) 860–871.

[21] Y.G. Ko, H.H. Oh, N. Kawazoe, T. Tateishi, G. Chen, J. Biomater. Sci. – Polym. Ed. 22 (2011) 123–138.

[22] G. Chen, T. Ushida, T. Tateishi, Biomaterials 22 (2001) 2563–2567.

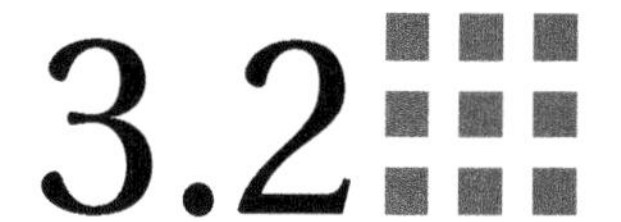

Cell Sheet Technologies

Jun Kobayashi, Teruo Okano
INSTITUTE OF ADVANCED BIOMEDICAL ENGINEERING AND SCIENCE, TOKYO WOMEN'S MEDICAL UNIVERSITY (TWINS), TOKYO, JAPAN

CHAPTER OUTLINE

3.2.1 Introduction

Recently, significant attention has been paid to exploring principles and developing techniques to regenerate damaged tissues and organs. Since proposing an epoch-making concept of "tissue engineering" by Langer and Vacanti in 1993 [1], it has been widely accepted as a promising method for the reconstruction of three-dimensional cellular tissues *in vitro*. In typical tissue engineering, biodegradable materials are used as a temporal scaffold to support the shape of desired tissues. To date, many biodegradable scaffolds including hydrogels [2] have been developed for tuning physical properties (e.g., elastic modulus of matrix), mass transport properties (e.g., diffusion of oxygen and nutrients toward cells), adhesiveness of cells on the scaffolds, and biological factors (e.g., cellular signaling).

By contrast, scaffold-free tissue engineering is performed by assembling cells into three-dimensional tissues. These approaches fundamentally have advantages in achieving proxemic connection between cells (e.g., the formation of gap junctions in myocardium [3]) and avoiding unfavorable host response to scaffolds (e.g., inflammatory reactions accompanied by the degradation of scaffolds [4]) over scaffold-based tissue engineering. Especially, our unique approach, referred to as "cell sheet engineering" [5], has achieved constructing transplantable tissues composed only of cells. Cell sheet engineering is a novel means of both creating transplantable cell sheets and constructing three-dimensional tissues from the cell sheets using a thermoresponsive cell culture dish, which is grafted with thermoresponsive polymer, poly(*N*-isopropylacrylamide) (PIPAAm), on the solid surface. Recently, other researches have reported on scaffold-free tissues through self-assembly of cells using a nanoscale coating of extracellular matrix (ECM) on cellular surfaces [6] or epithelial–mesenchymal interactions to form organ buds [7]. Although these approaches facilitate the formation of tissue constructs only by mixing the cells under appropriate conditions, cell sheet-based tissue engineering is a very flexible method to build any tissue constructs with precise space layout of heterotypic cells as desired.

This chapter focuses on the characteristics of thermoresponsive cell culture surfaces for preparing cell sheets and the applications for cell sheet-based regenerative therapies. Designing new types of thermoresponsive cell culture surfaces as the next generation for creating further functional and complex tissues is also described.

3.2.2 Nanostructure of Thermoresponsive Cell Culture Surfaces Facilitates Cell Sheet Formation and Manipulation

In 1990, our laboratory developed a thermoresponsive cell culture surface, which was grafted with thin PIPAAm by electron beam (EB) irradiation onto tissue culture polystyrene (TCPS) [8]. A grafted PIPAAm layer has a thickness of ca. 20 nm [9] and exhibits a reversible soluble/insoluble change with temperature in water across its phase transition temperature of 32°C [10]. At 37°C, grafted PIPAAm becomes hydrophobic [8] and enhances the adhesion of serum proteins such as fibronectin (FN) [9], leading to integrin-mediated adhesion of cells onto the surfaces (Fig. 3.2.1, left). When temperature is decreased from 37°C to 20°C, the shrunken, grafted PIPAAm layer becomes hydrated and swollen, resulting in reducing the interaction with the adhered proteins and cells and eventually triggering cell detachment [11] (Fig. 3.2.1, right). In other words, the cultured cells are harvested only by changing temperature without the use of digestive enzymes or chelating agents. Our laboratory found that this switching of cell attachment/detachment was observed only on an ultrathin PIPAAm layer with a thickness of ca. 20 nm on TCPS surfaces [9].

How is temperature-triggered switching of cell attachment/detachment on PIPAAm-grafted surfaces achieved? A schematic illustration of cell adhesion with different thickness of grafted PIPAAm is shown in Fig. 3.2.2. Cell attachment dramatically decreases on

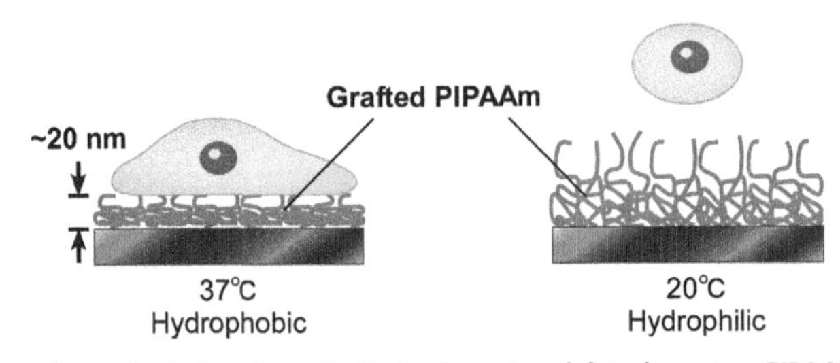

FIGURE 3.2.1 Temperature-dependent alteration of cell attachment and detachment on PIPAAm-grafted TCPS surface.

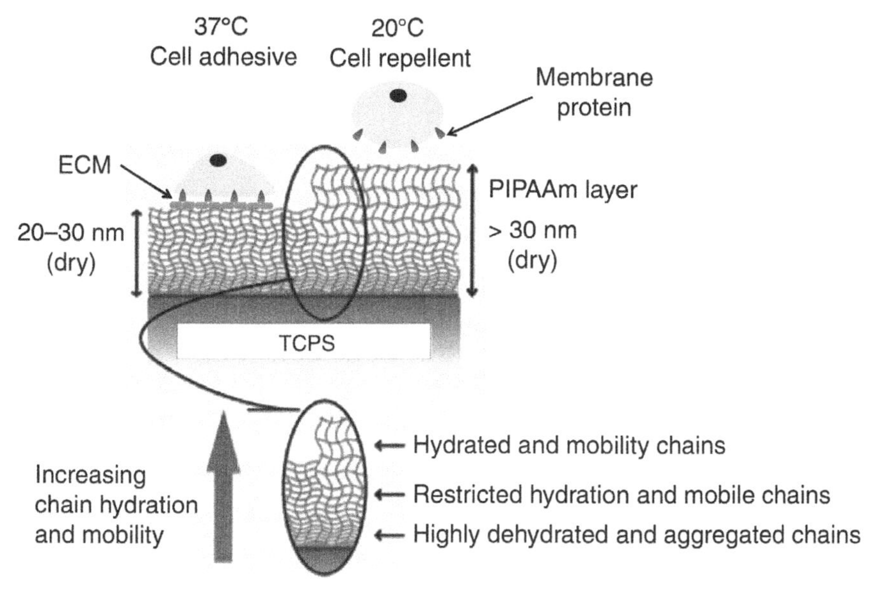

FIGURE 3.2.2 Schematic illustration of the effect of grafted PIPAAm thickness on cell adhesion. *Reprinted from Ref. [12], with permission.*

surfaces grafted with a thicker PIPAAm layer (>30 nm) or chemically cross-linked thick PIPAAm hydrogels at 37°C [9]. Partial hydration and mobility of PIPAAm chains within the thick layer would repeal the adhesion of adhesive proteins from serum-containing medium, although the temperature was at 37°C above the lower critical solution temperature. With decreasing thickness of PIPAAm (~20 nm), the motion of PIPAAm chains is strongly restricted due to the tethering of the chains on the TCPS surface. Additionally, the hydrophobicity in the vicinity of the polystyrene surface would decrease the hydration of grafted PIPAAm chains. These factors are considered to induce the aggregation and restricted mobility of grafted PIPAAm chains at 37°C, resulting in the attachment of proteins and cells on the grafted PIPAAm chains. By contrast, on PIPAAm with a thickness of >30 nm, the outermost layer of grafted PIPAAm chains has a protein-repealing property due to increased mobility of PIPAAm chains far from the hydrophobic polystyrene surface.

On PIPAAm brushes grafted on the solid surface, both grafting density and length of individual PIPAAm chains greatly govern the adhesiveness of proteins and cells. Recently, our group and other groups have investigated temperature-dependent cell adhesion/detachment on PIPAAm brushes, which are prepared by surface-initiated living radical polymerization techniques, such as atom transfer radical polymerization [13,14] and reversible addition-fragmentation chain transfer (RAFT) polymerization [15]. For example, PIPAAm brushes with a thickness of 1.8 nm on TCPS exhibited cell attachment when the temperature was 37°C, although the cells were unable to attach to thicker PIPAAm brushes [13]. In general, surface-initiated living radical polymerization provides dense PIPAAm chains compared with EB-induced grafting of PIPAAm. Also, densely grafted PIPAAm chains

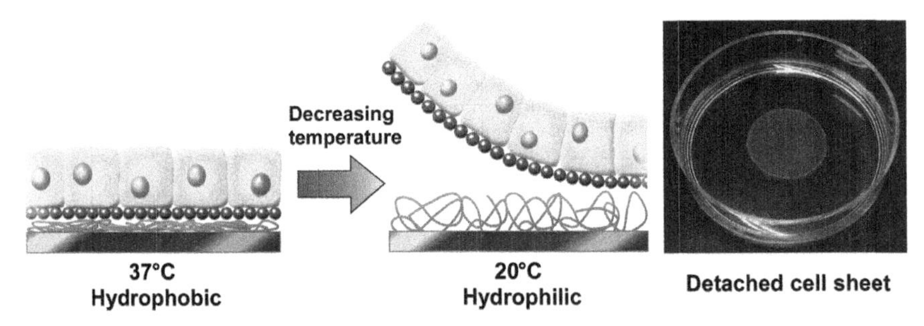

FIGURE 3.2.3 Cell sheet fabrication using thermoresponsive cell culture surface. By changing temperature from 37°C to 20°C, cultured cells were harvested as a contiguous cell sheet.

in aqueous media are more elongated than sparse chains. Therefore, the threshold of thickness for cell attachment on dense PIPAAm brushes is smaller than that of PIPAAm grafting by EB irradiation.

As the cultivation of cells on the thermoresponsive cell culture surfaces proceeds, the cells secrete proteins such as FN and create the ECM microenvironment. When the temperature of cultivation is decreased to 20°C, grafted PIPAAm becomes hydrophilic and confluently cultured cell monolayer is detached as a single cell sheet, which holds ECM on the bottom (Fig. 3.2.3). Fluorescent microscopy reveals that ECMs such as FN [16] and type IV collagen [17] were detected on the bottom of the recovered cell sheet after being stained with fluorescent-labeled antibodies. ECMs such as FN and type IV collagen are known to be major components of the basement membrane that underlies the epithelium. Therefore, the cell sheets easily attach to surfaces of body, tissues, and organs, facilitating the transplantation of the cell sheets on the targets. Furthermore, layering cell sheets results in the formation of three-dimensional thick tissues via ECM-mediated bonding between the layered cell sheets.

Cell sheet-based regenerative treatments have been successfully applied in the clinical setting. The current status of clinical applications is summarized in Table 3.2.1.

A successful clinical study was conducted by using limbal-derived cell sheets for the treatment of patients suffering from unilateral total corneal stem-cell deficiencies [18], which resulted from alkali burns or Stevens–Johnson syndrome. In the case of bilateral total corneal stem-cell deficiencies, an autologous oral mucosal epithelial cell sheet was transplanted onto the ocular surface [19]. A clinical trial in France for the treatment of a bilateral limbal stem-cell deficiency had been conducted by using autologous oral mucosal epithelial cell sheets [20]. Through this clinical trial, the treatment was safe and effective in 25 cases with a 1-year follow-up, although two patients experienced serious adverse events, which were not related to the transplantation of the cell sheets.

The treatment of dilated cardiomyopathy (DCM) and ischemic heart disease has been carried out by using autologous skeletal myoblast sheets [21]. After transplanting the myoblast sheets on the heart surface, the transplanted myoblasts were unable to differentiate into cardiomyocytes; the secretion of cytokines would induce the reduction of fibrosis,

Table 3.2.1 Clinical Applications Based on Single or Layered Cell Sheet-Based Tissues

Tissues/Organs	Target Illness	Cell Sheets	Implementation Site (Country)	Current Status
Corneal epithelium	Limbal stem-cell deficiency	Corneal limbal-derived cell or oral mucosal epithelial cell sheets [18,19]	Osaka University (Japan)	Started in 2003
		Oral mucosal epithelial cell sheet [19,20]	Les Hospices Civils de Lyon (France) Collaborator: Cellseed, Inc. (Japan)	Finished European clinical trial (25 cases with 1-year follow-up)
Myocardium	Severe cardiac disease including ischemic heart disease, DCM	Myoblast sheet [21]	Osaka University (Japan)	Started in May 2007
			Terumo Corporation (Japan); Collaborator: Cellseed, Inc. (Japan)	Approved in September 2015 by the Ministry of Health, Labor and Welfare, Japan, for marketing authorization
Esophagus	Prevention of stenosis after endoscopic submucosal dissection of esophageal cancer	Oral mucosal epithelial cell sheet [22]	Tokyo Women's Medical University (Japan)	Started in April 2008
	Barrett's esophagus		Karolinska Institute (Sweden)	Started in April 2012
Periodontal ligament	Periodontal disease	Periodontal ligament-derived cell sheet [23]	Tokyo Women's Medical University (Japan)	Started in November 2011
Cartilage	Knee cartilage injury	Cartilage cell sheet [24]	Tokai University (Japan)	Started in October 2011
Middle ear	Postoperative mucosal regeneration of middle ear cavity	Nasal mucosa epithelial cell sheet [25]	The Jikei University School of Medicine (Japan)	Started in 2014

angiogenesis, and the recruitment of hematopoietic stem cells. For marketing authorization, Japanese medical device company Terumo Corporation had applied the treatment of ischemic heart disease by transplanting autologous skeletal myoblast sheets to the Ministry of Health, Labor and Welfare, Japan, and approved in September 2015.

Other clinical studies based on cell sheet-based therapies have been conducted as follows: treatments in the fields of esophageal [22], periodontal [23], cartilage [24], and middle ear [25]. For the treatment of superficial esophageal cancer, a superficial neoplasm is removed by esophageal endoscopic submucosal dissection. Endoscopic transplantation of autologous mucosal epithelial cell sheets onto the ulcerations prevented stenosis [22]. Periodontitis is an inflammatory disease and irreversibly destroys the attachment between teeth and periodontal tissue including alveolar bone, cementum, and periodontal ligament. For the regeneration of damaged periodontal tissues, periodontal ligament-derived cell sheets have been transplanted in combination with porous β-tricalcium phosphate to fill bone defects [23]. Layered chondrocyte sheets were transplanted onto the knee joints to treat the defect of the knee cartilage by injury or osteoarthritis [24]. For enhancing postoperative mucosal regeneration of the middle ear cavity, autologous nasal mucosa epithelial cell sheets were transplanted to the surface of the bone of the middle ear [25]. Several preclinical investigations using cell sheet technology have been investigated to perform air leak sealant for lung punctures [26], and to create liver tissue [27], pancreatic islets [28], and endometrium [29] in animal models.

3.2.3 ECM-Mimicking Nanostructure on Thermoresponsive Cell Culture Surfaces for Creating Functional Cell Sheets

As mentioned in the previous section, the microenvironment around the cultured cells was formed by the secretion and deposition of FN. In other words, PIPAAm-grafted thermoresponsive cell culture surfaces lack any ECM components, which are composed of proteins, proteoglycans, and other soluble molecules. ECM provides a microenvironment to mediate the interactions between ligands and their receptors on the cellular membrane. Interactions between ligands and receptors play pivotal roles in regulating cellular adhesion, proliferation, migration, differentiation, and signal transduction. Therefore, installing bioactive ligands into thermoresponsive cell culture surfaces is essential for finely tuning cell proliferation, growth, and differentiation. Several EMC-mimicking thermoresponsive cell culture surfaces have been developed (listed in Table 3.2.2).

A peptide sequence Arg-Gly-Asp (RGD), which is found in FN, vitronectin, type I collagen, and other ECMs, is a common element for integrin-mediated cell adhesion. For covalent immobilization of bioactive ligands such as RGD peptide, poly(*N*-isopropylacrylamide-*co*-2-carboxyisopropylacrylamide) [poly(IPAAm-*co*-CIPAAm)] having carboxyl side chains, which were amine- or hydroxyl-reactive functional groups through condensing reaction, was grafted on TCPS [38]. Installing RGD peptide into the nanostructure of grafted poly(IPAAm-*co*-CIPAAm) provides ligands (Fig. 3.2.4a) to emulate cell adhesion on FN [31,32]. In serum-free medium at 37°C, endothelial cells were able to adhere to the RGDS-conjugated poly(IPAAm-*co*-CIPAAm)-grafted surfaces, where the RGDS moiety was considered to be exposed in the medium due to the shrinking of the grafted polymer chains. Coimmobilization of RGDS and Pro-His-Ser-Arg-Asn (PHSRN) peptides, which are found in the 10th and 9th type III repeats of FN, respectively, into the poly(IPAAm-*co*-CIPAAm)-grafted surfaces enhanced the number

Table 3.2.2 ECM-Mimicking Thermoresponsive Cell Culture Surfaces

Mimicked ECMs	ECM Components/Ligands
Fibronectin	RGD [30], RGDS [31–33], PHSRN and RGDS [34]
Proteoglycan	Heparin [35,36]
Collagen	Gelatin [37]

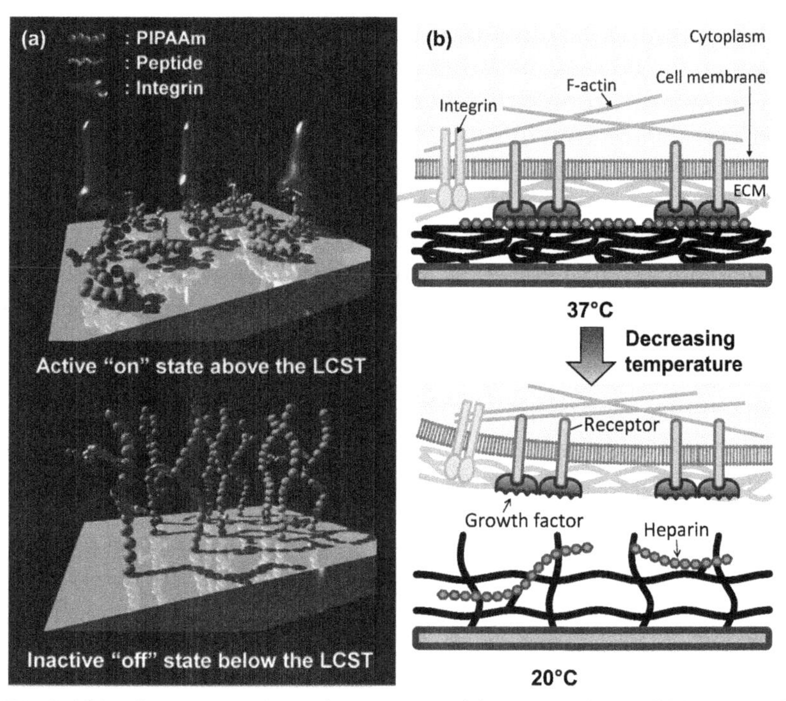

FIGURE 3.2.4 ECM-mimicking thermoresponsive surface containing (a) RGD peptides and (b) heparin molecules. *Reprinted from Ref. [34], with permission.*

of adhered/spread endothelial cells at 37°C[34]. This enhancement of cell adhesion and spreading is due to multivalent interaction of integrin receptor with adhesive RGDS peptide and synergy PHSRN peptide.

On the contrary, when temperature was lowered to 20°C, the adhered cells were detached from bioactive ligands-conjugated poly(IPAAm-*co*-CIPAAm)-grafted surfaces. The detachment of cells indicated that the affinity interaction between the cells and the immobilized bioactive ligands was reduced by the swelling of grafted polymer chains. Expanded, swollen PIPAAm chains were considered to increase their molecular motion and steric hindrance in the vicinity of the immobilized bioactive ligands, leading to dynamic reduction of the affinity interactions with the cells. Therefore, reversible swelling/deswelling of grafted PIPAAm chains can be used for regulating affinity interactions between bioactive ligands and their cell membrane receptors.

Kinetics of cell attachment/detachment from the bioactive ligand-immobilized thermoresponsive cell culture surfaces was greatly affected by the molecular architecture of immobilized ligands. Introduction of a spacer such as poly(ethylene glycol) between a bioactive peptide and a PIPAAm chain facilitates the access of integrin receptors on the cells [39]. When the temperature was changed from 37°C to 20°C, by contrast, the steric hindrance of swollen PIPAAm on spacer-inserted ligands was smaller than that on ligands without a spacer, resulting in delaying the detachment of cells. Moreover, immobilized

PHSRN-G_6-RGDS peptides also hindered the cell detachment because the length of G_6 (~3.5 nm) between the PHSRN and RGDS peptides was similar to spatial layout in native FN and the affinity interaction with integrin was reinforced via synergetic binding of PHSRN and RGDS peptides with integrin [34].

In addition to the above-mentioned one-on-one affinity binding with a receptor, multivalent binding with proteins can be also seen in proteoglycan for regulating cell functions. Proteoglycans, which are located on the cell surfaces and ECMs, possess negatively charged heparan sulfate chains. Heparin molecules, similar in structure and functions with heparan sulfate, interacts with various heparin-binding proteins such as basic fibroblast growth factor (bFGF), vascular endothelial growth factor, FN, and antithrombin III through multivalent binding [40]. In biology, the interaction between heparan sulfate and heparin-binding proteins plays important roles in regulating the stabilities and activities of the proteins: the stabilization of growth factors through the formation of complex, and the suppression of diffusion of growth factor. Therefore, the introduction of heparin molecules on thermoresponsive cell culture surfaces are able to mimic proteoglycan functions such as regulating cellular growth via heparin-binding proteins (Fig. 3.2.4b) [35,36].

For example, bFGF is able to bind to a heparin-functionalized thermoresponsive surface at 37°C. The activity of bound bFGF was higher than that of soluble and physisorbed bFGF, resulting in the acceleration of duration required for reaching confluence. Moreover, the confluent cells on the heparin-functionalized thermoresponsive surface detach themselves as a cell sheet by lowering the temperature to 20°C. Fluorescent staining of FN and bFGF after the detachment of the cell sheet revealed that both were localized on the cell sheet, while no FN and bFGF were observed on the heparin-functionalized temperature-responsive surface where the cell sheet had been removed. Therefore, bFGF was released and transferred from the heparin-functionalized surfaces to the cell sheet.

What is happing during cell detachment from heparin-functionalized thermoresponsive surfaces? When the temperature was lowered from 37°C to 20°C, the swelling of the grafted PIPAAm chains accompanied the dynamic motion of heparin molecules. Conformational changes in both PIPAAm chains and heparin molecules induced increased steric hindrance of the swollen PIPAAn chains in the vicinity of heparin and increased the dynamic motion of heparin, resulting in rupturing the complex among heparin, bFGF, and FGF receptor. Therefore, the heparin-functionalized thermoresponsive surface is able to regulate the switching of bFGF binding and separation by temperature change.

Moreover, heparin-functionalized thermoresponsive cell culture surfaces have an affinity interaction with heparin-binding EGF-like growth factor (HB-EGF), which is a potent mitogen for hepatocytes [41]. An HB-EGF-bound heparin-functionalized thermoresponsive surface was utilized for creating hepatocyte sheets with maintaining hepatic functions during cultivation [42]. The addition of HB-EGF in the cell culture media was essential for the survival of hepatocytes. When the medium contained less than 10 ng/cm^2 of soluble HB-EGF, the hepatocytes were not able to adhere and form their cell sheets. Hepatocytes adhered well and formed their sheets on the HB-EGF-bound heparin-functionalized thermoresponsive surface. The secretion of albumin was maintained and higher compared to that on PIPAAm-grafted surfaces with soluble HB-EGF. Higher expression of hepatocyte-specific genes was detected in hepatocyte sheets on affinity-bound HB-EGF compared with that on soluble HB-EGF. In addition, when lowering the temperature to 20°C, the cultured cell sheets were detached from the surface through the reduction of affinity binding between HB-EGF and immobilized heparin with increasing the mobility of heparin and the swollen PIPAAm. Therefore, ECM-mimicking heparin-functionalized thermoresponsive cell culture surfaces have a potential to create transplantable cell sheets with maintaining the functionality of the cell sheets.

3.2.4 Spatially Organized Three-Dimensional Tissue Reconstruction Using Cell Sheet Technologies

Two-dimensional cell sheets contain dense cells with ECMs on the bottom, facilitating the formation of cell-dense three-dimensional tissues simply by layering the cell sheets. The layered cell sheets are able to be functionally connected to each other: the layered cardiac cell sheets exhibit spontaneous pulsating, which is synchronized via electrical connection of connexions [3,43]. For further mimicking living tissues and organs, it is necessary to create complicated three-dimensional tissue architecture with the heterotypic cells. In large organs such as liver and kidneys, the society is formed by interactions among heterotypic cells for preserving differentiated cell functions. In addition, unique structures such as micrometer-scale organizations and alignment appear in liver, kidneys, and heart. Therefore, the reconstruction of spatially organized three-dimensional tissue is required for the creation of highly functional tissues and organs.

3.2.4.1 Creation of Heterotypic Cell Sheet-Based Tissues

The reconstruction of functional liver tissues is an important issue for the treatment of liver diseases such as hemophilia. Currently, to make these tissues, primary hepatocytes isolated from liver have been used. However, one big problem of liver tissue reconstruction is the reduction of hepatic functions *in vitro*. Healthy liver is anatomically divided into liver lobules, which are minimal functional units. Through the isolation process of hepatocytes, the microstructure such as cell–cell contacts and ECMs was destroyed, leading to reduced viability and reduced hepatic functions such as albumin secretion. Therefore, hepatocytes rapidly lose their viability and phenotypic functions after isolation.

To precisely mimic the microstructures of native tissues and organs, the manipulation of multiple cells and ECMs is essential. For maintaining the *in vitro* hepatic functions, several cell culture methods such as using sandwiched collagen [44] and coculture with nonparenchymal cells [45] have been previously developed. A two-dimensional alignment of hepatocyte/nonparenchymal cells is able to be precisely achieved by photolithographic [46] and soft lithographic techniques [47]. Although the hepatic functions on coculture systems were maintained compared with the monoculture of hepatocytes, the

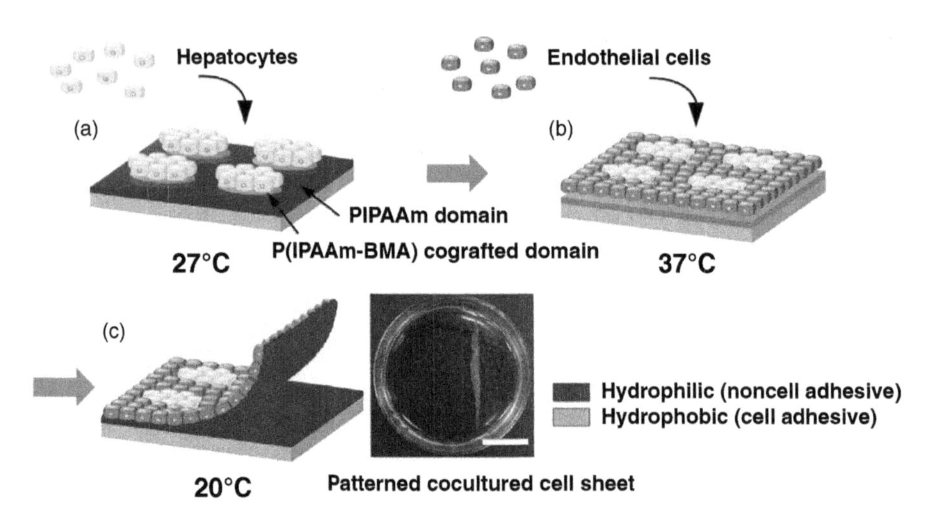

FIGURE 3.2.5 Fabrication of transplantable cocultured hepatic cell sheet. (a) Hepatocytes were selectively adhered to poly(IPAAm-BMA) cografted domains at 27°C. (b) After increasing temperature to 37°C, endothelial cells were adhered to PIPAAm domains. (c) When the temperature was changed from 37°C to 20°C, the cocultured hepatic cell sheet was recovered from the surface. *Reprinted from Ref. [50], with permission.*

cultured hepatocytes were not transplantable. By contrast, cell sheet-based technology facilitates the fabrication of transplantable, spatially aligned tissues because aligned two-dimensional cell sheets are allowed to be hierarchically stacked in a layered structure.

To make transplantable heterotypic cell sheets, we utilize micropatterned surfaces grafted with EB-induced polymerization of two types of temperature-responsive polymers, PIPAAm and *n*-butyl methacrylate (BMA)-*co*-grafted PIPAAm, which exhibit different phase transition temperatures (Fig. 3.2.5) [48]. As an alternative approach, microcontact printing (μCP) of fibronectin by using a patterned polydimethylsiloxane (PDMS) stamp on PIPAAm-grafted surfaces is also utilized to create cell-adhesive and nonadhesive regions [49]. Micropatterns prepared by μCP exhibited more accurate alignment than those by EB-induced polymerization. Moreover, μCP is relatively less time-consuming because micropatterned surfaces are obtained by using a uniformly grafted PIPAAm cell culture surface and PDMS stamps without a time-consuming process. Sequential seeding of hepatocytes and endothelial cells on the micropatterned surface with changing temperature or the medium enables two-dimensional alignment of the hepatocytes and endothelial cells. During cultivation at 37°C, higher hepatic functions including albumin secretion and urea synthesis were detected on micropatterned coculture compared with those on hepatocyte monoculture. By decreasing the size of micropatterns, the function was increased [50], probably due to increased boundary area between hepatocytes and endothelial cells. Eventually, the cocultured cells are harvested as a single micropatterned cell sheet by lowering the temperature and transferring onto another substrate such as a culture dish and a cell sheet using a gelatin-coated cell sheet manipulator [49].

In addition to two-dimensional alignment, layering an endothelial cell sheet onto a hepatocyte sheet creates three-dimensional tissues, where the endothelial cell sheet-derived ECMs are localized between the layered sheets [51]. Hepatic functions such as albumin secretion and urea synthesis in layered hepatocytes–endothelial cell sheets are highly maintained at least during 4 weeks. By contrast, the monoculture of hepatocytes on a collagen-coated dish shows remarkable dysfunction in albumin secretion and urea synthesis within 1 week. Higher expression of hepatocyte-specific genes such as albumin, hepatocyte nucleus factor 4, multidrug resistance-associated protein 2, and claudin-3 was detected more in the layered sheets than those in the hepatocyte monoculture. The maintenance of hepatic functions on the layered sheets was due to the coculture with nonparenchymal cells and the localization of ECMs around the hepatocytes. Moreover, the formation of bile canaliculi was clearly found between the hepatocytes within the layered sheets. These functional and morphological reconstructions were presumably considered to be attributed to mimicking a hepatic perisinusoidal space-like structure between the sheets of hepatocytes and endothelial cells with ECMs. Therefore, cell sheet technologies provide the creation of transplantable sheet-like liver tissues with maintaining hepatic functions.

3.2.4.2 Creation of Aligned Tissues by Using Anisotropic Cell Sheets

In native tissues such as skeletal muscle and myocardium, cells and ECMs are aligned in an anisotropic direction, resulting in the production of anisotropic forces. Therefore, mimicking an aligned structure within engineered tissues is a key issue for the creation of force-generating constructs. Micro/nanotechnologies including microgrooved substrate and electropinning scaffolds enable the orientation of cultured cells in the desired direction. By contrast, the combination of microfabrication and grafting with thin thermoresponsive polymer allows the aligned cells to detach themselves as a cell sheet, which is a transplantable and scaffold-free cellular monolayer.

For achieving the fabrication of cell sheets with alignment, two-dimensional micropatterns of thermoresponsive brushes, PIPAAm and PIPAAm-*b*-poly(*N*-acryloylmorpholine) (PAcMo), on the glass surfaces were prepared by surface-initiated RAFT polymerization (Fig. 3.2.6) [52]. Terminal grafting of PAcMo on PIPAAm brushes rendered the surface slightly hydrophilic compared with that on PIPAAm brushes: the attachment of seeded cells was delayed more on PIPAAm-*b*-PAcMo brushes than that on PIPAAm brushes. Eventually, spatioselective attachment of myoblasts on PIPAAm and PIPAAm-*b*-PAcMo brush domains (50/50 μm stripes) led to the alignment of attached myoblasts along the stripes. The aligned myoblasts were able to reach confluence, and were detached from the surface as an aligned myoblast sheet when lowering the temperature to 20°C. Additionally, the floating cell sheets detached from the micropatterned surface preferentially shrunk in a parallel direction with the stripes (Fig. 3.2.7a), although detached cell sheets from the PIPAAm brush surface exhibited isotropic shrinkage. These differences in the shrinkage of cell sheets were due to the anisotropy of cytoskeletal organization in the aligned cell sheets.

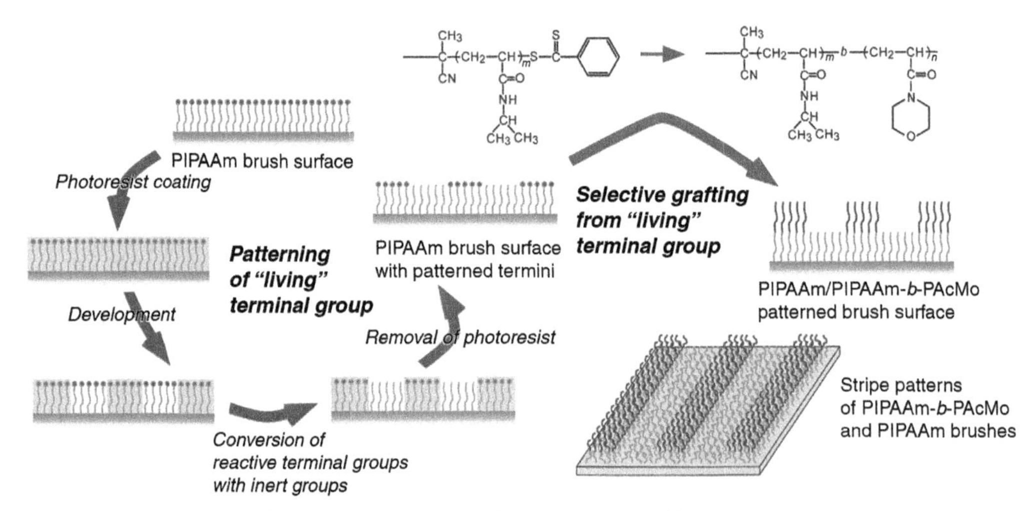

FIGURE 3.2.6 Micropatterned thermoresponsive surface for preparing aligned cell sheets. Hydrophilic poly (*N*-acryloylmorpholine) (PAcMo) segments were grafted on the terminal of PIPAAm brushes having chain-transfer active (living) terminal groups (circles [red in the web version]). Spatially selective grafting of PAcMo segments was performed through a photolithographic fabrication process. *Reprinted from Ref. [52], with permission.*

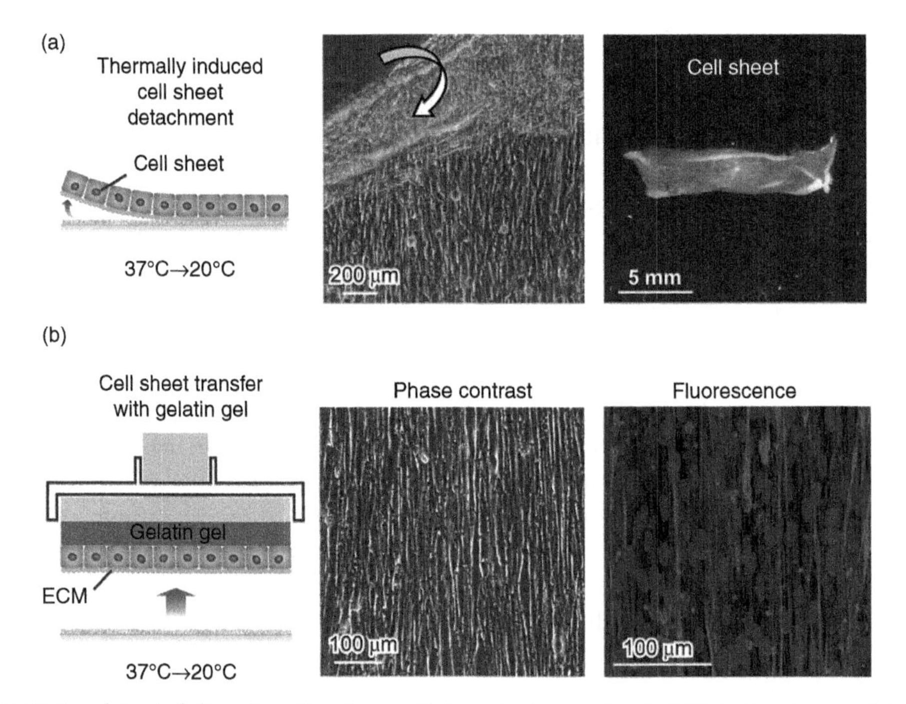

FIGURE 3.2.7 Detachment of aligned myoblast sheets with lowering temperature to 20°C. (a) Spontaneous detachment of the aligned myoblast sheet exhibited anisotropic shrinkage. (b) A gelatin-coated cell sheet manipulator facilitated the recovery and transfer of the aligned myoblast sheet without shrinkage. *Reprinted from Ref. [53], with permission.*

The aligned myoblast sheet was able to be transferred and stacked by using a gelatin-coated cell sheet manipulator, which facilitated the construction of three-dimensional tissues without the shrinkage of the cell sheets (Fig. 3.2.7b) [53]. Myotube formation along with the aligned orientation of myoblast sheets was found in differentiation media (e.g., 2% horse serum containing media). Compared with randomly oriented myoblasts, the aligned myoblasts formed longer myotubes. Therefore, the formed myotube from the aligned cellular sheets was able to be used as a layer of three-dimensional tissues with a well-organized cell orientation. Interestingly, this technology allowed us to create unique three-dimensional structures with parallel alignments. For example, when a randomly oriented myoblast sheet was layered beneath or above the aligned myoblast sheet, the randomly distributed myoblasts changed their orientation along the aligned myoblast sheet (Fig. 3.2.8a). When the aligned myoblast sheet was layered on another myoblast sheet, the orientation of myoblasts on the bottom was changed to the same direction as the alignment of the top sheet (Fig. 3.2.8b), regardless of whether the orientation of myoblasts on the bottom is random or orthogonal. Eventually, the layered myoblast sheets formed a parallel anisotropic structure, where the direction of aligned myoblasts on the top was dominant. Although the mechanism of this reorganization of myoblasts has remained unclear, the reorganization was induced by a number of factors including the aligned ECMs on the top of the cell sheet.

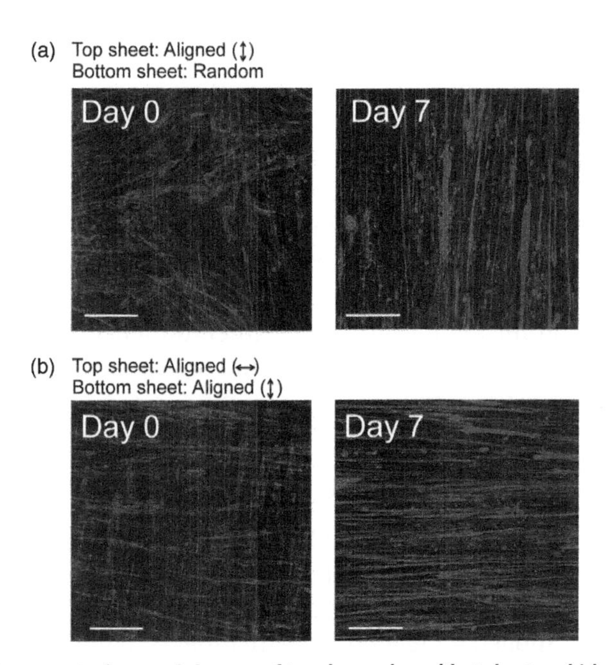

FIGURE 3.2.8 Confocal fluorescent microscopic images of two-layered myoblast sheets, which were layered by using a gelatin-coated cell sheet manipulator. (a) An aligned myoblast sheet was transferred onto randomly oriented myoblast sheet. (b) Two aligned myoblast sheets were orthogonally layered. Day on the upper-left corner indicate incubation time after layering the sheets. Actin fibers were stained with AlexaFluor 568-conjugated phalloidin. Scale bars: 100 μm. *Reprinted from Ref. [53], with permission.*

Additionally, tissue engineering technology using self-reorganization of myoblasts facilitates rapid formation of anisotropically oriented three-dimensional tissue. Only an aligned myoblast sheet on the top of multilayered cellular sheets commands all of the myoblasts to be aligned along the orientation on the top [53]. The reorganization of the orientation of myoblasts rapidly occurs within 24 h after layering. Therefore, this cell sheet-based manipulation technology has a potential for quick construction of complex tissues composed of natively oriented three-dimensional tissues including skeletal muscle tissue.

In order to mimic further functional muscle tissues, a key factor is the formation of networks of blood vessels and nerves, which are required for interactive connection of the implanted tissues with the host. However, the creation of functional cellular networks within the engineered tissues is still a challenging issue in tissue engineering technologies. In particular, it is difficult to manipulate the cellular microstructures such as capillary and neural networks in scaffold-free and cell-dense tissues. Here, cell sheet-based manipulation technologies enable the cellular microstructures to be incorporated within three-dimensional tissues. One approach is the combination of micropatterned cells and other types of cell sheets [54]. The micropatterned cells were constructed on thermoresponsive micropatterned surfaces, which were fabricated by a maskless photolithography method [55]. Recovered micropatterns of endothelial cells from the thermoresponsive surfaces by lowering the temperature were sandwiched between fibroblast sheets using a gelatin-coated cell sheet manipulator. The fidelity of the micropatterned endothelial cells within the multilayered tissue was temporarily maintained after assembly. During 5-day cultivation, the endothelial cells self-organized and eventually formed capillary-like random networks. To precisely form the cellular networks as designed, self-organization behavior within layered anisotropic myoblast sheets is used [56,57]. When human neurons [57] and endothelial cells [56,57] were sandwiched between two of the aligned myoblast sheets, the self-organization of the cells in the direction of the anisotropic myoblast sheet, resulting in the formation of cellular networks mimicking their structures in native muscle tissue. These techniques are promising for fabricating three-dimensional tissues with complex and multicellular architectures, and useful in future regenerative medicine as well as the development of an *in vitro* tissue model.

3.2.5 Conclusions and Future Trends

Thermoresponsive cell culture surfaces grafted with a nanoscale PIPAAm layer on solid surfaces facilitate cell sheet formation and manipulation with changing culture temperature. Cell sheet-based tissue engineering using thermoresponsive cell culture surfaces have been successfully applied for regenerative treatments in the clinical setting. As a next generation of cell sheet-based tissue engineering, ECM mimicking on thermoresponsive cell culture surfaces is essential for creating functional cell sheets such as hepatic cellular tissues. Cell sheet-based tissue engineering has also contributed to the establishment of three-dimensional tissues with complex and multicellular structures. In addition, self-organization of multilayered tissues using aligned cell sheets has a potential to quickly engineer complicated and functional tissue structures. Eventually, the advancement of tissue engineering such as cell sheet technologies may realize the creation of functional tissues and organs.

References

[1] R. Langer, J.P. Vacanti, Science 260 (1993) 920–926.

[2] J.L. Drury, D.J. Mooney, Biomaterials 24 (2003) 4337–4351.

[3] T. Shimizu, M. Yamato, Y. Isoi, T. Akutsu, T. Setomaru, K. Abe, A. Kikuchi, M. Umezu, T. Okano, Circ. Res. 90 (2002) E40–E48.

[4] J. Yang, M. Yamato, C. Kohno, A. Nishimoto, H. Sekine, F. Fukai, T. Okano, Biomaterials 26 (2005) 6415–6422.

[5] M. Yamato, T. Okano, Mater. Today 7 (2004) 42–47.

[6] M. Matsusaki, K. Kadowaki, Y. Nakahara, M. Akashi, Angew. Chem. Int. Ed. Engl. 46 (2007) 4689–4692.

[7] T. Takebe, K. Sekine, M. Enomura, H. Koike, M. Kimura, T. Ogaeri, R.R. Zhang, Y. Ueno, Y.W. Zheng, N. Koike, S. Aoyama, Y. Adachi, H. Taniguchi, Nature 499 (2013) 481–484.

[8] N. Yamada, T. Okano, H. Sakai, F. Karikusa, Y. Sawasaki, Y. Sakurai, Makromol. Chem. Rapid Commun. 11 (1990) 571–576.

[9] Y. Akiyama, A. Kikuchi, M. Yamato, T. Okano, Langmuir 20 (2004) 5506–5511.

[10] M. Heskins, J.E. Guillet, J. Macromol. Sci. A 2 (1968) 1441–1455.

[11] M. Yamato, C. Konno, A. Kushida, M. Hirose, U. Mika, A. Kikuchi, T. Okano, Biomaterials 21 (2000) 981–986.

[12]J. Kobayashi, Y. Akiyama, M. Yamato, T. Okano, Biomaterials: temperature-responsive polymer, in: M.-Y. Murray (Ed.), Comprehensive Biotechnology, second ed., Oxford, Academic Press, 2011, pp. 51–64.

[13] A. Mizutani, A. Kikuchi, M. Yamato, H. Kanazawa, T. Okano, Biomaterials 29 (2008) 2073–2081.

[14] K. Nagase, M. Watanabe, A. Kikuchi, M. Yamato, T. Okano, Macromol. Biosci. 11 (2011) 400–409.

[15] H. Takahashi, M. Nakayama, M. Yamato, T. Okano, Biomacromolecules 11 (2010) 1991–1999.

[16] A. Kushida, M. Yamato, C. Konno, A. Kikuchi, Y. Sakurai, T. Okano, J. Biomed. Mater. Res. 45 (1999) 355–362.

[17] T. Ide, K. Nishida, M. Yamato, T. Sumide, M. Utsumi, T. Nozaki, A. Kikuchi, T. Okano, Y. Tano, Biomaterials 27 (2006) 607–614.

[18] K. Nishida, M. Yamato, Y. Hayashida, K. Watanabe, N. Maeda, H. Watanabe, K. Yamamoto, S. Nagai, A. Kikuchi, Y. Tano, T. Okano, Transplantation 77 (2004) 379–385.

[19] K. Nishida, M. Yamato, Y. Hayashida, K. Watanabe, K. Yamamoto, E. Adachi, S. Nagai, A. Kikuchi, N. Maeda, H. Watanabe, T. Okano, Y. Tano, N. Engl. J. Med. 351 (2004) 1187–1196.

[20] C. Burillon, L. Huot, V. Justin, S. Nataf, F. Chapuis, E. Decullier, O. Damour, Invest. Ophthalmol. Vis. Sci. 53 (2012) 1325–1331.

[21] Y. Sawa, S. Miyagawa, T. Sakaguchi, T. Fujita, A. Matsuyama, A. Saito, T. Shimizu, T. Okano, Surg. Today 42 (2012) 181–184.

[22] T. Ohki, M. Yamato, M. Ota, R. Takagi, D. Murakami, M. Kondo, R. Sasaki, H. Namiki, T. Okano, M. Yamamoto, Gastroenterology 143 (2012) 582–588 e581-e582.

[23] T. Iwata, M. Yamato, H. Tsuchioka, R. Takagi, S. Mukobata, K. Washio, T. Okano, I. Ishikawa, Biomaterials 30 (2009) 2716–2723.

[24] G. Ebihara, M. Sato, M. Yamato, G. Mitani, T. Kutsuna, T. Nagai, S. Ito, T. Ukai, M. Kobayashi, M. Kokubo, T. Okano, J. Mochida, Biomaterials 33 (2012) 3846–3851.

[25] T. Hama, K. Yamamoto, Y. Yaguchi, D. Murakami, H. Sasaki, M. Yamato, T. Okano, H. Kojima, J. Tissue Eng. Regen. Med. 2015 Apr 7. doi: 10.1002/term.2012. [Epub ahead of print]

[26] M. Kanzaki, M. Yamato, J. Yang, H. Sekine, R. Takagi, T. Isaka, T. Okano, T. Onuki, Eur. J. Cardiothor. Surg. 34 (2008) 864–869.

[27] K. Ohashi, T. Yokoyama, M. Yamato, H. Kuge, H. Kanehiro, M. Tsutsumi, T. Amanuma, H. Iwata, J. Yang, T. Okano, Y. Nakajima, Nat. Med. 13 (2007) 880–885.

[28] H. Shimizu, K. Ohashi, R. Utoh, K. Ise, M. Gotoh, M. Yamato, T. Okano, Biomaterials 30 (2009) 5943–5949.

[29] G. Kuramoto, S. Takagi, K. Ishitani, T. Shimizu, T. Okano, H. Matsui, Hum. Reprod. 30 (2015) 406–416.

[30] R.A. Stile, K.E. Healy, Biomacromolecules 2 (2001) 185–194.

[31] M. Ebara, M. Yamato, T. Aoyagi, A. Kikuchi, K. Sakai, T. Okano, Biomacromolecules 5 (2004) 505–510.

[32] M. Ebara, M. Yamato, T. Aoyagi, A. Kikuchi, K. Sakai, T. Okano, Tissue Eng. 10 (2004) 1125–1135.

[33] M. Nishi, J. Kobayashi, S. Pechmann, M. Yamato, Y. Akiyama, A. Kikuchi, K. Uchida, M. Textor, H. Yajima, T. Okano, Biomaterials 28 (2007) 5471–5476.

[34] M. Ebara, M. Yamato, T. Aoyagi, A. Kikuchi, K. Sakai, T. Okano, Adv. Mater. 20 (2008) 3034–3038.

[35] Y. Arisaka, J. Kobayashi, M. Yamato, Y. Akiyama, T. Okano, Biomaterials 34 (2013) 4214–4222.

[36] Y. Arisaka, J. Kobayashi, M. Yamato, Y. Akiyama, T. Okano, Organogenesis 9 (2013) 125–127.

[37] N. Morikawa, T. Matsuda, J. Biomater. Sci. Polym. Ed. 13 (2002) 167–183.

[38] M. Ebara, M. Yamato, M. Hirose, T. Aoyagi, A. Kikuchi, K. Sakai, T. Okano, Biomacromolecules 4 (2003) 344–349.

[39] M. Ebara, M. Yamato, T. Aoyagi, A. Kikuchi, K. Sakai, T. Okano, Biomaterials 29 (2008) 3650–3655.

[40] I. Capila, R.J. Linhardt, Angew. Chem. Int. Ed. 41 (2002) 390–412.

[41] N. Ito, S. Kawata, S. Tamura, S. Kiso, H. Tsushima, D. Damm, J.A. Abraham, S. Higashiyama, N. Taniguchi, Y. Matsuzawa, Biochem. Biophys. Res. Commun. 198 (1994) 25–31.

[42] Y. Arisaka, J. Kobayashi, K. Ohashi, K. Tatsumi, K. Kim, Y. Akiyama, M. Yamato, T. Okano, Regen. Ther. (submitted).

[43] Y. Haraguchi, T. Shimizu, M. Yamato, A. Kikuchi, T. Okano, Biomaterials 27 (2006) 4765–4774.

[44] J.C. Dunn, M.L. Yarmush, H.G. Koebe, R.G. Tompkins, FASEB J. 3 (1989) 174–177.

[45] Y. Nahmias, R.E. Schwartz, W.S. Hu, C.M. Verfaillie, D.J. Odde, Tissue Eng. 12 (2006) 1627–1638.

[46] S.N. Bhatia, M.L. Yarmush, M. Toner, J. Biomed. Mater. Res. 34 (1997) 189–199.

[47] S.R. Khetani, S.N. Bhatia, Nat. Biotechnol. 26 (2008) 120–126.

[48] Y. Tsuda, A. Kikuchi, M. Yamato, A. Nakao, Y. Sakurai, M. Umezu, T. Okano, Biomaterials 26 (2005) 1885–1893.

[49] I.E. Hannachi, K. Itoga, Y. Kumashiro, J. Kobayashi, M. Yamato, T. Okano, Biomaterials 30 (2009) 5427–5432.

[50] Y. Tsuda, A. Kikuchi, M. Yamato, G. Chen, T. Okano, Biochem. Biophys. Res. Commun. 348 (2006) 937–944.

[51] K. Kim, K. Ohashi, R. Utoh, K. Kano, T. Okano, Biomaterials 33 (2012) 1406–1413.

[52] H. Takahashi, M. Nakayama, K. Itoga, M. Yamato, T. Okano, Biomacromolecules 12 (2011) 1414–1418.

[53] H. Takahashi, T. Shimizu, M. Nakayama, M. Yamato, T. Okano, Biomaterials 34 (2013) 7372–7380.

[54] Y. Tsuda, T. Shimizu, M. Yamato, A. Kikuchi, T. Sasagawa, S. Sekiya, J. Kobayashi, G. Chen, T. Okano, Biomaterials 28 (2007) 4939–4946.

[55] K. Itoga, J. Kobayashi, M. Yamato, T. Okano, Methods Cell Biol. 119 (2014) 141–158.

[56] M. Muraoka, T. Shimizu, K. Itoga, H. Takahashi, T. Okano, Biomaterials 34 (2013) 696–703.

[57] H. Takahashi, T. Shimizu, M. Nakayama, M. Yamato, T. Okano, Adv. Healthcare Mater. 4 (2015) 356–360.

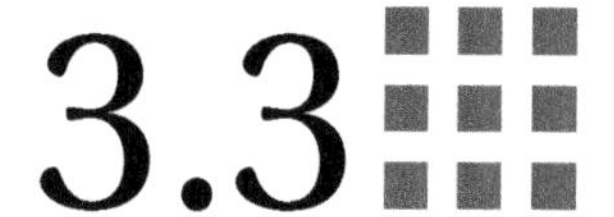

Cell Manipulation Technologies

Jun Nakanishi

INTERNATIONAL CENTER FOR MATERIALS NANOARCHITECTONICS (MANA), NATIONAL INSTITUTE FOR MATERIALS SCIENCE (NIMS), TSUKUBA, JAPAN

CHAPTER OUTLINE

3.3.1 Introduction

Activities of cells are regulated not only by soluble factors such as growth factors and cytokines, but also by interactions with surrounding cells and extracellular matrices (ECMs) (Fig. 3.3.1). Moreover, these insoluble regulatory factors change quite dynamically in living bodies through the active production and decomposition of proteins. This dynamic feature of insoluble factors is important for the expression of biological activities. When we look at the situation of *in vitro* cell culture, the culture medium and substrates serve as substitutes for extracellular aqueous milieu and ECMs, respectively. Soluble factors are rather easy to control their concentration and timing of administration, and hence we already know many things about their impact on cellular activities and fates. On the other hand, the insoluble factors are basically uncontrollable. What we can do is to let the cells adapt to the originally set environments and observe cellular response passively. Therefore, there exist technical limitations to understand the contribution of the insoluble environmental factors to the regulation of biological processes.

From this viewpoint, dynamic substrates, whose surface chemical and physical characteristics can be controlled by an extracellular stimulus, such as heat, voltage, and light, are promising research tools to address such issues and they have attracted the attention of material scientists [1]. These tools enable us not only to mimic dynamic changes of extracellular niches, but also to resolve the processes of how the cells gain and change their phenotypes in response to the changes in the niches. Moreover, they are useful for cell manipulation, such as coculturing heterotypic cell types, cell migration and processes extension, and cell sheet peeling by spatially and/or temporally controlled application of

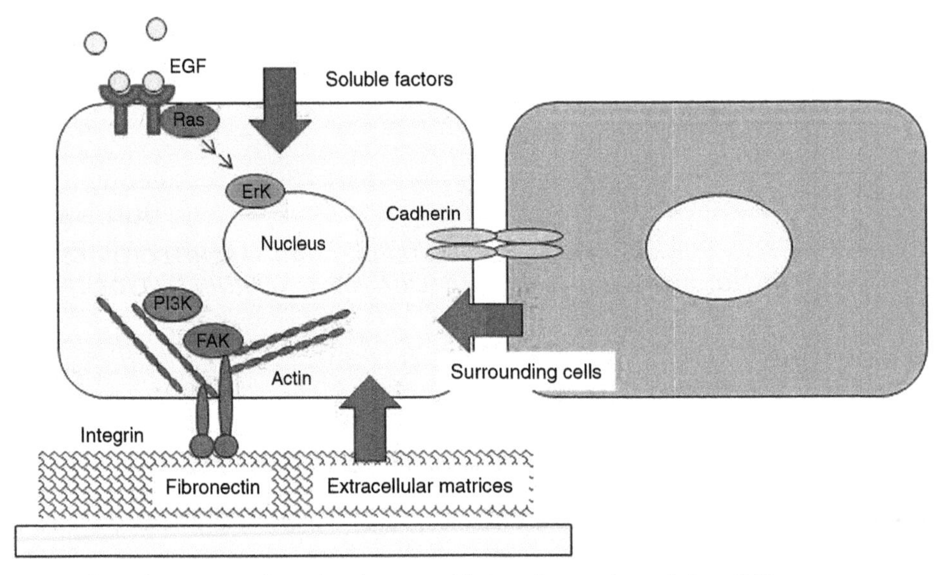

FIGURE 3.3.1 Schematic representations of environmental factors that regulate cellular activities.

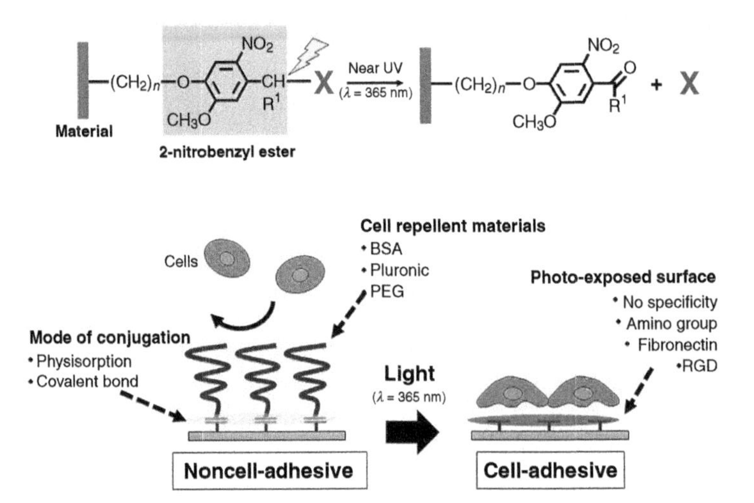

FIGURE 3.3.2 Schematic representations of the basic concept of photoactivatable substrates.

the external stimulus. These aspects open new paradigms in drug testing and cell/tissue engineering for pharmaceutical and medical applications.

Our group has developed for the first time photoactivatable dynamic substrates based on the photocleavage reaction of 2-nitrobenzyl ester (Fig. 3.3.2) [2] and have been made various technical and conceptual innovations. The common feature is that the surface is initially noncell adhesive, but changes to cell adhesive in response to near-UV irradiation. On these substrates, we are able not only to pattern cells in arbitrary geometries, but also to induce their migration by the secondary irradiation. One of the biggest advantages of the photochemical approach is its high spatiotemporal controllability. However, it is technically challenging to make the surface switchable between two completely opposite states – noncell adhesive versus cell adhesive – keeping the contrast region-selective for a wide timeframe in culture environments. This chapter will summarize how we designed and developed the photoactivatable substrates in terms of the conceptual and technical innovations to fulfill these requirements. Some of the biological applications, especially on cell migration studies, will be discussed to demonstrate the potentials of such material biological research tools for fundamental biological studies.

3.3.2 Development History of Photoactivatable Substrates

The basic principle of the photoactivatable substrates is depicted in Fig. 3.3.2. Protein- and cell-repellent materials, blocking agents in other words, are physically or chemically adsorbed on a surface functionalized with a molecule bearing photocleavable 2-nitrobenzyl ester to make the entire surface inert for cell adhesion at the beginning. Upon irradiation of the substrate, the blocking agents are dissociated from the surface, resulting in the conversion of the surface from a state preventing cell adhesion to a state promoting cell adhesion. We have developed various kinds of photoactivatable substrates by modifying the cell-repellent materials, the mode of conjugation of the materials, and the surface chemistry of the photoexposed surfaces.

3.3.2.1 First Generation: Photoactivatable Substrates Based on Physisorbed Blocking Agents

3.3.2.1.1 Development of Substrates

For the first photoactivatable dynamic substrates, we synthesized a silane-coupling agent bearing 2-nitrobenzyl ester, 1-(2-nitrophynyl)ethyl-5-trichlorosilylpentanoate (**1**), and functionalized the surface of a glass coverslip with this reagent. The photochemical reaction of this glass substrate was translated to the cell adhesiveness change via two commonly used proteins, bovine serum albumin (BSA) and fibronectin, both of which prevent or promote cell adhesion, in the following procedure (Fig. 3.3.3a). At first BSA is physically adsorbed to the substrate to make the entire surface inert for cell adhesion. Upon irradiation of the surface with near-UV light, the 2-nitrobenzyl group photocleaves to yield a carboxyl group dissociating BSA from the surface via the surface hydrophilization. Finally, fibronectin is adsorbed to the surface to fill in the vacancy of the dissociated BSA and make the surface cell adhesive. Later studies demonstrated that triblock copolymer Pluronic F108 substitutes for BSA with a better photoswitchability in terms of long-term persistence of cellular patterns. The medium is kept serum free until the final fibronectin addition step in order to prevent exchange adsorption of BSA with protein included in serum. This treatment reduces the nonspecific cell adhesion to nonirradiated regions.

The photocleavage reaction proceeds in the cell culturing environments in response to near-UV light at 365 nm. We can use a mercury arc lamp as a light source equipped on standard fluorescence microscopes. Although it depends on the magnification of the

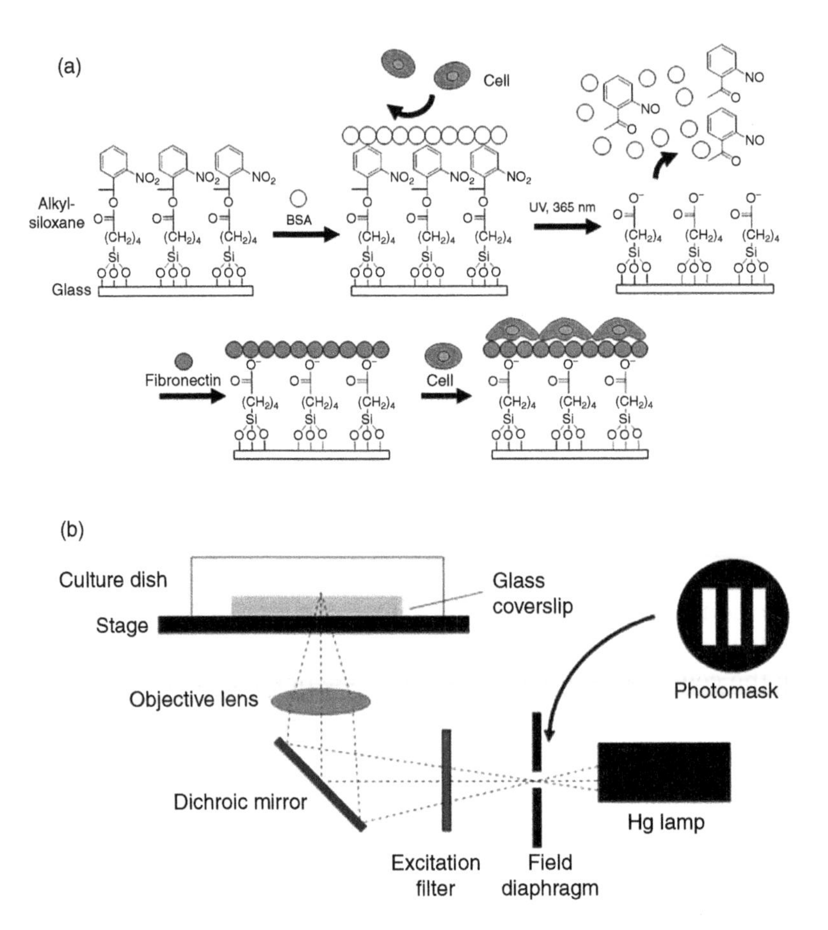

FIGURE 3.3.3 (a) The working principle of the first-generation photoactivatable substrates and (b) the projection exposure by using a fluorescence microscope.

objective lens, basically the reaction completes within several seconds. Moreover, in this configuration, we are able to place a photomask at the field diaphragm to control irradiation regions by the projection exposure (Fig. 3.3.3b). This way of patterned irradiation enables us to selectively dissociate BSA corresponding to the designs of the photomasks, deposit fibronectin thereon, and eventually form the same cellular pattern (Fig. 3.3.4a–e). Thanks to the high spatial resolution of the photocontrol, arbitral cell arraying as well as precise shape control of single cells becomes possible (Fig. 3.3.4f, g) [3]. Moreover, when we reduce the irradiation regions to the subcellular size, we are able to control the positions of focal adhesion, which can been seen as cellular morphologies with nodal structures (Fig. 3.3.4h) [4].

The most characteristic feature of the dynamic substrates is that they can be used to change the cellular pattern during cell cultivation. Two representative proof-of-concept experiments are shown in Fig. 3.3.5. By repeating the irradiation and cell seeding, we can

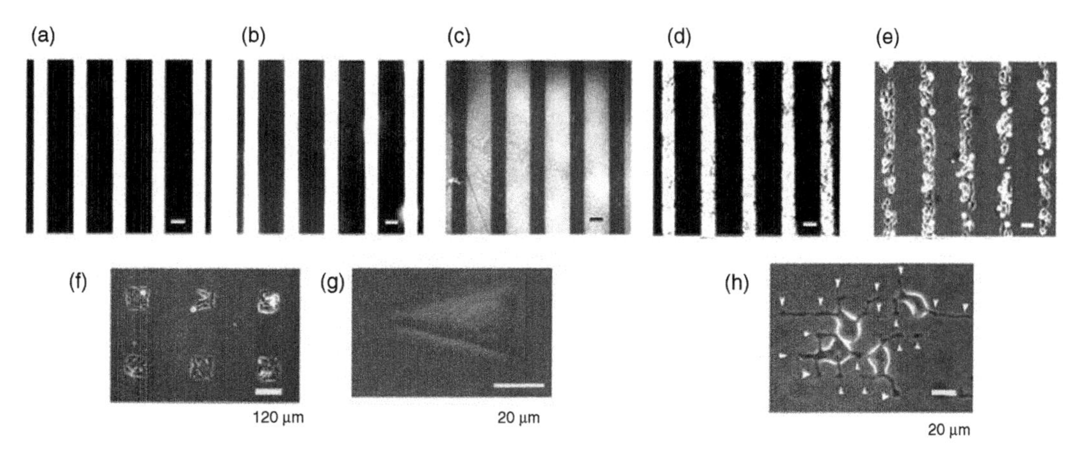

FIGURE 3.3.4 (a–e) Processes and (f–h) performances of cell patterning on the first-generation photoactivatable substrates.

sequentially array heterotypic cells even at the single cell levels (Fig. 3.3.5a) [2,5]. On the other hand, when we irradiate the region alongside the initially patterned cells, we are able to induce their migration to the newly irradiated regions (Fig. 3.3.5b) [4]. This cell migration induction technology was further applied to study the geometrical dependence of the migration of single fibroblast cells (Fig. 3.3.6a) [6]. After arraying single NIH3T3 cells in a square spot of 25 × 25 μm^2, we induced their migration by irradiating either a wide (25 μm) or a narrow (5 μm) path alongside the arrayed cells. The cells extended wide lamellipodium-like protrusions over wide paths, but they extended filopodium-like or neurite-like protrusions along the narrow paths. It should be noted that such cell migration induction can be performed in the array format via patterned irradiation by using a corresponding photomask. By taking advantage of this feature, we collected ample time profiles of single cells migrating along the wide and narrow paths and compared the migration rates between them (Fig. 3.3.6b). Interestingly, the cells migrated faster along the wide paths than along narrow paths, presumably because of the mechanical obstruction of cytoskeletal elongation and/or subcellular organelles. Whatever the reason might be, the results clearly represent that cell migration in a restricted micrometer space is different from normal soft matters.

The success in the induction of the neurite-like protrusions in fibroblast cells inspired us to apply this technique to the induction and navigation of neurites in real neuronal cells (Fig. 3.3.7). The technique allowed us not only to induce the neurite extension in desired directions (Fig. 3.3.7a, b), but also to either branch or bend the neurites by repeated irradiation (Fig. 3.3.7c, d). By taking advantage of this feature, we tried to generate autapse-like structures (Fig. 3.3.7e). In the autapse circuit of neurons, the axon projects back to its own dendrite or cell soma to form synaptic connections between themselves. Autapses have attracted the interest of neuroscientists; why they form and how they function. However,

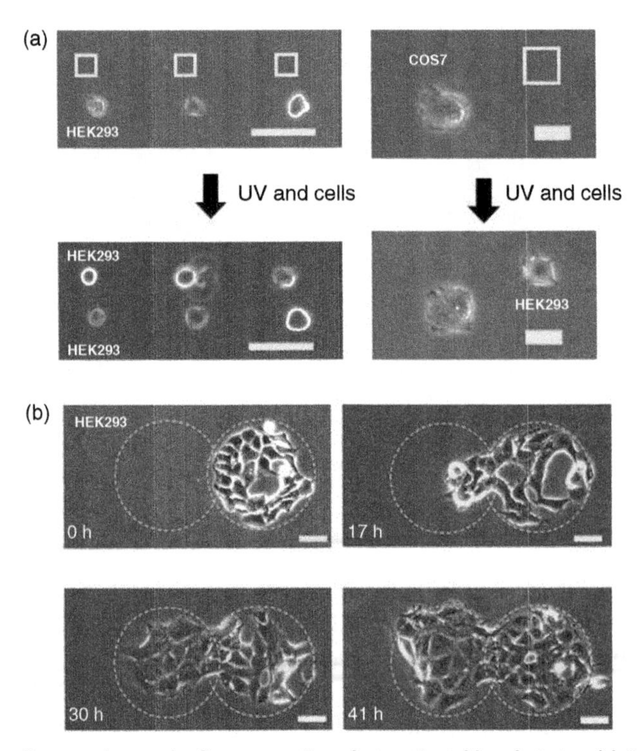

FIGURE 3.3.5 Dynamic cell patterning on the first-generation photoactivatable substrates. (a) Coculturing and (b) migration induction.

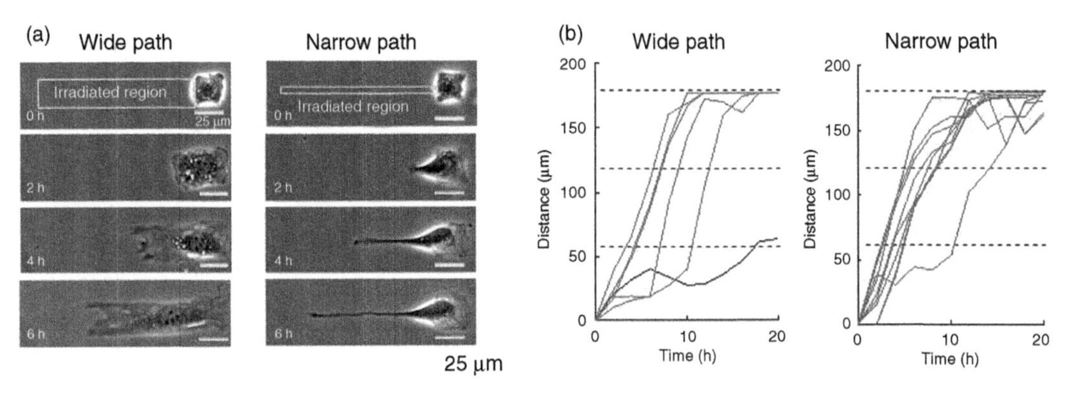

FIGURE 3.3.6 Applications of a first-generation photoactivatable substrate to single cell migration studies.

there were no rational approaches to generate such unique structures, so the researchers had to study autapse formed by chance in sparsely seeded neuronal cells. On the other hand, the current strategy to use photoactivatable dynamic surfaces enables researchers to rationally form autaptic structures at any desired locations in appropriate timings by controlled irradiation. The spatiotemporal controllable feature of this method will help in the understanding of the roles of autapses in neural transmission.

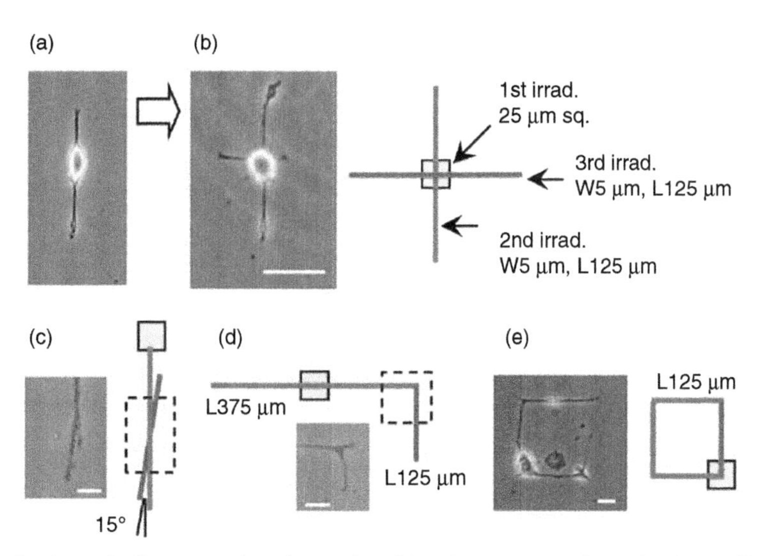

FIGURE 3.3.7 Applications of a first-generation photoactivatable substrate to neurite navigation studies.

3.3.2.1.2 Mechanism Study

In order to elucidate the working principle of photoswitching of cell adhesion on the first-generation photoactivatable substrates, we looked at the protein/polymer adsorption and dissociation processes before and after photoirradiation through surface physicochemical analyses. For this purpose, new silane-coupling agents, which produce an NH_2, OH, or SH group, have been synthesized (**2–4**, Fig. 3.3.8a, b) [5]. Hereafter, we will call these surfaces caged NH_2, OH, and SH surfaces and the states after photoirradiation uncaged surfaces. The three new surfaces, together with the original caged COOH surface, possess similar responses against photoirradiation, which can be seen from the contact angle measurements (Fig. 3.3.8c). Therefore, we coated the caged surfaces with BSA in the same way as we did in the first report [2] and evaluated their changes in cell adhesiveness in response to near-UV irradiation under serum-free conditions. Among the four surfaces, only the caged NH_2 surface became cell adhesive for COS7, NIH3T3, and HEK293 cells by photoirradiation (Fig. 3.3.8d). The caged COOH surface became slightly cell adhesive, but it did not become sufficiently adhesive unless fibronectin was added to promote cell adhesion, as we did in the first report [2]. On the other hand, no cell adhesion was observed for caged OH and SH surfaces. It is noteworthy that the cells strongly adhere to all of the four pristine uncaged surfaces without protein coating (Fig. 3.3.9a). Therefore, it seems that only a small portion, if any, of BSA is dissociated from the surface in response to photoirradiation, although the immunofluorescence data shows obvious photoinduced BSA desorption (Fig. 3.3.4a). Then, we evaluated the amount of adsorbed BSA at each step more quantitatively by its *in situ* staining with SYPRO Ruby dyes (Invitrogen). The results indicate only 10–30% of BSA dissociated by photoirradiation from caged COOH and NH_2 surfaces, whereas there was no change in the adsorbed BSA amounts on caged OH and SH surfaces (Fig. 3.3.9d,

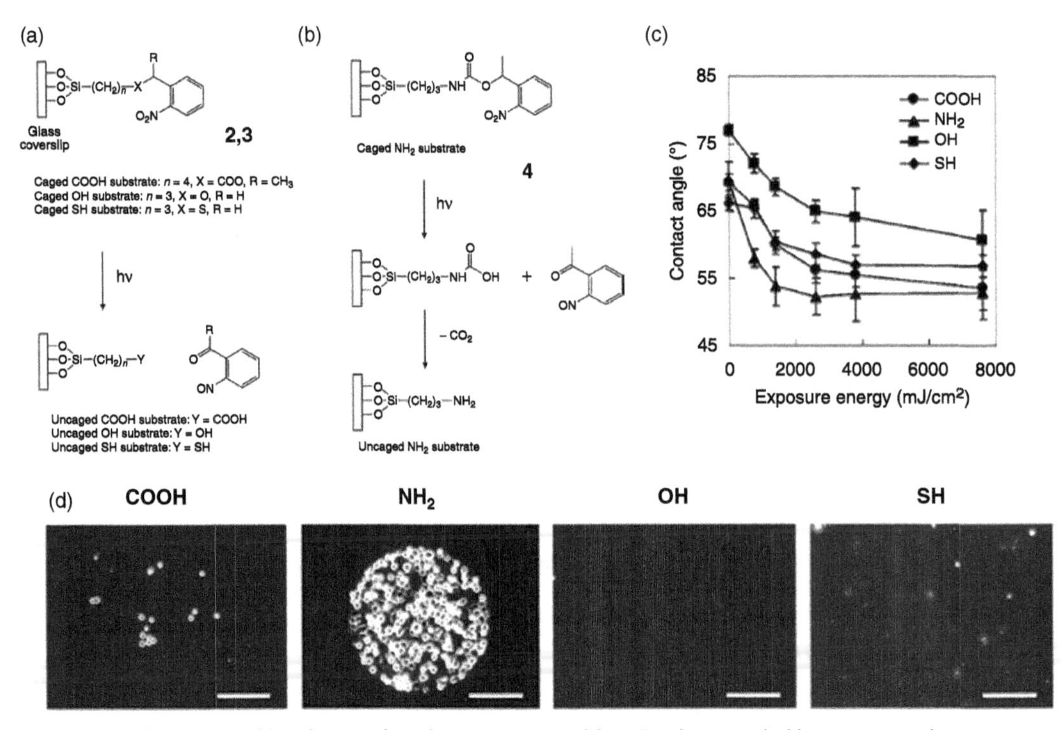

FIGURE 3.3.8 Photoactivatable substrates based on various caged functional groups. (a, b) Structures and photocleavage reactions. (c) Wettability profile. (d) Cell adhesion test, COS7.

F_{I} vs. F_{II}). By considering the fact that the surface wettability changes were similar for all four caged surfaces (Fig. 3.3.8c), photoinduced BSA desorption probably requires the generation of charged species in addition to the surface wettability change. This is the major reason why the cells did not adhere onto caged OH and SH surfaces (Fig. 3.3.8d). Another important fact for these surfaces is that the uncaged NH_2 surface allows cell adhesion even after BSA is adsorbed to the surface (Fig. 3.3.9b). Altogether we are able to lead the following mechanism of photoswitching of cell adhesion on our first-generation photoactivatable substrates: (1) only a small portion of the surface-adsorbed BSA is dissociated from caged COOH and caged NH_2; (2) since BSA adsorbed on the uncaged COOH retains the ability to prevent cell adhesion (Fig. 3.3.8d, COOH), it requires subsequent addition of fibronectin to covert the surface into a cell-adhesive state (Fig. 3.3.4a); (3) on the other hand, the remaining BSA of the caged NH_2 surface after photoirradiation does not possess sufficient cell-repelling ability, and hence the uncaged NH_2 surface becomes cell adhesive without the addition of fibronectin (Fig. 3.3.8d, NH_2); (4) in the case of caged OH and SH surfaces, the surface-adsorbed BSA stays on the surface by photoirradiation and does not lose its original cell-repelling ability. So these surfaces are not photoswitchable (Fig. 3.3.8d, OH and SH).

We also examined the impact of the surface wettability change before and after photoirradiation on the adsorption of Pluronic to the surfaces. For this study, we synthesized another silane-coupling agent, 1-(2-nitropheny) ethyl 11-trichlorosilylundecanoate (**5**),

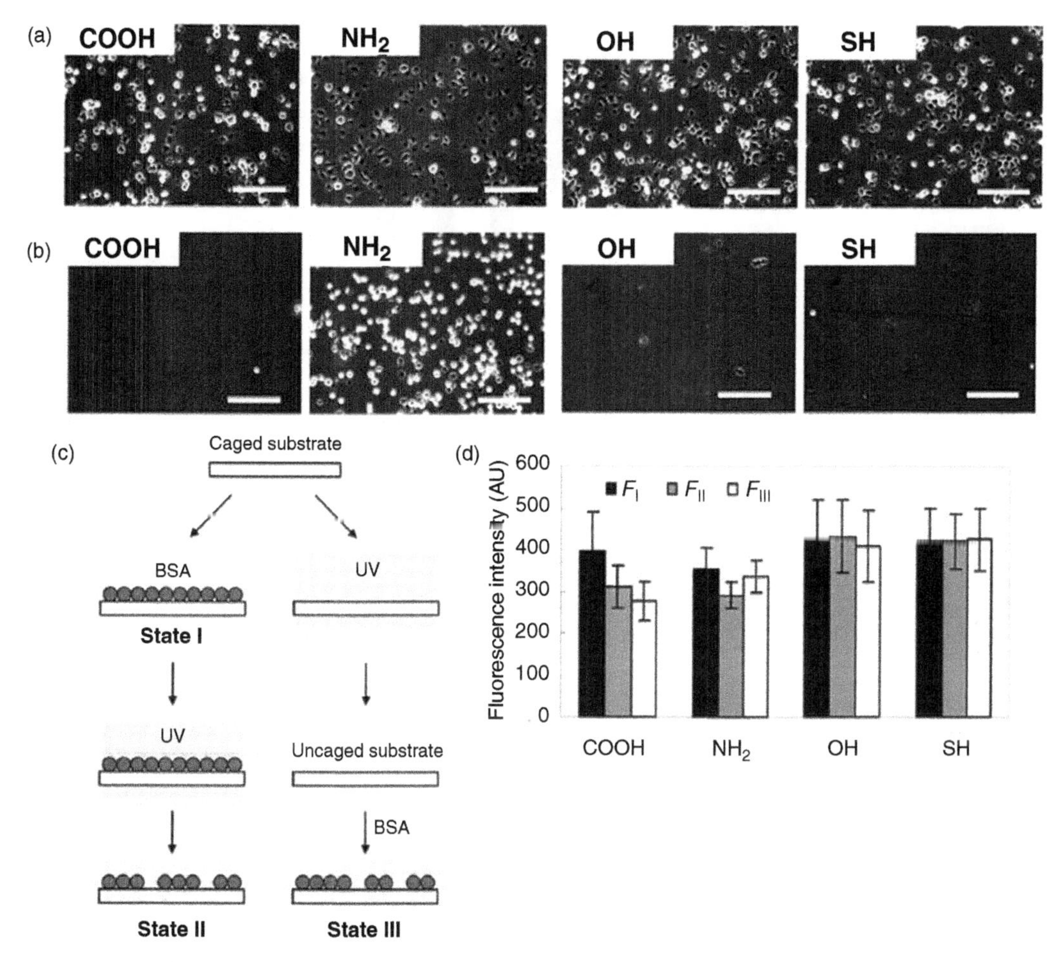

FIGURE 3.3.9 Mechanism studies of the first-generation photoactivatable substrate: impact of the type of functional groups. Cell adhesion tests to (a) bare and (b) bovine serum albumin (BSA)-coated surfaces. (c, d) BSA adsorption quantification in various states.

bearing a longer alkyl chain in between the silane group and the 2-nitrobenzyl group, both yielding a COOH group by photoirradiation (Fig. 3.3.10a). The alkyl chain length changes the dynamic ranges of surface wettability change in response to photoirradiation; the surface bearing the longer alkyl chain ($n = 10$) is more hydrophobic than that of the original shorter one ($n = 4$) and the wettability change is smaller for the former (Fig. 3.3.10b). Hereafter, we call these surfaces $n10$ and $n4$ surfaces. When we examined the adsorption of Pluronic to these surfaces in the caged and uncaged states by using its fluorescently labeled conjugate, the adsorption amount showed good correlation with the surface wettability (Fig. 3.3.9c, d). The following addition of fibronectin to these surfaces resulted in its good adsorption to the uncaged surfaces, but very weak adsorption to the caged surfaces (Fig. 3.3.9e). When the protein adsorption amount was compared between the uncaged

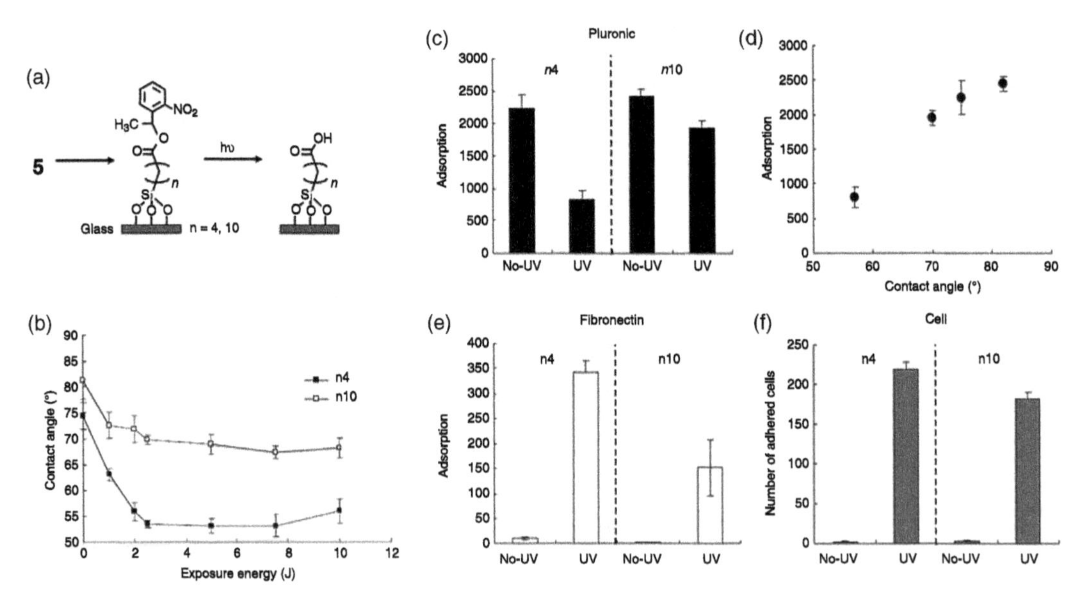

FIGURE 3.3.10 Mechanism study of the first-generation photoactivatable substrate: impact of surface wettability. (a) Chemistry. (b) Wettability change. (c, d) Pluronic and (e) fibronectin adsorption. (f) Cell adhesion.

*n*4 and *n*10 surfaces, more fibronectin adsorbed to the *n*4 surface than to the *n*10 surface. On the contrary, the caged *n*10 surface had higher fibronectin repelling ability than the *n*4 surface, which is probably suitable to resist cell and protein fouling to the nonirradiated regions. These results agree well with the relationship between the adsorption amount of Pluronic and surface wettability. Moreover, the cell seeded on these surfaces showed good selective adhesion to the irradiated regions with slightly more adhesion on the uncaged *n*4 surface. It should be noted that although the uncaged *n*4 surface only showed a slightly less adsorption of BSA than on the caged *n*4 surface (~70%, Fig. 3.3.9d, COOH F_{I} vs. F_{III}), the adsorption of Pluronic on the uncaged surface was much less (~30%) than on the caged surface. Therefore, adsorption/desorption equilibrium of Pluronic is simpler than BSA; it is highly dependent on the surface wettability. The results are reasonable by considering the fact that proteins have various heterogeneous side chains – hydrophilic, hydrophobic, and charged – and they have various quasi-stable three-dimensional structures, whereas synthetic polymers, especially for block copolymers like Pluronic, possess discrete domains with homogeneous chemistry.

3.3.2.2 Second Generation: Photoactivatable Substrates Based on Covalently Conjugating a Cell-Repellent Polymer

The first-generation photoactivatable substrates demonstrated a wide range of applications based on their dynamic features with high spatiotemporal resolutions. However, there was a big technical limitation regarding the cell-repelling ability of the nonirradiated surfaces. The cell-repelling ability of the nonirradiated regions does not last for more than

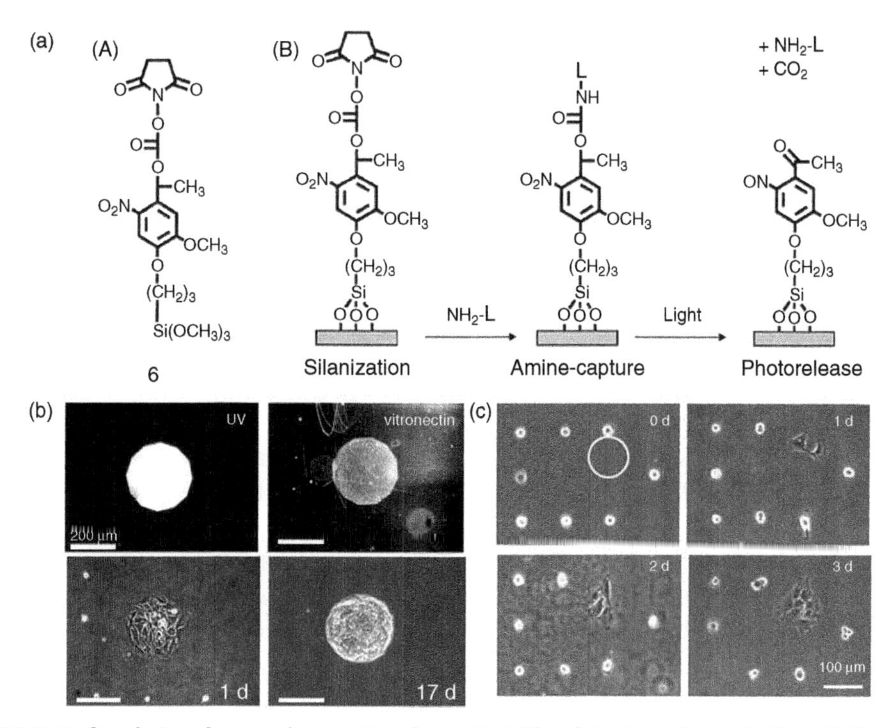

FIGURE 3.3.11 Surface design of a second-generation photoactivatable substrate and its applications. (a) Chemistry. (b) Static patterning. (c) Dynamic patterning.

2–3 days and hence the patterned cells can fall into these regions via migration and proliferation. Such insufficient ability of the geometrical cell confinement is not suitable for application of the surfaces to biological processes that need long-term cell culturing, such as cell proliferation and differentiation studies. Therefore, there was a strong demand for technical innovation.

The time-dependent loss of the cell-repelling ability of the first-generation photoactivatable substrates was mainly due to the susceptibility of the physically adsorbed blocking agents to undergo exchange adsorption with proteins involved in culture media. Therefore, one straightforward solution to overcome this drawback is to covalently immobilize the blocking agent to the photocleavable 2-nitrobenzyl group functionalized on the substrate. A new silane-coupling agent, 1-[3-methoxy-6-nitro-4-(3-trimethoxysilylpropyloxy)phenyl]ethyl *N*-succinimidyl carbonate (**6**, Fig. 3.3.11a), has been designed and synthesized based on this idea [7]. It has a photocleavable 2-nitrobenzyl ester bearing a trimethoxysilyl group at one end and a succinimidyl carbonate at the other end. Each group reacts with hydroxyl groups of inorganic oxides and primary amines, respectively. Therefore, the molecule can be functionalized on the glass surface, exposing succinimidyl carbonate via the photocleavable linker. Amines can be grafted to the surface via the reaction with the activated ester, but their linkage can be subsequently cleaved by the following photocleavage reaction of the 2-nitrobenzyl ester. With this surface design, we are able to introduce certain chemical and physical characteristics depending on the type of ligand molecules to be immobilized, but restore the surface by the following photoirradiation. The point is that the second restoring step is based on the photocleavage reaction, and therefore the region-specific restoration can be achieved by simply controlling the phoroirradiating regions. We took advantage of this feature to make a glass surface photoswitchable for cell adhesion by using an amino derivative of cell-repellent poly(ethylene glycol) (PEG) as an immobilized ligand. This method of covalent conjugation of the blocking agent elongated the timeframe of the cells confined within the initial patterns by up to more than 17 days (Fig. 3.3.11b). The dynamically switchable feature of the substrate was demonstrated by photoinduced cell migration induction. Especially, the long-term persistence of initial cellular patterns opened up a new paradigm in the applications of the dynamic substrates. In Fig. 3.3.11c, the single cell array was formed at first, followed by the selective induction of migration of a chosen single cell by controlled irradiation. Thanks to the long-lasting cell-repelling feature of the nonirradiated surfaces, the other single cells stayed within the initial spot, and only small populations proliferate therein to form small aggregates. On the other hand, the cell chosen to migrate proliferated more efficiently and formed a new colony within the newly irradiated region. All the cells proliferated in this region originated from the specific single cell. This means that we are able to induce selective proliferation of specific single cells. This technique can be used for a new cell cloning method, and its efficiency in terms of the number of parent populations is much higher than commonly used conventional cloning methods such as the limiting dilution method and that based on penicillin cups.

Another important feature for the second-generation photoactivatable substrates is that the degree of the restoration can be tuned by controlling the dose of photoirradiation [8]. In other words, we are able to produce a surface where the surface physical and/or chemical characteristics are partially restored toward the original surface at a certain intermediate level from the state before irradiation. Figure 3.3.12 clearly demonstrates the feature of the surface, where amino-biotin was used as a model ligand. The immobilized biotinyl ligand exhibited irradiation time-dependent dissociation from the substrate surface (Fig. 3.3.12a, b). Since the rate constant of the photochemical reaction is almost constant regardless of the ligand types [8], we are able to quantitatively tune the surface ligand density once we know the surface ligand density before photoirradiation with the help of other surface analysis methods such as ellipsometry. Moreover, we are able to construct surface chemical density gradients by controlling irradiating regions as well as doses. Figure 3.3.12c and d show stepwise decrease of the surface biotin ligand densities. By diluting initial load biotin ligand with an inert ethylene glycol ligand, we have succeeded in the initial biotin ligand density before irradiation, and hence lowering the dynamic range of the surface chemical gradient (Fig. 3.3.12e and the lower profile in Fig. 3.3.12f). Thus, formed fine-tunable surface ligand gradients will be useful to study how cell migration directionally depends on the juxtacrine stimulation, which means the stimulation of chemical ligands presented as an immobilized state in ECM and the surface of surrounding cells.

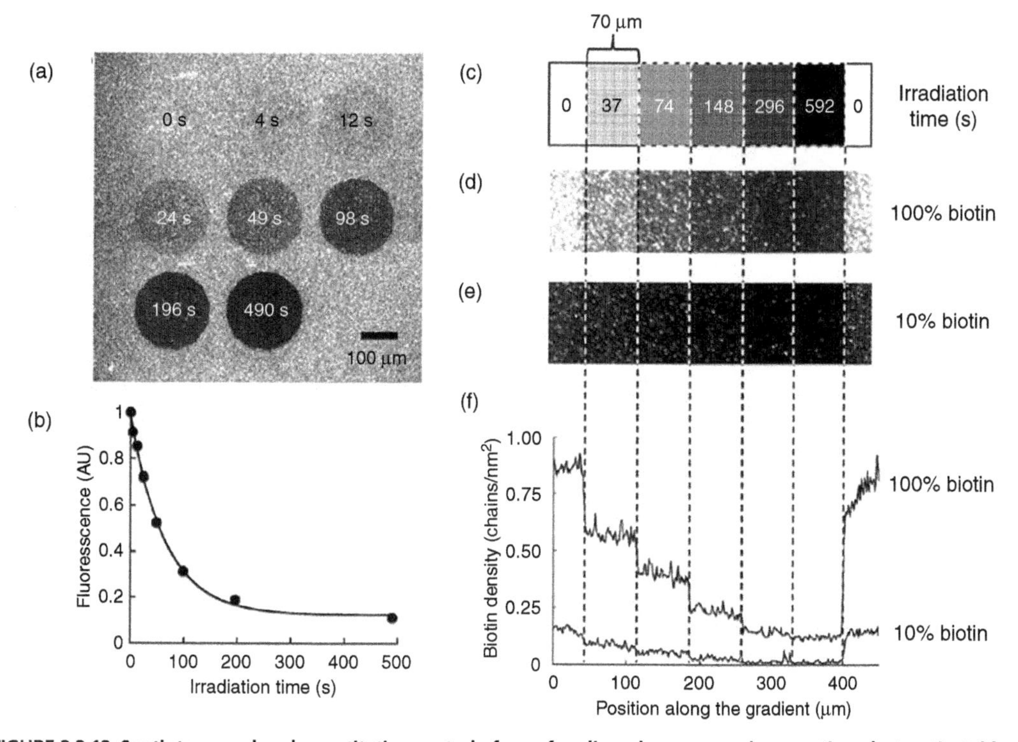

FIGURE 3.3.12 Spatiotemporal and quantitative control of a surface ligand on a second-generation photoactivatable substrate. (a, b) Dose-dependent dissociation. (c–f) Chemical gradient formation.

3.3.2.3 Third Generation: Photoactivatable Substrates Based on Photocleavable Poly(ethylene Glycol)

3.3.2.3.1 Development of Substrates

The second-generation photoactivatable substrates elongated the applicable time window up to more than 2 weeks. However, the surface generated after the photoirradiation is not well designed for cell adhesion; the product nitrosobenzophenone does not have any specific chemical affinity for proteins and cells. In fact, the cell adhesiveness of the surface is not high enough and it takes several hours for the cells to adhere and spread over the surface after irradiation. Moreover, the methods described above are designed to control cell adhesion on artificial inorganic or organic substrates because we used silane-coupling agents bearing a photocleavable 2-nitrobenzyl group to make the surfaces photoswitchable. It is known that some cell types show physiologically relevant biological activities only on the surfaces coated with natural ECM, such collagen and laminin. To address these issues, we have developed a new method for making amino-bearing surfaces photoswitchable for cell adhesion. The reason why we chose an amino group as a target is that most cells adhere well on the functional group (see Fig. 3.3.8d, for example). Moreover,

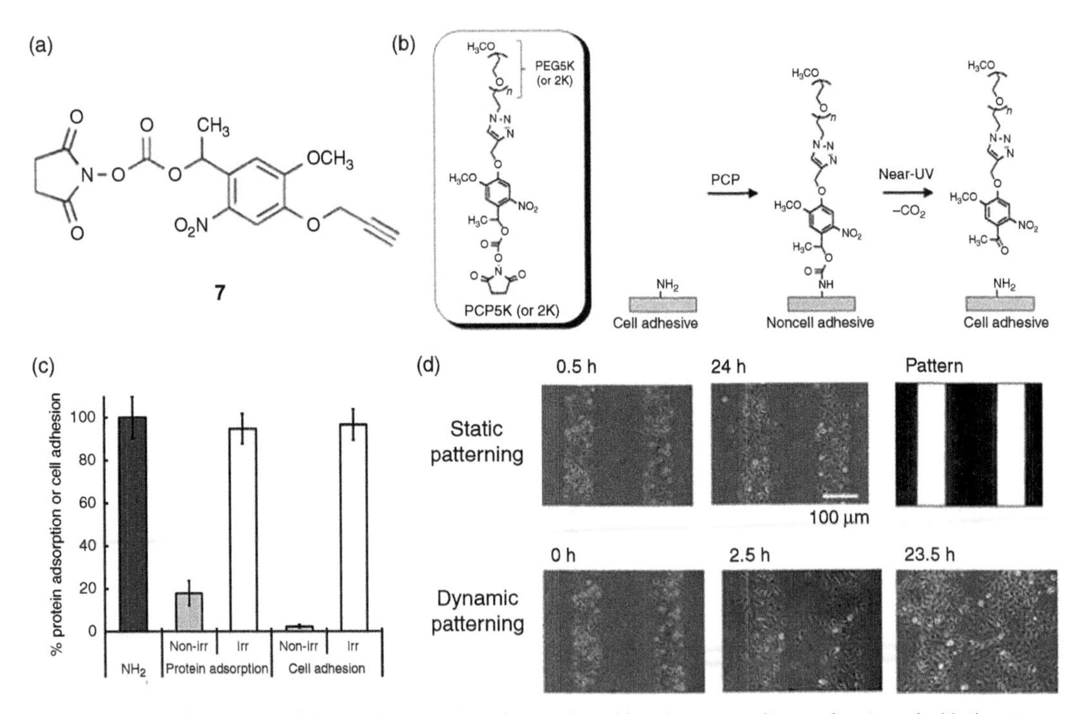

FIGURE 3.3.13 Surface design of the third generation photoactivatable substrate and its applications. (a, b) Chemistry. (c) Bovine serum albumin (BSA) adsorption and cell adhesion. (d) Static and dynamic cell patterning.

the amino group exists abundantly in biological substances, hence the photoswitching method has a potential to be applied to protein-based scaffolds.

To this end, we synthesized a new photocleavable linker, 1-(5-methoxy-2-nitro-4-prop-2-ynyloxyphenyl)ethyl *N*-succinimidyl carbonate (**7**, Fig. 3.3.13a) [9]. This molecule bears two orthogonal chemical functional groups at each end linked by 2-nitrobenzyl ester: succinimidyl carbonate and an alkynyl group. The alkynyl group can undergo Cu(I)-catalyzed Huisgen 1,3-dipolar cycloaddition (click chemistry) [10], whereas the succinimidyl carbonate reacts with primary amines. An azide derivative of PEG was first reacted with this photocleavable linker in the presence of Cu(I) ion to yield PEG bearing a photocleavable succinimidyl group (**8**, Fig. 3.3.13b). Thus, synthesized photocleavable PEG (PCP) reacts with amino-bearing surfaces to make the surface inert for cell adhesion. Upon photoirradiation of the substrate with near-UV light, the 2-nitrobenzyl undergoes the photocleavage reaction being PEG dissociated from the substrate surface, resulting in the retrieval of the original cell-adhesive feature of the amino-bearing surfaces (Fig. 3.3.13b). Figure 3.3.13c demonstrates the results on the change in cell adhesiveness on an aminosilanized surface. The surface modification with PCP almost completely passivated the aminosilanized surface for cell adhesion, whereas its protein- and cell-adhesive features were restored to indistinguishable levels of its original state

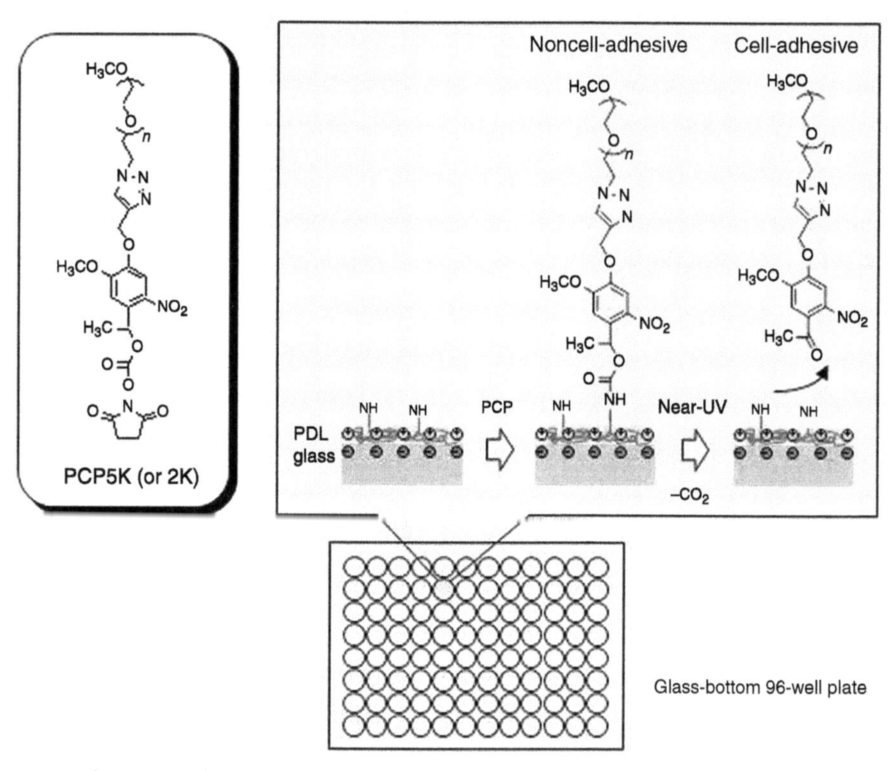

FIGURE 3.3.14 A photoactivatable multiwell plate based on the third generation photoactivatable substrate.

after photoirradiation. Figure 3.3.13d shows static and dynamic cell patterning on this surface. Altogether we have succeeded in making the amino-bearing surface photo-switchable for cell adhesion.

By following the same strategy, we have also succeeded in making a photoactivatable surface on a commercial glass bottom 96-well plate through mild treatment of the material surface with aqueous and ethanol solutions of poly-D-lysine (PDL) and PCP, respectively (Fig. 3.3.14) [11]. This method opens up the possibility for the development of a versatile and multiplex cell migration assay platform since pharmaceutical treatment of cell migration is considered as a promising strategy to block cancer invasion and metastasis at the early stage of tumor expansion [12]. It should be emphasized that cell migration is highly dependent on their migrating microenvironments. Nevertheless, this aspect is undervalued in conventional cell migration assays, such as wound healing assays and exclusion zone assays. In contrast, the dynamic substrate-based cell migration assay enables robust control over cell migrating environments. Therefore, it will become a promising candidate for a high-throughput cell migration assay for drug candidates as well as for functional genomics, like siRNA screening [13], to identify essential proteins involved in cell migration behaviors.

Another important point in this methodology is that the residual carbamate group after the photocleavage reaction spontaneously undergoes decarboxylation and yields the original amino-bearing surface. Looked at from another standpoint, we could say the modification of the amino-bearing surfaces by PCP is, in principle, reversible. This feature is useful for future applications to prepare photoswitchable not only for aminosilanized glass surface and PDL-coated surfaces, but also for protein-based scaffolds, as their biological activities are expected to be fully restored to the original ones after the cycle of PEGylation and photoirradiation.

3.3.2.3.2 Mechanism Study

However, there still exists a critical problem with this substrate shown in Figure 3.3.13. The cellular pattern can be maintained for only 1 day and the cells migrate and proliferate out to the nonirradiated regions even though PEG is conjugated through a covalent bond. This undesired outcome is somewhat expectable when we focused on the insufficient protein-repelling ability of the PEGylated surface (Fig. 3.3.13c). To overcome this issue, we further analyzed the surface physicochemical properties by the contact angle measurements, ellipsometry, and the zeta potential measurements, complemented with protein adsorption observation [14]. In addition, we prepared the surface with varied amino densities by preparing mixed siloxane layers and considered the impact of a mixed PEG approach [15] on biocompatibility (Fig. 3.3.15a). The ellipsometric measurements indicated that the PEG densities of the first PEGylation reaction with PCP5K were almost identical for all the surfaces, whereas the density of backfilling PEG was highly dependent on the surface amino group density (Fig. 3.3.15b). The surface zeta potentials became closer to neutral by the sequential PEGylation (Fig. 3.3.15c) and the amount of protein adsorption showed good correlation with these zeta potentials (Fig. 3.3.15d). Furthermore, variation in the surface composition, such as densities of the amino group and PEG chains, had almost no effect on the surface photoswitching efficiency for cell adhesion, whereas it became more significant after culturing cells for a longer time (Fig. 3.3.15e). Altogether, this study elucidated that the surface zeta potential is an essential factor for the long-term persistence of cellular patterns. Such detailed physicochemical analyses of the interfacial nanoarchitectures, composed of PEG brushes and charged base materials, provide useful insight into how these parameters affect the biocompatibility of the photoactivatable substrates.

3.3.2.4 Fourth Generation: Photoactivatable Substrates with Molecularly Defined Cell–Substrate Interactions

On the photoactivatable substrates discussed so far, the cells adhere to the photoirradiated regions via the interaction with proteins physically adsorbed onto the surface after photoirradiation. These proteins originally existed in the culture medium, but we are not able to specify which proteins mediate cell adhesion. This fact obscures the molecular level discussion of the signaling originated from the cell–substrate interactions. To tackle this issue, we have developed two new photoactivatable substrates, where the photoexposed surface presents molecularly controlled cell-adhesive ligand.

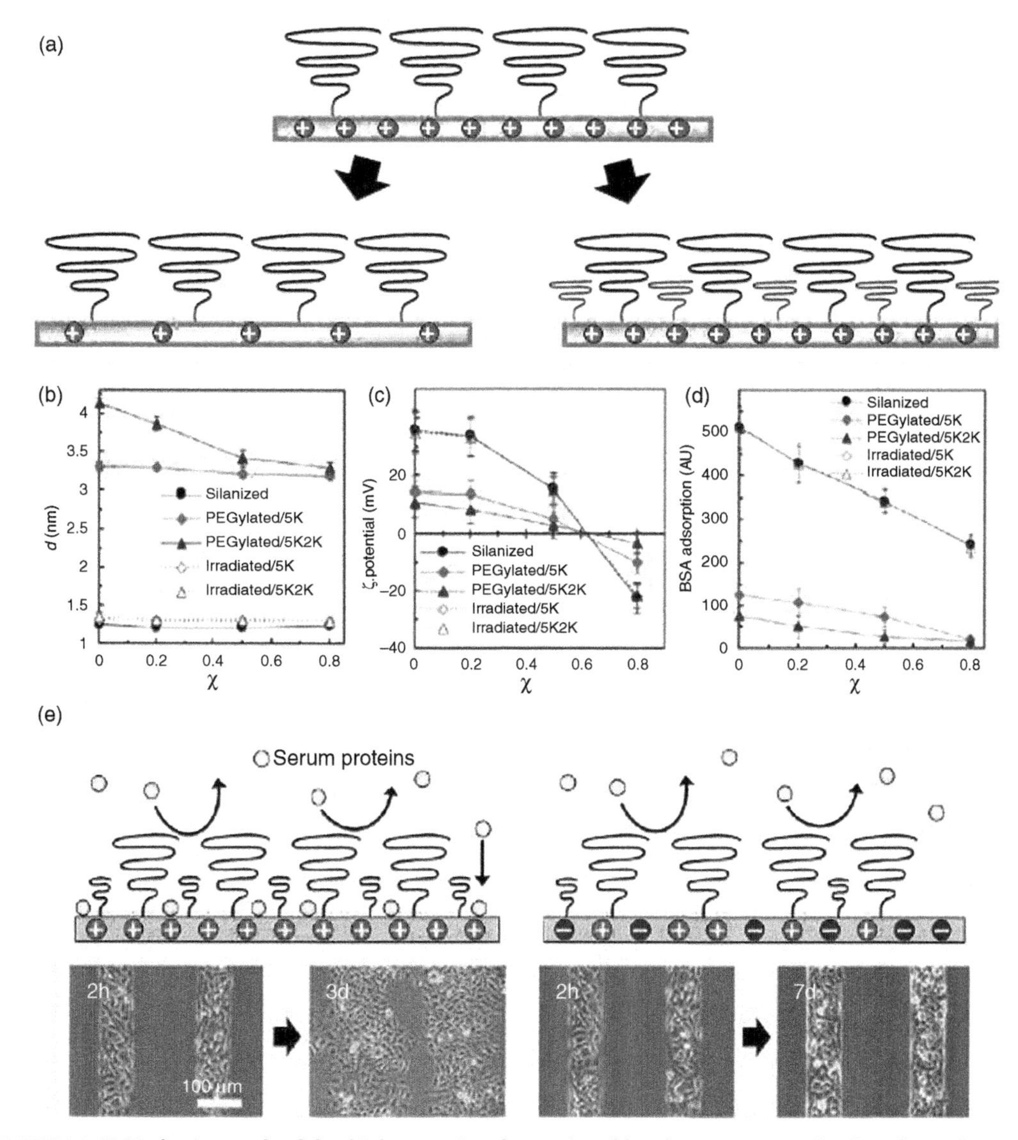

FIGURE 3.3.15 Mechanism study of the third generation photoactivatable substrate: impact of surface charge density and PEG backfilling. (a) Experimental design. (b) Ellipsometry. (c) Zeta potential. (d) BSA adsorption. (e) Long-term persistence of cellular patterns.

On the first surface, we coimmobilized a nitrilotriacetic acid (NTA) group with the photocleavable PEG to a gold substrate (Fig. 3.3.16a). The NTA group is a commonly used group for protein purification and its Ni^{2+}-ion complex interacts with a genetically introduced oligohistidine tag (His-tag). Before irradiation the NTA group is hidden under the bulky PEG chains, and hence His-tagged proteins cannot interact with the NTA. Upon irradiation of near-UV light to cleave the PEG umbrella, the NTA group becomes accessible

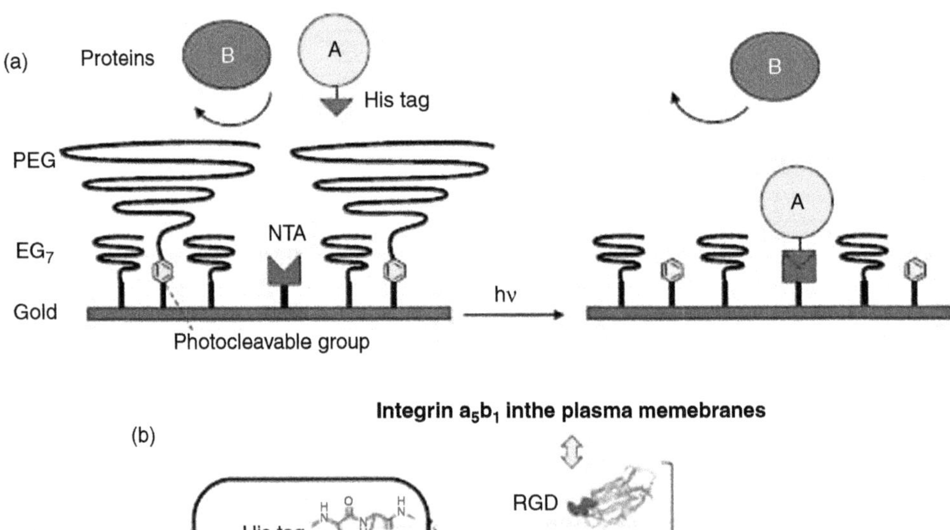

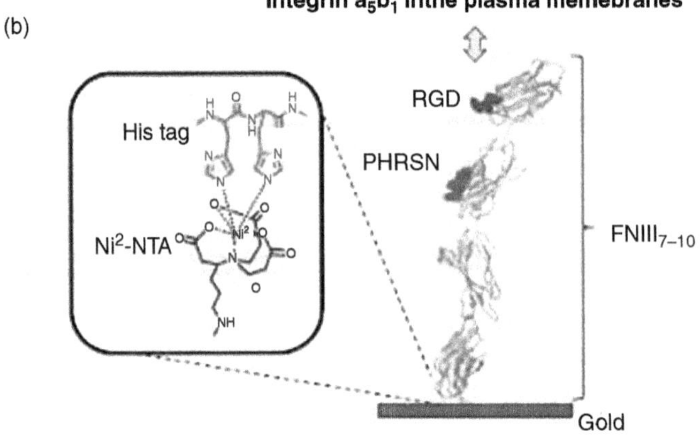

FIGURE 3.3.16 Surface design of the fourth generation photoactivatable substrate. (a) Surface and (b) molecular designs.

to the His-tagged proteins. The surface permits selective capturing of the His-tagged proteins, since additional oligoethyleneglycol ligands prevent nonspecific protein adsorption to the surface after photoirradiation. We prepared a His-tagged fusion protein of a fibronectin fragment ($FNIII_{7-10}$), which encompasses the integrin $\alpha_5\beta_1$ binding domain including Arg-Gly-Asp (RGD) and Pro-His-Ser-Arg-Asn sequences. This substrate enabled us to photoinduce cell patterning and their specific cell–substrate adhesion mediated by the interaction between $FNIII_{7-10}$ (Fig. 3.3.16b) and type $\alpha_5\beta_1$ integrin was confirmed by the immunofluorescence study.

Another surface is prepared on a gold nanoparticles array prepared by block copolymer nanolithography [16], where 10-nm gold nanoparticles were arrayed with 57-nm spacing on the glass surface in a hexagonal arrangement. The gold nanoparticles were functionalized with cyclic RGD peptide together with photocleavable PEG12K, whereas remaining glass regions were passivated by PEG2K silane to develop a photoactivatable nanopatterned substrate (Fig. 3.3.17a) [17]. The size of gold nanoparticles is

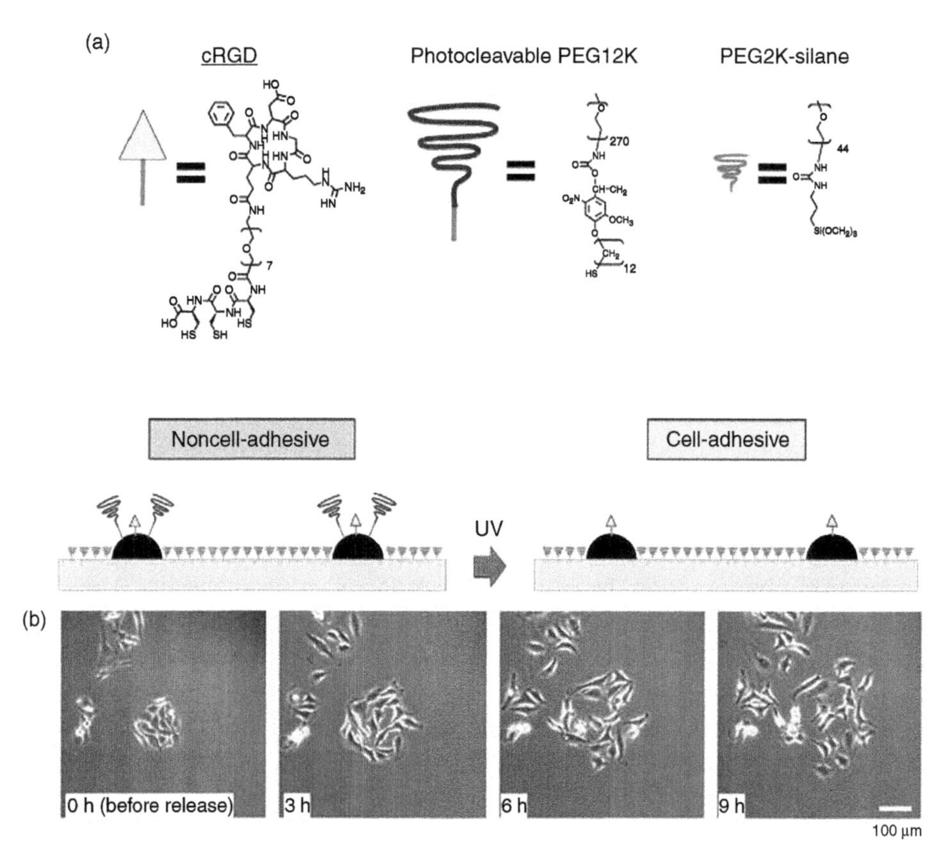

FIGURE 3.3.17 (a) Photoactivatable nanopatterned substrate based on the fourth generation photoactivatable substrate and (b) its applications.

small enough that it is unlikely that ECM proteins, like fibronectin, physisorb thereon. In addition, their size is compatible to a single integrin heterodimer. Therefore, we can expect that cell adhesion is mainly mediated by interaction of the cRGD ligand with $\alpha_v\beta_3$ integrin, with only a single heterodimer accommodated on each gold nanoparticle. Since interparticle separation can be tuned by changing the surface preparation conditions in block copolymer nanolithography, we are able to control cell–substrate interactions in "nanodigital" resolution [18]. By taking advantage of these features, we found the HeLa cells lost collective motion by decreasing cell–ECM interactions (Fig. 3.3.17b), which is opposite to that expected based on conventional soft matter theory [19]. Moreover, we found the reduced phosphorylation at a specific tyrosine residue of focal adhesion kinase on the nanopattern.

These results clearly demonstrated that these surfaces provide more physiologically relevant scaffolds for dissecting the nano- and microscopic regulation of cell migration machinery together with the molecular level discussion.

3.3.3 Conclusions and Future Trends

In this chapter, we described a series of dynamic substrates based on the photocleavable 2-nitrobenzyl group and their design rationales. Since the single substrate has to convert between completely opposite states, that promoting and preventing cell adhesion, in response to light, achieving both a high-switching efficiency between the two states and keeping their difference for a long period of time is technically challenging. These difficult requirements stimulate us to develop the various photoactivatable substrates introduced here. Still, there are pros and cons for each generation at present. Depending on the first priority of the experiments, we use different substrates. For example, we use the second generation when long-term cell confinement is the topmost demand, but we use the third generation if the cellular responses at a very early stage are the major interest in the study. The fourth generation is used in case we need a molecular level discussion. The first generation is beneficial in terms of mass production. Further conceptual and technical innovation is demanded to achieve all the things in a single photoactivatable substrate. We have already succeeded in revealing various biological and mechanical insights, especially in cell migration phenomenon, by using the photoactivatable substrates. However, only a few of them were introduced here because of the limitation of space. Readers who are interested in further details in this aspect should read the original papers. We believe cell manipulation technology based on the photoactivatable substrates provides biological insight, which cannot be addressed by conventional molecular biological technologies, and both of them serve as complementary research tools to elucidate biology and life.

Acknowledgments

This work was supported in part by the World Premier International Research Centre Initiative (WPI) on Materials Nanoarchitectonics, JST PRESTO, and JSPS Kakenhi. All the work was done in collaboration with Prof. K. Yamaguchi (Kanagawa University).

References

[1] J. Nakanishi, Chem. Asian J. 9 (2014) 406.

[2] J. Nakanishi, Y. Kikuchi, T. Takarada, H. Nakayama, K. Yamaguchi, M. Maeda, J. Am. Chem. Soc. 126 (2004) 16314.

[3] J. Nakanishi, Y. Kikuchi, Y. Tsujimura, H. Nakayama, S. Kaneko, T. Shimizu, K. Yamaguchi, H. Yokota, Y. Yoshida, T. Takarada, M. Maeda, Y. Horiike, Supramol. Chem. 22 (2010) 396.

[4] J. Nakanishi, Y. Kikuchi, T. Takarada, H. Nakayama, K. Yamaguchi, M. Maeda, Anal. Chim. Acta 578 (2006) 100.

[5] Y. Kikuchi, J. Nakanishi, T. Shimizu, H. Nakayama, S. Inoue, K. Yamaguchi, H. Iwai, Y. Yoshida, Y. Horiike, T. Takarada, M. Maeda, Langmuir 24 (2008) 13084.

[6] J. Nakanishi, Y. Kikuchi, S. Inoue, K. Yamaguchi, T. Takarada, M. Maeda, J. Am. Chem. Soc. 129 (2007) 6694.

[7] Y. Kikuchi, J. Nakanishi, H. Nakayama, T. Shimizu, Y. Yoshino, K. Yamaguchi, Y. Yoshida, Y. Horiike, Chem. Lett. 37 (2008) 1062.

[8] H. Nakayama, J. Nakanishi, T. Shimizu, Y. Yoshino, H. Iwai, S. Kaneko, Y. Horiike, K. Yamaguchi, Colloids Surf. B 76 (2010) 88.

[9] S. Kaneko, H. Nakayama, Y. Yoshino, D. Fushimi, K. Yamaguchi, Y. Horiike, J. Nakanishi, Phys. Chem. Chem. Phys. 13 (2011) 4051.

[10] V.V. Rostovtsev, L.G. Green, V.V. Fokin, K.B. Sharpless, Angew. Chem. – Int. Ed. 41 (2002) 2596.

[11] M. Kamimura, O. Scheideler, Y. Shimizu, S. Yamamoto, K. Yamaguchi, J. Nakanishi, Phys. Chem. Chem. Phys. 17 (2015) 14159.

[12] N. Kramer, A. Walzl, C. Unger, M. Rosner, G. Krupitza, M. Hengstschläger, H. Dolznig, Mutat. Res./ Rev. Mutat. Res. 752 (2013) 10.

[13] K.J. Simpson, L.M. Selfors, J. Bui, A. Reynolds, D. Leake, A. Khvorova, J.S. Brugge, Nat. Cell Biol. 10 (2008) 1027.

[14] S. Kaneko, K. Yamaguchi, J. Nakanishi, Langmuir 29 (2013) 7300.

[15] K. Uchida, Y. Hoshino, A. Tamura, K. Yoshimoto, S. Kojima, K. Yamashita, I. Yamanaka, H. Otsuka, K. Kataoka, Y. Nagasaki, Biointerphases 2 (2007) 126.

[16] T. Lohmuller, D. Aydin, M. Schwieder, C. Morhard, I. Louban, C. Pacholski, J.P. Spatz, Biointerphases 6 (2011) MR1.

[17] Y. Shimizu, H. Boehm, K. Yamaguchi, J.P. Spatz, J. Nakanishi, PLoS ONE 9 (2014) e91875.

[18] M. Arnold, M. Schwieder, J. Blummel, E.A. Cavalcanti-Adam, M. Lopez-Garcia, H. Kessler, B. Geiger, J.P. Spatz, Soft Matter 5 (2009) 72.

[19] D. Gonzalez-Rodriguez, K. Guevorkian, S. Douezan, F. Brochard-Wyart, Science 338 (2012) 910.

4

Diagnostics Technologies

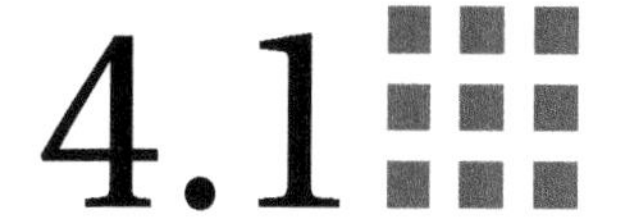

4.1 Point-of-Care Diagnostics

Nuttada Panpradist, James J. Lai

DEPARTMENT OF BIOENGINEERING, UNIVERSITY OF WASHINGTON, SEATTLE, WA, USA

CHAPTER OUTLINE

4.1.1 Introduction

Infectious diseases such as influenza and HIV/AIDS are leading causes of mortality and morbidity globally [1,2]. Pathogen detection can utilize tests such as cell culture, nucleic acid amplification test, and enzyme-linked immunosorbent assay (ELISA). For example, ELISA can detect disease-specific protein biomarkers in human bodily fluids to provide both diagnostic and prognostic value [3]. While these tests might help to diagnose infected patients, they do not necessarily facilitate timely treatments or medical attention because these tests require significant health care infrastructure, and are often laborious and time consuming [4]. The situation is even worse in resource-limited settings (e.g., developing countries) where the need for rapid and accurate diagnosis of disease is the greatest. In order to address the challenges, the World Health Organization (WHO) has established a set of criteria to guide the development of point-of-care (POC) diagnostic tools in resource-limited settings, which are: (1) affordable, (2) sensitive, (3) specific, (4) user friendly, (5) rapid and robust, (6) equipment free, and (7) deliverable to end-users, abbreviated "ASSURED" [5]. These criteria can be used to guide the development of suitable diagnostic methodologies for use in low-resource settings.

Nanotechnologies have allowed the field of the POC diagnostic test to advance rapidly during the past decades by improving clinical diagnostic assays (e.g., sensitivity) [6,7]. For example, immunosensors improve their performance by employing biomolecules (e.g., antibody), integrated with nanomaterials, including carbon [8–11], metal [11,12], silica [13,14], and quantum dots [15,16]. The focus of this chapter is to introduce few recently developed technologies, which can potentially address some of the critical challenges for two major clinical diagnostic tests - immunoassays and nucleic acid amplification tests.

4.1.2 Diagnostics Targeting Proteins

Immunoassays have been utilized for various clinical applications since the mid-1960s and have revolutionized the care of patients [17]. The ability to detect trace amounts of certain proteins in human plasma has enabled clinicians to identify harmful populations of cells and troublesome cellular processes and change management. Immunoassays detect biomarkers in the sample fluid via recognition using the immobilized antibodies at solid surfaces. They are performed in central laboratories using a variety of instrument-based technologies as well as on-site via rapid test techniques, primarily lateral-flow assays [18]. For example, HIV diagnosis has been utilizing immunoassays in both centralized hospitals and POC settings [19,20]. Improved assay analytical sensitivity can help identify those individuals that need immediate intervention and effectively rule out disease, and as a result is very useful in screening situations where a second-line diagnostic strategy can be used to diagnose disease. Therefore, manufacturers are constantly improving the assay sensitivity on their immunoassay analyzers. The overall immunoassay workflow includes sample processing (target analyte recognition/separation) and detection/readout.

4.1.2.1 Sample Processing

The performance of immunoassays is intrinsically associated with specimen quality and quantity because the biomarker concentration and the specimen volume define the absolute number of available target molecules for detection. Immunoassay utilizes antibodies immobilized on solid surfaces for recognizing the specific biomarkers in the sample fluid, so the antibody-biomarker binding occurs at a solid–liquid interface. The solid surfaces enable the biomarker separation but also result in mass transport limitations, which lead to slow reaction kinetics [21,22], because the biomarkers have to diffuse to the surfaces for recognition. In order to address the kinetic challenge, immunoassays can utilize significantly higher amounts (≥10-fold) of antibodies [23]. However, a large solid surface area increases the nonspecific binding, which raises the assay background noise and compromises the limit of detection [24]. Additionally, the rarity of a disease biomarker in a broad sample background can lead to crippling signal-to-noise problems because the rare antigens themselves can be lost at various places when they are adsorbed nonspecifically to the device surfaces. Therefore, chromatography has been employed for purifying and concentrating biomarkers prior to diagnostic testing [25,26]. For example, magnetic microbeads have been utilized to enhance immunoassays via biomarker purification [27,28]. Here we would like to discuss two different sample-processing approaches for POC diagnostic applications.

4.1.2.1.1 Aqueous Two-Phase System

Lateral flow assay (LFA) is a rapid assay for diagnosing various infectious diseases [29,30]. Compared to common laboratory techniques such as ELISA, LFA exhibits significantly lower sensitivity, which results in numerous false negatives [31]. Therefore, LFA cannot be widely utilized for early disease diagnosis. One of the major reasons for the low sensitivity is extremely low concentrations of the biomarkers in a sample fluid. In order to regain the clinical utilities for LFA, approaches for concentrating biomarkers prior to detection have been employed to enhance the LFA sensitivity [32,33].

Aqueous two-phase systems (ATPS) have been utilized for concentrating biomarkers via liquid–liquid extraction format [34,35]. For example, some aqueous micellar systems, under appropriate solution conditions, can spontaneously separate into two water-based, yet immiscible, liquid phases [36]. The approach has been utilized to concentrate genomic DNA [37,38]. When the solution phase separated, genomic DNA partitions almost exclusively in the micelle-poor phase because the molecules experience greater steric, repulsive, excluded-volume interactions with the larger and more abundant micelles. The final DNA concentration can be controlled by adjusting the volume ratio between the micelle-poor and -rich phases [35,38]. For example, the final DNA concentration can be approximately 10 times higher by using a volume ratio of 1:9, which reduces the micelle-poor phase to one-tenth of the initial volume. The Kamei group has done some pioneering work to employ ATPS for protein marker enrichment to enable detection via LFA. Because of the small size, protein markers such as transferrin (Tf) partition pretty evenly in both micelle-rich and -poor phases. However, gold nanoparticles with ~40 nm diameter partition extremely well into the micelle-poor phase by experiencing greater excluded-volume interactions with the larger and more abundant micelles in the micelle-rich phase [39]. In order to concentrate protein markers such as Tf using ATPS, the Kamei group developed an affinity reagent – gold nanoparticles (GNPs) conjugated with Tf antibodies for recognizing Tf before the separation [39]. The GNP-bound Tf molecules were concentrated in the micelle-poor phase, and then the concentrated Tf was applied to LFA for detection. The resulting assays show about a 10-fold improvement for enhancing the detection limit of Tf [39].

In order to utilize ATPS in conjunction with LFA for POC diagnostic applications, the Kamei group also engineered the system to reduce the sample processing time, and streamlined the interface between sample preparation and LFA detection [40,41]. To reduce the long processing time (e.g., 18 h [38]) associated with micellar ATPS, the Kamei group employed an ATPS using polyethylene glycol (PEG)–potassium phosphate salt (PEG–salt ATPS) [42,43]. The system exhibits two phases that are rich and poor with PEG, respectively. PEG–salt ATPS can concentrate protein markers such as Tf 10 times within 30 min using dextran-coated GNPs (DGNPs). DGNPs are utilized to preferentially partition Tf in the PEG-poor phase rapidly by experiencing excluded-volume interactions with the greater number of PEG molecules in the PEG-rich phase [44]. Additionally, the PEG–salt ATPS solution that is well mixed with DGNPs and Tf can be directly applied to an LFA for detection without waiting for the phase separation because the PEG-poor domains, containing Tf-bound DGNPs, were able to move quickly up the strip, whereas the PEG-rich domains appeared to be held back [26,40]. This new approach significantly streamlines the interface between ATPS enrichment and LFA detection.

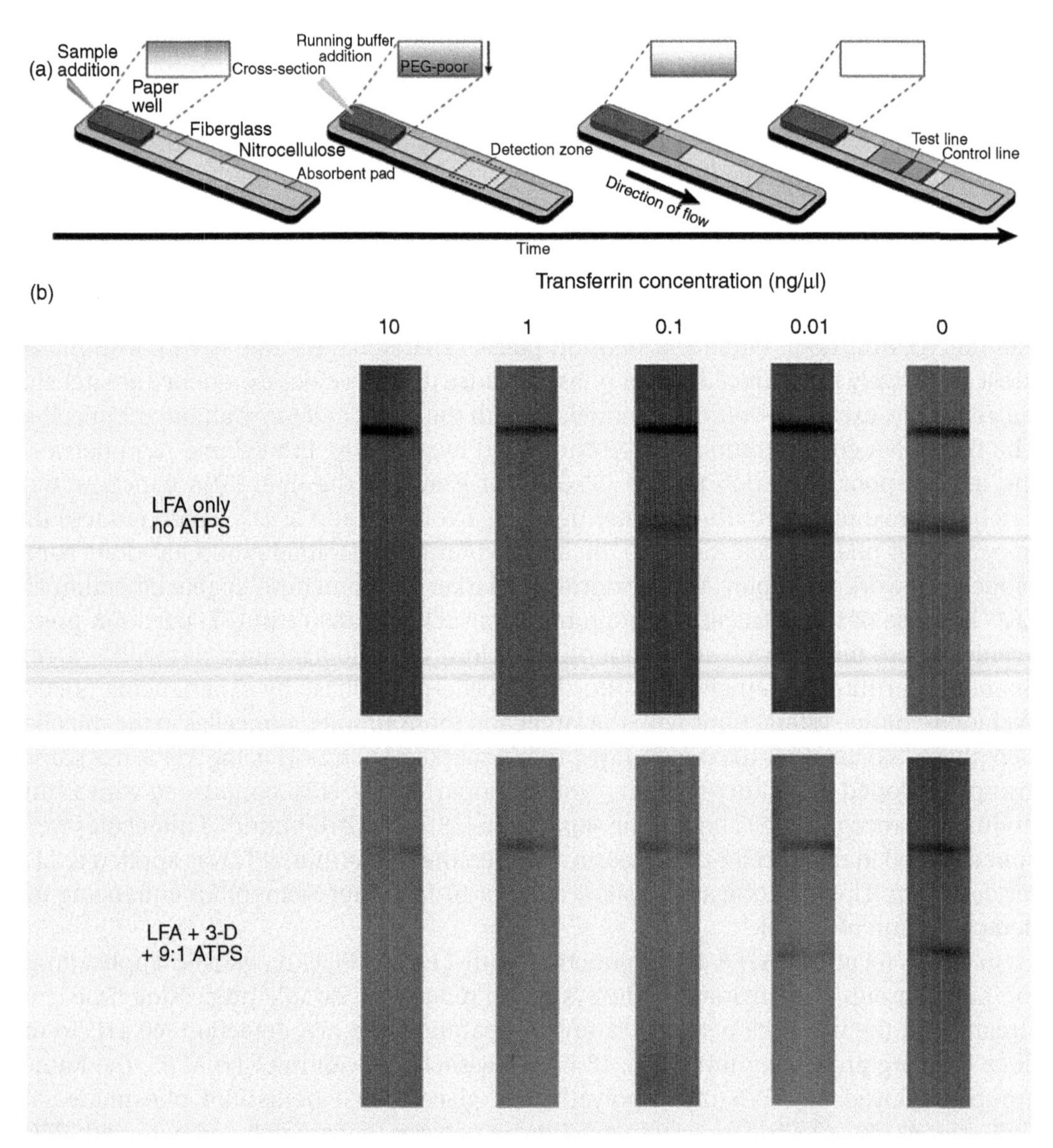

FIGURE 4.1.1 (a) The three-dimensional paper well was combined with ATPS and LFA for Tf competition assay on nitrocellulose paper. (b) Conventional LFA detected Tf at 1 ng/μL. A 9:1 volume ratio ATPS with the three-dimensional paper well successfully detected Tf at 0.1 ng/μL. *Reproduced from Ref. [40], with permission from the Royal Society of Chemistry.*

The Kamei group improved Tf detection on a three-dimensional paper device that utilized the rapid PEG–salt ATPS biomarker enrichment. This all-in-one device allows phase separation, concentration, and detection to simultaneously and seamlessly occur on paper. The paper device contains a well consisting of layers of stacked paper (Fig. 4.1.1a), which significantly increases the cross-sectional area perpendicular to the fluid flow. Therefore, the phase separation process was significantly enhanced by increasing the retention of the PEG-rich phase in the top layers of the well and simultaneously concentrating the PEG-poor phase in the paper strip below. Additionally, the well design can accommodate solutions with larger volumes, which provide more biomarkers to improve the detection. This new approach is suitable for POC diagnostic applications because it reduces time for the biomarker enrichment process from multihour down to several minutes and removes the need for having trained personnel to extract the concentrated biomarkers from ATPS to LFA for detection. The new device has demonstrated an improvement in the detection limit of Tf 10-fold, 0.1 ng/mL, in less than 25 min (Fig. 4.1.1b) [40].

4.1.2.1.2 Stimuli-Responsive Reagents

Stimuli-responsive reagents such as polymer–antibody conjugates have been utilized in achieving liquid-phase/homogeneous affinity separation of target molecules to facilitate chromatography and immunoassays [45,46]. Stimuli-responsive polymers sharply and reversibly respond to physical or chemical stimuli by changing their conformation and physical–chemical properties, that is, changing from a hydrophilic state to a more hydrophobic state. Poly(*N*-isopropylacrylamide), pNIPAAm, the most extensively studied and utilized stimuli-responsive polymer, exhibits a lower critical solution temperature (LCST) behavior [47]. Below a defined temperature designated as the LCST, it is hydrophilic and highly solvated, while above the LCST, it is more hydrophobic and aggregated. This temperature transition is completely reversible and notably sharp around 32°C. When the biomolecules such as proteins conjugated with the polymer, the stimuli-responsive transition properties are conferred to the biomolecules. The biggest impact of stimuli-responsive polymers has been in the biomedical field, where the versatility and usefulness of these polymers as molecular engineering tools have been demonstrated in the development of biological sensors, drug delivery vehicles, and tissue engineering.

Stimuli-responsive bioconjugates have been utilized for biomolecule separation to improve clinical diagnostic tests and life science research. Biomolecules containing stimuli-responsive polymers such as pNIPAAm–antibody conjugates also exhibit reversible temperature responsiveness. These conjugates have been utilized to enable enzyme-based immunoassay for detecting a wide range of clinical analytes such as hepatitis B surface antigen with analytical sensitivity comparable to conventional ELISA [48,49]. The overall assay process starts from mixing the polymer conjugates with the patient specimens and assay detection reagents (e.g., enzyme–antibody conjugates) in a homogeneous solution to rapidly form sandwich immunocomplexes. These polymer conjugates overcome the mass transport limitations associated with heterogeneous immunoassays by enabling biomarker recognition in a homogeneous solution where molecular diffusion of the reagents facilitates rapid mass transport equilibration. Then, the bound biomarkers can be rapidly isolated by aggregating immune complexes and polymer conjugates above the polymer LCST to enable separation (e.g., centrifugation, membrane, magnetic field) [49,50].

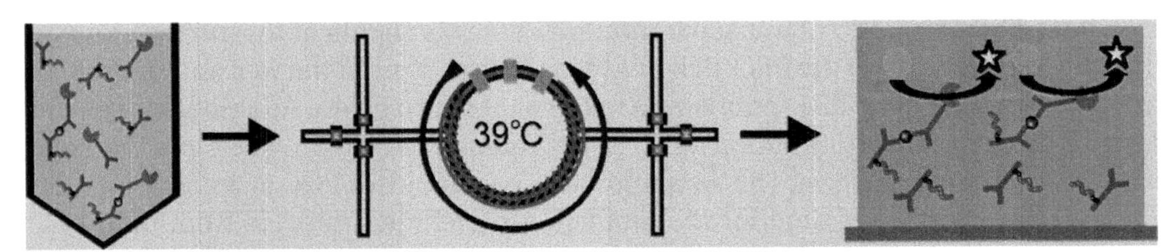

FIGURE 4.1.2 Immunocomplexes, composed of antibody–poly(*N*-isopropylacrylamide) (Ab–PNIPAAm) conjugates, antibody–alkaline phosphatase (Ab–AP) conjugates, and PSA, are formed in a 50% human plasma solution. Samples are loaded into the microfluidic device and the surface is heated to 39°C. Above 39°C, immunocomplexes are separated from the human plasma solution by immobilization on the microfluidic device sidewalls through hydrophobic interactions. To enrich samples, the microfluidic device is washed to remove nonimmobilized material and an additional sample is injected with the temperature at 39°C. Once the sample is separated, enzyme substrate is loaded into the microfluidic device and turned over into a fluorescent product by immobilized Ab–AP conjugates for detection. *Reproduced from Ref. [51], with permission from the American Chemical Society.*

Therefore, assay incubation times can be reduced from hours to minutes. The purified biomarkers can be detected via the enzyme–antibody conjugates without compromising sensitivity. Since a large bulk solid phase is not present during the immunospecific capture step, nonspecific binding is also minimized, which can reduce the assay background noise to improve the limit of detection.

Hoffman et al. recently utilized pNIPAAm–antibody conjugates in a microfluidic immunoassay to enable rapid prostate-specific antigen (PSA) purification and enrichment as well as sensitive detection in human plasma specimens (Fig. 4.1.2) [51]. The polymers were conjugated to antibodies via carbodiimide chemistry. The carboxyl end-groups of semitelechelic pNIPAAm synthesized by reversible addition–fragmentation chain transfer polymerization were modified with tetrafluorophenol to yield amine-reactive ester groups for conjugation to lysine residues of antibodies. The assay used anti-PSA IgG-polymer conjugates in conjunction with an alkaline phosphatase-linked antibody to form sandwich immunocomplexes via PSA binding. The complexes in human plasma specimens were loaded into a recirculating poly(dimethylsiloxane) microreactor, equipped with micropumps and transverse flow features, for subsequent separation, enrichment, and quantification. The overall assay took 25 min. In one approach, the assay resulted in a 37 pM PSA limit of detection, which is comparable to a plate ELISA employing the same antibody pair, when utilizing ca. 80 nL immunocomplex solution (microreactor volume) that was loaded at room temperature before separation at 39°C. In another approach, immunocomplex solution was flowed through the reactor that was preheated to 39°C. The capture process was repeated multiple times to process a larger specimen volume, 7.5 μL. The resulting assay limit of detection was 0.5 pM, which is two orders of magnitude lower than the plate ELISA. Both approaches generate an antigen-specific signal over a clinically relevant range. The sample processing capabilities and subsequent utility in a biomarker assay demonstrate the opportunity for stimuli-responsive polymer–protein conjugates in novel diagnostic technologies.

4.1.2.2 Detection Reagents

In addition to the sample preparation, technologies associated with detection and readout have also made significant progress. Nanoparticles have been widely utilized as labels for detecting analytes using various techniques (e.g., color) because of their unique electronic, magnetic, and optical properties, attributed to their nanoscale dimension [52,53]. For example, magnetic nanoparticles [54,55] and quantum dots [56,57] have been utilized to facilitate detection by labeling the target analytes.

4.1.2.2.1 Plasmonic ELISA

Gold nanoparticles (GNPs), which exhibit SPR-related optical phenomena, can be utilized as the reagent for detecting the presence or absence of target biomarkers. For example, GNPs with immobilized antibodies have been widely used as detection reagents for POC diagnostic tests such as lateral flow immunoassay [58,59] because gold colloids can be prepared in bulk quantities with narrow size distributions, are readily functionalized with affinity ligands using various conjugation approaches, exhibit long shelf-life, and can be stored in a dry format [60].

Surface plasmon resonance (SPR) is the basic principle for many colorimetric assays and is induced when the frequency of incident photons complements the natural frequency of surface electron oscillations against the attraction to the positive nuclei. GNPs exhibit a pronounced absorbance peak in the visible light wavelength range, which is caused by localized SPR and the optical excitation of surface plasmons. Changing the morphology of gold nanostructures leads to the color change of gold solution by changing the SPR wavelength. In addition to morphology, the GNP optical properties are also closely associated with the interparticle distances. For example, when dispersed particles in solution become aggregated, reducing the interparticle distance, the particle solution shifts from red to blue. Some agglutination immunoassays utilize the particle aggregation-based color change for detecting biomarkers [61,62].

Stevens et al. developed plasmonic ELISA – an ultrasensitive immunoassay that utilizes the growth of GNPs in conjunction with the biocatalytic cycle of the enzyme label for detection [63,64]. The immunocomplex for plasmonic ELISA is the same as the conventional sandwich assay, which consists of a target molecule, captured with specific antibodies on a solid-phase support and subsequently labeled with an enzyme–antibody conjugate. Conventional ELISA utilizes enzymes such as horseradish peroxidase to generate assay signals by converting enzyme substrates into color, light, or fluorescent molecules. The signal from assays with low concentration analytes can be detected using instruments with sophisticated optics but cannot be confidently distinguished by the naked eye.

The plasmonic ELISA links the color of plasmonic nanoparticles to the presence or absence of the analyte. The assay uses enzymes to control the particle synthesis for generating plasmonic particles with different sizes [65,66], which exhibit distinct solution colors caused by different localized SPR. In one of the demonstrations that utilize p24 as the target analyte, the assay incorporates catalase to regulate the hydrogen peroxide concentration,

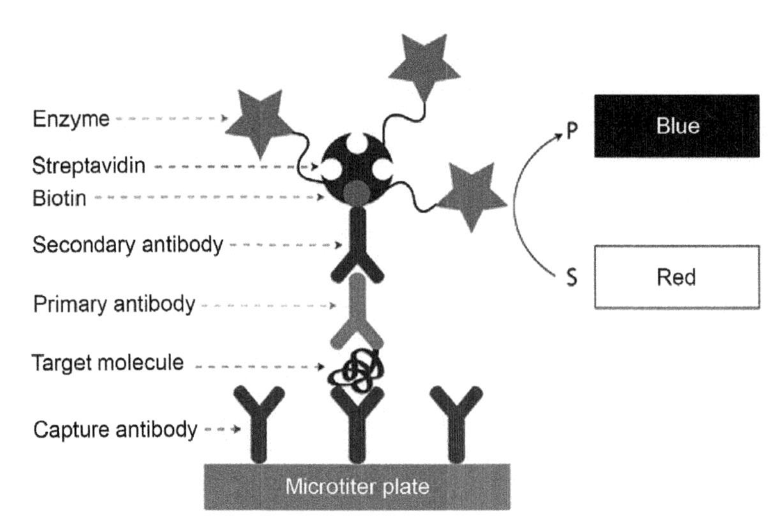

FIGURE 4.1.3 In plasmonic ELISA the biocatalytic cycle of the enzyme generates colored nanoparticle solutions of characteristic tonality. S, substrate; P, product; NP, nanoparticle. *Reproduced from Ref. [64], with permission from the Nature Publishing Group.*

which controls the growth of GNPs, for obtaining blue- or red-colored solutions in the presence or absence of the analyte, respectively.

When the specimen does not contain target analyte, the assay results in a red-colored solution because the hydrogen peroxide solution concentration is high, which reduces gold ions rapidly to form quasispherical, nonaggregated GNPs. In the presence of the analyte, the assay results in a blue-colored solution because the enzyme catalase catalyzes the decomposition of hydrogen peroxide. Low hydrogen peroxide concentration slows down the kinetics of GNP nucleation and results in aggregated nanoparticles. The blue and red colors are easily distinguishable at a glance, therefore facilitating the detection of the analyte with the naked eye. The plasmonic ELISA was utilized for detecting HIV-1 capsid antigen p24 in whole serum at the ultralow concentration of 10^{-18} g/mL, which is several orders of magnitude lower than the clinically utilized ELISA. p24 was also detected with the naked eye in the sera of HIV-infected patients showing viral loads undetectable by a gold standard nucleic acid-based test [64] (Fig. 4.1.3).

4.1.3 Diagnostics Targeting Nucleic Acids

Key advantages of nucleic acid targeting technologies over protein targeting are that often they can provide earlier diagnosis as well as identification of disease-associated alleles. These allow health care providers to select effective treatment for an individual (e.g., personalized medicine) in a timely fashion. As a result, there has been a strong push to expand the accessibility of nucleic acid targeting technologies worldwide. Unfortunately, nucleic acid targeting tests are much more complicated than protein targeting tests, and often they require trained personnel. To illustrate, the main steps for the assays targeting nucleic acid biomarkers include sample preparation (cell lysis to expose nucleic acid, purification and concentration of nucleic acid), amplification of targeted nucleic acid, and detection of the amplified products. To date, several commercially available nucleic-acid targeting technologies have been developed to offer easy-to-use, (nearly) autonomous options. Examples are Cepheid GeneXpert™, IDBox™, BioFire™, Roche IQuum™, Nanosphere™, Xagenic™, iCubate™, Curetis™, Meridian Illumigene™, Biocartis Idylla™, and Alere i™. Below, we highlight some applications of nanostructured materials that have improved efficiency, simplicity, and speed of these steps in POC molecular diagnostics over the traditional bench-top approaches.

4.1.3.1 Nanostructured Materials for Point-of-Care Nucleic Acid Sample Preparation

In the sample preparation step, the nucleic acid content from the sample is extracted, concentrated, and purified to meet the quality required by the downstream amplification process. Sample preparation of nucleic acid targeting technologies involves several processes. In most cases, lysis is an initially required process to break open intact structures of targeted species (e.g., cell wall, membrane, and capsules) and to release nucleic acids. Additional purification or extraction of the released nucleic acids from the lysate may be conducted to minimize inhibitory effects on downstream amplification. Following the lysis step, the chemicals introduced (e.g., membrane-solubilizing ionic detergents or proteinases), cell debris, and other interferents that come with samples are removed. For diluted specimens (i.e., urine), nucleic acid concentration may be required in order to reduce the limit of detection of amplification and detection assays.

The advancement of nanostructured materials has facilitated the development of POC lysis tools. Traditional mechanical lysis relies on shear forces that are created by several means to disrupt cells and to release amplifiable nucleic acid. The gold standard bench-top mechanical lysis, bead beaters, relies on large, expensive equipment and trained personnel. To enable the use of mechanical lysis at the POC, bench-top bead beaters have been modified into low-powered units that drive bead movement in the sample reservoir (e.g., omnilyse [68], audiolyse [69], miniaturized bead beater [70], μbead beater [71]). Besides moving beads to create shear force, nanostructures have allowed alternatives to shear forces; nanoscaled patterns integrated in the microfluidic channel can lyse cells as they pass through these nanoscaled patterns. Examples are nanoblade [72], filter-like nanoknives [73], nanospike membrane [74], high-aspect ratio nanowires [75]. Furthermore, lysis can be made pathogen specific. For example, a nanorod coated with the antibody targeting the specific pathogen can be used for photothermal lysis. When the cells pass through the microchannel, target pathogens are captured onto the gold nanorod selectively and subsequently lysed with near-infrared radiation [76].

Sequence-specific or nonspecific nucleic acids can be further extracted to purify and in some cases concentrate biomarker nucleic acid targets for subsequent amplification. A common approach relies on the use of positively charged matrices to capture negatively charged nucleic acid, followed by a washing step to remove other components of lysate and finally elution of the purified nucleic acid targets. Alternatively, specific sequences of nucleic acids can be captured via hybridization. Below we highlight two examples of nucleic acid extraction nanostructured technologies: Nanobind™ and salicylic acid coated magnetic nanoparticles (SAMNPs) for genomic DNA extraction.

4.1.3.1.1 Nanobind – Hierarchical Silica Nanomembranes for Nucleic Acid Extraction

The chemistry of Nanobind is similar to traditionally solid-phase silica-based nucleic acid extraction; however, the Nanobind technology has a nanostructure that enables a highly efficient nucleic extraction. Fabrication of Nanobind relies on the deposition of silica (silicon dioxide, SiO_2) on heat-inducing self-wrinkled films. Prestretched thermoplastic polymer substrates (i.e., polymethacrylate, polycarbonate, polystyrene, and cyclic polyolefin) are deposited with silica via electron-beam evaporation on both sides of the substrate. For cyclic polyolefin-coated polymer substrates, heat treatment at 250°F for 3 min results in shrunk films (approximately 10% of its original size) with a nanoscaled silica structure (ranging from tens of nm to μm in size) [77]. This process creates nanoscaled structures with large surface areas of silica. The large surface areas increase DNA binding capacity and DNA recovery yield. The binding capacity of Nanobind is more than 180 μg of DNA yield from 25 million cells input. Recovery from Nanobind is two-fold higher than the commonly used commercial products (e.g., Qiagen minispin column and Qiagen magnetic particles). This extraction method has been shown to yield long DNA fragments >48 kbp comparable to the gold strand phenol–chloroform extraction. Nanostructured membrane Nanobind holds DNA molecules on a single substrate. In contrast, the magnetic particle beads (large or small particle sizes) usually result in short DNA fragments; multiple particles binding to the same DNA molecule shear the DNA into small fragments during particle mixing.

4.1.3.1.2 Salicylic Acid-Coated Magnetic Nanoparticles for One-Step DNA Extraction

SAMNPs [78] are synthesized by vigorously stirring a mixture of salicylic acid (SA) and sodium hydroxide solution (pH 11) under argon gas. Subsequently, Fe(III)/Fe(II) salts are added to the mixture at a ratio of 2Fe(III):1Fe(II):4SA prior to a 4-h reflux at 90°C. SA is a chemical ligand used as the modifier in chelating resins that has been shown to have excellent sorption properties. The pH 11 of sodium hydroxide avoids liquid flooding that occurs when using ammonium hydroxide. This synthesis method yields particles with a hydrodynamic radius of 122.7 nm (Fig. 4.1.4a). Although nanoparticles with a zeta potential from −30 mV to +30 mV tend to aggregate, SAMNPs synthesized by this method with a zeta potential of 38.1 mV are water soluble [79]. An explanation of this phenomenon could be that SA symmetrically binds to an Fe_3O_4 nanoparticle surface, permitting SAMNPs to be water soluble via the exposed hydroxyl groups.

Synthesized SAMNPs, in conjunction with basic chemistry for standard nucleic extraction and purification, can be used to capture both the crude cells during prelysis (to concentrate the targeted cells) and subsequently capture genomic DNA for postlysis (to purify

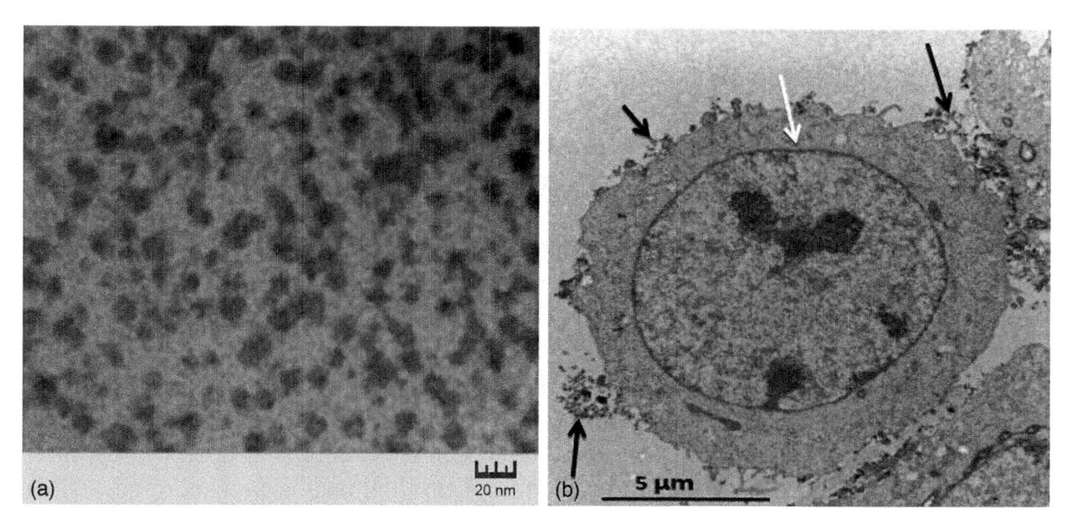

FIGURE 4.1.4 (a) Transmission electron microscope (TEM) image of SAMNPs with a scale bar of 20 nm. Note that the estimated size by dynamic light scattering is 127.7 nm in diameter (b) TEM image of mammalian cells captured by SAMNPs with a scale bar of 5 μm. *Reproduced from Ref. [78], with permission from Elsevier.*

and concentrate the targeted nucleic acids, Fig. 4.1.4b). Briefly, crude cells are introduced to SAMNPs and incubated for 5 min to form complexes. These complexes are then separated from the supernatant by magnet immobilization. The supernatant is then discarded, and the immobilized cells are lysed and incubated for another 5 min. Isopropanol is added to permit the released DNA to bind to SAMNPs during a 3-min incubation. DNA–SAMNP complexes are then pulled down via magnetic absorption. Seventy percent ethanol is then used to elute the DNA from the magnetic beads. After ethanol evaporates, the DNA is purified and ready for downstream purification.

SAMNP-mediated genomic DNA extraction is relatively simple (free from filtration and centrifugation), fast (30 min), and environmental friendly (free of toxic chemicals). It can be used to extract genomic DNA from crude cell culture media without shearing, and is ideal for use in genomic sequencing applications.

4.1.3.2 Nanostructured Materials for Point-of-Care Nucleic Acid Amplification

Amplification is the most crucial step for nucleic acid targeting assays, especially for samples containing low copy numbers of the sequence of interest. The gold standard for nucleic acid amplification is polymerase chain reaction (PCR), which requires a thermal cycler to create the changes in temperatures to allow for nucleic acid dehybridization, primer annealing, and extension of polymerase enzyme. Over the past decades, several commercial isothermal nucleic acid amplification techniques have been developed and commercialized [80–84]. These techniques are chemically designed to operate at a fixed temperature and thus avoid the need for a thermal cycler, increasing access of molecular assays at the POC. In the context of nucleic acid amplification, nanoscale materials have been used to improve both traditional PCR and isothermal amplification. Here we present two amplification technologies that utilize nanostructured and nanoscaled materials to enable an improved performance of nucleic acid amplification: nanodroplet digitalized amplification and nanoparticle-assisted PCR.

4.1.3.2.1 Nanodroplet Digital Amplification

Bench-top digital PCR amplification has demonstrated a high accuracy of nucleic acid quantitation over traditional quantitative PCR [85]. Digitalized PCR permits quantitative amplification by the creating the small micro/nanosized droplets for zero or single target amplification. This allows 20,000 reactions of PCR to occur all at once in a single PCR run. The droplets, either with or without amplified sequences, flow through the sensor that detects the nanodroplets containing amplified targets. This system has been incorporated into POC microfluidic chips such as the PCR SlipChip [86], self-digitalized chip [87,88], and self-priming compartmentalization chip [89]. In these chips, nanopatterns permit the generation of small droplets.

4.1.3.2.2 Nanoparticle-Assisted Polymerase Chain Reaction

GNPs can improve the performance of PCR as well as other isothermal amplification methods via several roles: polymerase absorption, primer absorption, and amplified product absorption [90–92]. GNPs can be used to absorb polymerases, enabling "hot-start polymerization." In hot-start polymerization, the polymerase enzyme is inactive at room temperature and becomes active upon heat activation (e.g., 95°C during the nucleic acid denaturing step in PCR). Hot-start polymerization eliminates nonspecific polymerization from a primer–dimer complex that normally occurs when PCR reactions are set up at room temperature. However, optimization of polymerase-absorbed GNPs is necessary for each specific amplification assay, because the affinity and kinetics of polymerase absorption depend on the isoelectric points of polymerases, PCR buffer, and PCR conditions. In some cases, amplification can be inhibited if the heat activation temperature is too low and polymerases remain absorbed onto the GNPs. The required optimization of polymerase-absorbed GNPs adds complexity compared to alternative hot-start polymerization: wax-coated polymerase microbeads (e.g., Ampliwax™ and TaqBead™). These wax-coated polymerases use nonpolar wax as a physical barrier between the polymerase and the reaction mixture that melts and releases polymerase at a specific temperature with great robustness across the PCR buffer conditions.

In addition to polymerase-absorbed GNPs, primer and amplified products can be absorbed onto GNPs. Primer-absorbed GNPs can differentiate single nucleotide polymorphisms (SNPs) in the target, based on the different melting temperatures of the primer to the SNP-containing nucleic acid target sequence and to the nontarget sequence. Similarly to the case of primers, GNPs can be designed to absorb one strand of amplified product, assisting nucleic acid denaturation at a lower temperature that the 95°C required in a typical PCR.

4.1.3.3 Nanostructured Materials for Nucleic Acid Detection

In addition to amplification, another key step for nucleic acid assay is the detection of products from the amplification. Nanostructured materials provide a substrate and labeling system for nucleic acid detection. For example, nanoparticles such as quantum dots [93] and metal nanoparticles (silver, gold) have been used as a means to generate signal for molecule recognition. This detection step can happen during or post amplification. During nucleic acid amplification, molecular beacon and hydrolysis probes with quenchers and fluorophores can be used to track the amount of amplified product generated in real time. Alternatively, amplified nucleic acid targets can be analyzed after amplification via visual readout using lateral flow strips. The synthesis methods of these detection molecules were introduced in Section 4.1.2.2. Below we present two examples of technologies that are specific to nucleic acid targets: nanopore for high-throughput DNA sequencing and nanowire that recognizes a sequence of interest via hybridization.

4.1.3.3.1 Nanopore

As an alternative for the gold standard Sanger sequencing, nanopore-based technology (e.g., MinION™) has proven its capability as the pocket-sized POC nucleic acid sequencer that can identify the order of bases without requiring an amplification step. Nanopores contain ionic current across the diameter, induced by the two surrounding ultra-thin membranes that are connected to an external electric field. As the nucleic acid strand moves through the pore, the conductivity across the diameter changes and creates the electrical signal that can be interpreted to the unique bases that pass through the pore.

Nanopores can be classified into two categories based on how they are fabricated: pore-forming biological protein and solid-state nanopores. Protein-based nanopores are limited by modifications of sizes of channels in natural proteins such as alpha-hemolysin or mycobacterium smegmatis porin A [94]. In contrast, solid-state nanopores can be mass-produced using silicon- or graphene-based microfabrication. A common fabrication approach starts with the deposition of a low-stress, 30-nm silicon nitride layer on a silicon substrate using low-pressure chemical vapor deposition. Focus ion beam (FIB) is then used to create the nanoscaled pores through the silicon nitride later. To create the size of pores applicable for sequencing applications, the atomic layer deposition of titanium dioxide is then introduced to reduce the size of the nanopores that have been created by the FIB to <10 nm. As an alternative to titanium dioxide, single-wall carbon nanotubes can be grown inside the pore to achieve desirable size [95]. Some customized ion beam systems can create pores <5 nm in diameter [96]. The pores below 5-nm size can linearize long nucleic acid coils and potentially can scan long genomic DNA in minutes.

In addition to the fabrication of nanopores, a key challenge is to control the speed of the nucleic acid strand as it moves through the pore to the level that can be detected. Excessively rapid movement of nucleic acid strand (1–5 μS per one base) results in noisy reads and thus requires multiple passes (1000 times) for successful identification of the base sequence. This challenge can be addressed either using a high-speed recording technology or feeding the strand of nucleic acid into the pore more slowly by using protein modification (such as exonuclease).

4.1.3.3.2 Nanowire

Nanowire is a label-free, electrical tool that can sensitively detect the binding events of small molecules, peptide nucleic acid (PNA)–DNA as well as DNA–DNA hybridization [97]. Sensing occurs when there is the change of charge density (inducing the change of electric field on the nanowire surface) upon binding of biomolecules (negatively charged molecules bind to the n-type field-effect transistor).

Nanowires are fabricated in two ways [98]. In the bottom-up process, or semiconductor nanowire growth method, crystals grow into the desirable structures. This process allows the addition of dopant during the crystal growth to create intrinsic charge carrier properties, eliminating the need for subsequent ion implantation. In contrast, top-down processes utilize optical lithography or electron beam lithography to create nanowires. After the nanowire structure has been created, it must be attached to the probe to allow recognition of the DNA target. A common method to attach the probes to nanowires uses silane chemistry (e.g., 3-aminopropyltriethozysilane) or phosphonate derivatives (for attaching PNA) that react with native oxide naturally grown on silicon nanowire. Applications of nanowire in diagnostics include microRNA detection (PNA–DNA, Fig. 4.1.5 [99]), dengue virus detection (PNA–DNA), and on-chip flu A detection using Si nanowire.

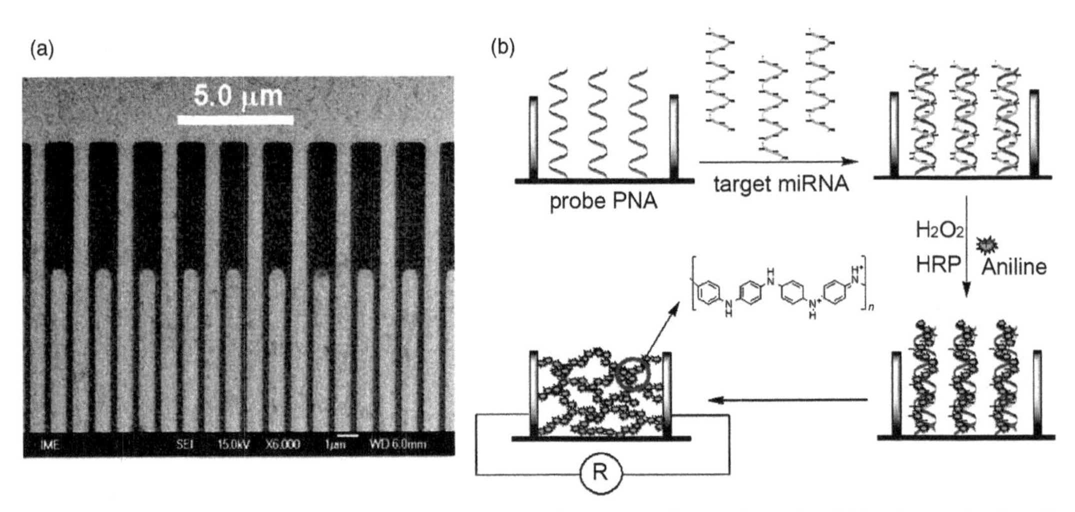

FIGURE 4.1.5 (a) Scanning electron microscope (SEM) image of nanogapped microelectrodes. (b) Sensing mechanism of probe PNA. PNA–miRNA bound to mixture of hydrogen peroxide and horseradish peroxidase (H_2O_2/HRP) initiates the polymerization of polyanaline nanowire that increases conductance in the nanogaps. *Reproduced from Ref. [99], with permission from the IEEE.*

4.1.4 Conclusions and Future Trends

In vitro diagnostic assays with improved sensitivity and specificity have been utilized to facilitate health care and patient treatment decisions. In order to improve the clinical utilities for these assays in resource-limited settings (e.g., developing countries), POC diagnostic tests and related technologies are being developed by following WHO's ASSURED guideline. Nanotechnologies have been utilized for POC diagnostic tests by addressing some of the challenges such as sample preparation, amplification, and detection. Implementation of POC diagnostic tests requires more than the standard evaluation of sensitivity and specificity. Therefore, all new technologies have to be further evaluated in the field, for example, resource-limited locations, as well as compared with the current gold standard assays.

References

[1] Centers for Disease Control. Cdc.gov, 2015. Estimating Seasonal Influenza-Associated Deaths in the United States: CDC Study Confirms Variability of Flu| Seasonal Influenza (Flu) | CDC [WWW Document]. URL http://www.cdc.gov/flu/about/disease/us_flu-related_deaths.htm (accessed 10. 30. 15).

[2] World Health Organization. Who.int, 2015. WHO | HIV/AIDS [WWW Document]. URL http://www.who.int/gho/hiv/en/ (accessed 10. 30. 15).

[3] N.L. Anderson, Clin. Chem. 56 (2010) 177.

[4] P. Yager, G.J. Domingo, J. Gerdes, Annu. Rev. Biomed. Eng. 10 (2008) 107.

[5] R.W. Peeling, K.K. Holmes, D.S Ronald, A. Mabey, Sex. Transm. Infect. 5 (82 Suppl.) (2006) v1.

[6] M.M. Stevens, P.D. Howes, S. Rana, Chem. Soc. Rev. 43 (2014) 3035.

[7] D. Yang, Q. Zhang, N. Li, J. Yang, P.A. Raju, M. Peng, Y. Luo, W. Hui, C. Chen, Y. Cui, Anal. Chem. 85 (2013) 6688.

[8] K. Zhu, R. Dietrich, A. Didier, D. Doyscher, E. Märtlbauer, Toxins (Basel) 6 (2014) 1325.

[9] Y. Song, H. Yu-Yen, X. Liu, X. Zhang, M. Ferrari, L. Qin, Trends Biotechnol. 32 (2014) 132.

[10] A. Rutebemberwa, M.J. Stevens, M.J. Perez, L.P. Smith, L. Sanders, G. Cosgrove, C.E. Robertson, R.M. Tuder, J.K. Harris, PLoS One 9 (2014) e111150.

[11] D. Liu, J. Yang, H. Wang, Z. Wang, X. Huang, Z. Wang, G. Niu, A.R.H. Walker, X. Chen, Anal. Chem. 86 (2014) 5800.

[12] L. He, T. Nan, Y. Cui, S. Guo, W. Zhang, R. Zhang, G. Tan, B. Wang, Malar. J. 13 (2014) 1.

[13] Y. Wu, C. Chen, S. Liu, Anal. Chem. 81 (2009) 1600.

[14] L. Yuan, X. Hua, Y. Wu, X. Pan, S. Liu, Anal. Chem. 83 (2011) 6800.

[15] D. Du, W. Chen, W. Zhang, D. Liu, H. Li, Y. Lin, Biosens. Bioelectron. 25 (2010) 1370.

[16] J. Wang, G. Liu, H. Wu, Y. Lin, Small 1 (2008) 82.

[17] B.R.S. Yalow, S.A. Berson, J. Clin. Invest. 39 (1960) 1157.

[18] G.A. Posthuma-Trumpie, J. Korf, Anal. Bioanal. Chem. 393 (2009) 569.

[19] K.P. Delaney, B.M. Branson, A. Uniyal, S. Phillips, D. Candal, S.M. Owen, P.R. Kerndt, HIV/AIDS 52 (2011) 257.

[20] B. Weber, L. Gürtler, R. Thorstensson, U. Michl, A. Mühlbacher, P. Bürgisser, R. Villaescusa, A. Eiras, C. Gabriel, H. Stekel, S. Tanprasert, S. Oota, M. Silvestre, C. Marques, M. Ladeira, J. Clin. Microbiol. 40 (2002) 1938.

[21] K.V. Klenin, W. Kusnezow, J. Langowski, J. Chem. Phys. (2005) 214715.

[22] R.W. Glaser, Anal. Biochem. 213 (1993) 152.

[23] K. Okano, S. Takahashi, K. Yasud, D. Tokinaga, K. Imai, M. Koga, Anal. Biochem. 202 (1992) 120.

[24] T. Soukka, H. Härmä, J. Paukkunen, T. Lövgren, Anal. Biochem. 73 (2001) 2254–2260.

[25] M. Krishnan, V. Namasivayam, R.S. Lin, R. Pal, M.A. Burns, Curr. Opin. Biotechnol. 12 (2001) 92.

[26] G. Ocvirk, E. Verpoorte, A. Manz, M. Grasserbauer, H.M. Widmer, Anal. Methods Instrum. 2 (1995) 74.

[27] R. Sista, Z. Hua, P. Thwar, A. Sudarsan, V. Srinivasan, A. Eckhardt, M. Pollack, V. Pamula, Lab Chip 8 (2008) 2091.

[28] J. Choi, K.W. Oh, J.H. Thomas, W.R. Heineman, H. Brian, J.H. Nevin, A.J. Helmicki, H. Thurman, H. Chong, Lab Chip 2 (2002) 27.

[29] G. Zhou, X. Mao, D. Juncker, Anal. Chem. 84 (2012) 7736.

[30] C. Quach, D. Newby, G. Daoust, E. Rubin, J. Mcdonald, Clin. Diagn. Lab. Immunol. 9 (2002) 925.

[31] A.C. Cêtre-Sossah, B.A. Billecocq, A.R. Lancelot, C.C. Defernez, C.J. Favre, B.M. Bouloy, A.D. Martinea, A.E. Albina, Prev. Vet. Med. 90 (2009) 146.

[32] M.K.M. Kehrel, N. Dassinger, S. Merkl, D. Vornicescu, Phys. Status Solidi 209 (2012) 917.

[33] M.A. Nash, J.N. Waitumbi, A.S. Hoffman, P. Yager, P.S. Stayton, ACS Nano (2012) 6776.

[34] H. Johansson, J. Persson, F. Tjerneld (1999).

[35] C. Liu, Y.J. Nikas, D. Blankschtein, Biotechnol. Bioeng. 52 (1996) 185.

[36] G. Thurston, G.M. Blankschtein, D. Fisch, M.R. Benedek, J. Chem. Phys. 85 (1986) 4558.

[37] S.C. Ribeiro, G.A. Monteiro, J.M.S. Cabral, D.M.F. Prazeres, Biotechnol. Appl. Biochem. 78 (2002) 376.

[38] F. Mashayekhi, A.S. Meyer, S.A. Shiigi, V. Nguyen, D.T. Kamei, Biotechnol. Bioeng. 102 (2009) 1613.

[39] F. Mashayekhi, A.M. Le, P.M. Nafisi, B.M. Wu, D.T. Kamei, Anal. Bioanal. Chem. 404 (2012) 2057.

[40] R.Y. Chiu, E. Jue, A.T. Yip, A.R. Berg, S.J. Wang, A.R. Kivnick, P.T. Nguyen, D.T. Kamei, Lab Chip 14 (2014) 3021.

[41] E. Jue, C.D. Yamanishi, R.Y.T. Chiu, B.M. Wu, D.T. Kamei, Biotechnol. Bioeng. 111 (2014) 2499.

[42] A.S. Schmidt, A.M. Ventom, J.A. Asenjo, Enzym. Microb. Tech. 16 (1994) 131.

[43] J.C. Merchuk, B.A. Andrews, J.A. Asenjo, J. Chromatogr. B 711 (1998) 285.

[44] R.Y. Chiu, P.T. Nguyen, J. Wang, E. Jue, B.M. Wu, D.T. Kamei, Ann. Biomed. Eng. 42 (2014) 2322.

[45] A.S. Hoffman, Clin. Chem. 1486 (2000) 1478.

[46] R.B. Fong, Z. Ding, C.J. Long, A.S. Hoffman, P.S. Stayton, Bioconjug. Chem. 10 (1999) 720.

[47] H.G. Schild, Prog. Polym. Sci. 17 (1992) 163.

[48] P. Lin, H. Zheng, H.H. Yang, W. Yang, C.G. Zhang, J.G. Xu, Chem. J. Chinese Univ. 24 (2003) 1198.

[49] N. Monji, C.A. Cole, M. Tam, L. Goldstein, R.C. Nowinski, A.S. Hoffman, Biochem. Biophys. Res. Commun. 172 (1990) 652.

[50] N. Monji, C.A. Cole, A.S. Hoffman, J. Biomater. Sci. Ed. 5 (1994) 407.

[51] M. Hoffman, P.S. Stayton, A.S. Hoffman, J.J. Lai, Bioconjug. Chem. 26 (2015) 29.

[52] P.C. Chen, S.C. Mwakwari, A.K. Oyelere, Nanotechnol. Sci. Appl. 1 (2008) 45.

[53] G. Liu, Y. Lin, Talanta 74 (2007) 308.

[54] L. Gao, J. Zhuang, L. Nie, J. Zhang, Y. Zhang, N. Gu, T. Wang, J. Feng, D. Yang, S. Perrett, X. Yan, Nat. Nanotechnol. 2 (2007) 577.

[55] Y.R. Chemla, H.L. Grossman, Y. Poon, R. Mcdermott, R. Stevens, M.D. Alper, J. Clarke, PNAS 97 (2000) 14268.

[56] L. Yang, Y. Li, Analyst 131 (2006) 394.

[57] R. Cui, H. Pan, J. Zhu, H. Chen, Anal. Chem. 79 (2007) 8494.

[58] T.R.J. Holford, F. Davis, S.P.J. Higson, Biosens. Bioelectron. 34 (2012) 12.

[59] K. Omidfar, S. Kia, S. Kashanian, Appl. Biochem. Biotechnol. 160 (2010) 843.

[60] M.Q. Zhu, L.Q. Wang, G.J. Exarhos, A.D.Q. Li, J. Am. Chem. Soc. 126 (2004) 2656.

[61] S. Gupta, H. Andresen, J.E. Ghadiali, M.M. Stevens, Small 6 (2010) 1509.

[62] R. Elghanian, J.J. Storhoff, R.C. Mucic, R.L. Letsinger, C.A. Mirkin, Science 277 (1997) 1078.

[63] L. Rodríguez-Lorenzo, R. De Rica, R.A. Álvarez-Puebla, L.M. Liz-Marzán, M.M. Stevens, Nat. Mater. 11 (2012) 10.

[64] R. De Rica, M.M. Stevens, Nat. Nanotechnol. 7 (2012) 821–824.

[65] C. Pejoux, R. De Rica, H. Matsui, Small 6 (2010) 999.

[66] D. Kisailus, J.H. Choi, J.C. Weaver, W.J. Yang, D.E. Morse, Adv. Mater. 17 (2005) 314.

[67] R. de la Rica, L.W. Chow, C.-M. Horejs, M. Mazo, C. Chiappini, E. Thomas Pashuck, R. Bittonb, M.M. Stevens, Chem. Commun. 50 (2014) 10648.

[68] P.E. Vandeventer, K.M. Weigel, J. Salazar, B. Erwin, B. Irvine, R. Doebler, A. Nadim, G.a. Cangelosi, A. Niemz, J. Clin. Microbiol. 49 (2011) 2533.

[69] J.R. Buser, A. Wollen, E.K. Heiniger, S. Byrnes, P.C. Kauffman, P.D. Ladd, P. Yager, Lab Chip 15 (2015) 1994–1997.

[70] L.J.A. Beckers, M. Baragona, S. Shulepov, T. Vliegenthart, A.R. Van Doorn, Methods (2010) 85.

[71] R.W. Doebler, B. Erwin, A. Hickerson, B. Irvine, D. Woyski, A. Nadim, J.D. Sterling, JALA – J. Assoc. Lab. Autom. 14 (2009) 119.

[72] S.-S. Yun, S.Y. Yoon, M.-K. Song, S.-H. Im, S. Kim, J.-H. Lee, S. Yang, Lab Chip 10 (2010) 1442.

[73] D. Di Carlo, K.-H. Jeong, L.P. Lee, Lab Chip 3 (2003) 287.

[74] H. So, K. Lee, Y.H. Seo, N. Murthy, A.P. Pisano, ACS Appl Mater Interfaces. 6 (2014) 6993–6997.

[75] J. Kim, J.W. Hong, D.P. Kim, J.H. Shin, I. Park, Lab Chip 12 (2012) 2914.

[76] R. Sean Norman, J.W. Stone, A. Gole, C.J. Murphy, T.L. Sabo-Attwood, Nano Lett. 8 (2008) 302.

[77] T.-H. Wang, Y. Zhang, Fabrication of hierarchical silica nanomembranes and uses thereof for solid phase extraction of nucleic acids, US 2015/0,037,802 A1, 2015.

[78] Z. Zhoua, U. Kadam, J. Irudayaraj, Anal. Biochem. 442 (2013) 249.

[79] G. Liu, P. Liu, Colloids Surfaces A 354 (2010) 377.

[80] M. Goto, E. Honda, A. Ogura, A. Nomoto, K.I. Hanaki, Biotechniques 46 (2009) 167.

[81] T. Edwards, P.A. Burke, H.B. Smalley, L. Gillies, G. Hobbs, J. Clin. Microbiol. 52 (2014) 2163.

[82] S. Kersting, V. Rausch, F.F. Bier, M. von Nickisch-Rosenegk, Microchim. Acta (2014) 1.

[83] L. An, W. Tang, T. a Ranalli, H.-J. Kim, J. Wytiaz, H. Kong, J. Biol. Chem. 280 (2005) 28952.

[84] A. Niemz, T.M. Ferguson, D.S. Boyle, Trends Biotechnol. 29 (2013) 240.

[85] C.M. Hindson, J.R. Chevillet, H.A. Briggs, E.N. Gallichotte, I.K. Ruf, B.J. Hindson, R.L. Vessella, M. Tewari, Nat. Methods 10 (2013) 1003.

[86] F. Shen, W. Du, J.E. Kreutz, A. Fok, R.F. Ismagilov, Lab Chip 10 (2010) 2666.

[87] A.M. Thompson, A. Gansen, A.L. Paguirigan, J.E. Kreutz, J.P. Radich, D.T. Chiu, Anal. Chem. 86 (2014) 12308.

[88] D.E. Cohen, T. Schneider, M. Wang, D.T. Chiu, Anal. Chem. 29 (2012) 997.

[89] Q. Zhu, L. Qiu, B. Yu, Y. Xu, Y. Gao, T. Pan, Q. Tian, Q. Song, W. Jin, Q. Jin, Y. Mu, Lab Chip 14 (2014) 1176.

[90] X. Lou, Y. Zhang, ACS Appl. Mater. Interfaces 5 (2013) 6276.

[91] X. Ma, Y. Cui, Z. Qiu, B. Zhang, S. Cui, J. Virol. Methods 193 (2013) 374.

[92] B.V. Vu, D. Litvinov, R.C. Willson, Anal. Chem. 80 (2008) 5462.

[93] D.A.I. Zhao, Chin. J. Ch. E. 15 (2007) 791.

[94] A. Studer, X. Han, F.K. Winkler, L.X. Tiefenauer, Colloids Surfaces B 73 (2009) 325.

[95] E.-H.S. Sadki, G. Slaven, D. Vlassarev, J.A. Golovchenko, D. Branton, J. Vac. Sci. Technol. B 29 (5) (2015).

[96] R. dela Torre, J. Larkin, A. Singer, A. Meller, Nanotechnology 23 (2012) 385308.

[97] G.J. Zhang, Y. Ning, Anal. Chim. Acta 749 (2012) 1.

[98] R.G. Hobbs, N. Petkov, J.D. Holmes, Chem. Mater. 24 (2012) 1975.

[99] Y. Fan, X.T. Chen, C.H. Tung, J.M. Kong, Z.Q. Gao, Transducers Eurosensors'2007–4th International Conference Solid-State Sensors, Actuators Microsystems, 2007, pp. 1887.

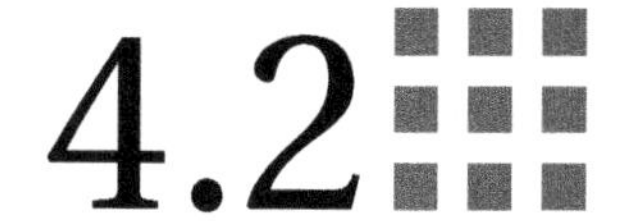

Biosensors

Akifumi Kawamura, Takashi Miyata

DEPARTMENT OF CHEMISTRY AND MATERIALS ENGINEERING, KANSAI UNIVERSITY, OSAKA, JAPAN

CHAPTER OUTLINE

Monitoring biological or biochemical processes are of utmost importance for medical and biological applications. The development of highly sensitive, specific, and cost-effective biosensors is in considerable demand because they contribute to the realization of highly precise diagnosis and individualized medicine. Therefore, a variety of biosensors has been extensively studied since the development of the first-generation biosensors using glucose oxidase in 1962. In general, biosensors typically consist of a biorecognition component for selective/specific binding with target analytes and a transducer component for converting the binding event to electrical or optical signals (Fig. 4.2.1). Because enzymes, antibodies, and DNA recognize target biomolecules selectively, they are immobilized as biorecognition components on the sensor substrate. In biosensors, the biorecognition events are generally transduced to electrical or optical signals through electrochemical or fluorescence techniques. Therefore, the development of smart materials to improve both biorecognition and transduction processes is key in designing biosensors with higher sensitivity, higher selectivity, rapid responsiveness, and low limits of detection. Thus, biosensor-related research is multidisciplinary and requires divergent knowledge in science and technology including electrochemistry, surface chemistry, biochemistry, solid-state physics, etc. This chapter will provide an overview of conventional biosensors and biosensing techniques that detect the small biomolecules, proteins, DNAs, and RNAs. Important research into the development of biosensors and biosensing techniques by utilizing surface plasmon resonance sensor (SPR), field-effect transistor (FET), and gold nanoparticles (AuNPs) will also be described.

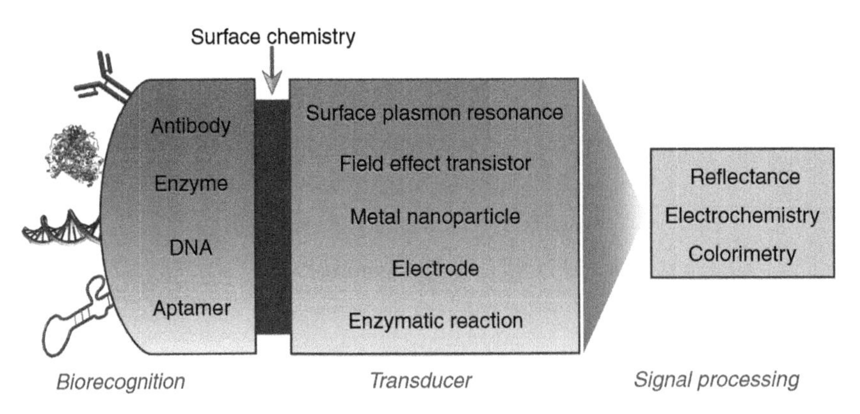

FIGURE 4.2.1 Schematic illustration of typical biosensor components.

4.2.1 Conventional Biosensors and Biosensing Techniques

4.2.1.1 Enzyme-Based Electrochemical Biosensors for Measuring Relatively Small Biomolecules

Enzyme-based electrochemical biosensors are constructed by the combination of an immobilized enzyme and a transducer. The immobilized enzyme recognizes a target molecule and catalyzes the reaction using hydrolysis and redox reactions. In a typical electrochemical biosensor, the molecular recognition events by enzymes were transduced into changes in current (*amperometric*), potential (*potentiometric*), or conductive properties of a medium (*conductometric*) induced by the enzymatic reactions. By combining enzymatic reactions with electrochemical transducers, numerous electrochemical biosensors have been developed and used in the medical fields. For example, glucose sensors are the most typical and basic enzyme-based electrochemical biosensors. Measurement of glucose concentration in the blood is the most common routine analysis in clinical chemistry. In 1962, Clark and Lyons proposed the concept of enzyme electrodes for monitoring glucose concentration [1]. The glucose sensor devices by Clark and Lyons were constructed by entrapping a thin layer of glucose oxidase (GOD) within a glucose permeable membrane on an oxygen electrode (Fig. 4.2.2). In the glucose sensor devices, monitoring the oxygen consumed in the GOD-catalyzed reactions is a key principle for the detection of glucose. Since the basic principle proposed by Clark and Lyons was successful, many research and commercial biosensors to monitor not only glucose but also other biomolecules have been produced using the concepts that utilize both enzymatic reactions and electrochemical transducers. Hundreds of biosensors have been constructed by combining various enzymatic reactions with their transducers into analytical signals. Detailed principles, constructions, and applications of other electrochemical biosensors can be found in a number of review articles [2–4].

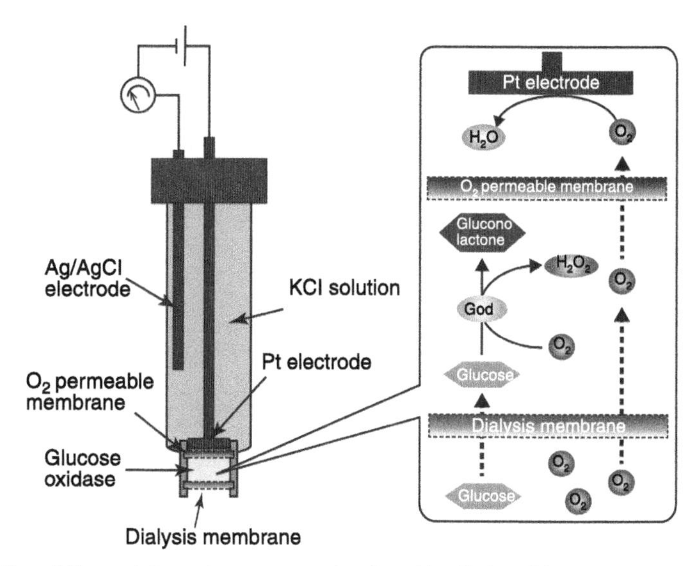

FIGURE 4.2.2 Illustration of the prototype glucose sensor developed by Clark and Lyons.

4.2.1.2 Enzyme-Linked Immunosorbent Assay (ELISA) for Measuring Proteins

Recently, the progress in proteomics accelerated the discovery of novel marker proteins that are useful signals for monitoring body conditions and diseases. In biological and medicinal fields, ELISA is the gold standard for measuring the amount of protein expression. The ELISA technique was conceptualized and developed by Perlmann's group and Schuurs' group in 1971 [5,6]. The key principle of ELISA is the complex formation between an analyte and an enzyme-conjugated antibody, followed by the enzymatic reaction that transduces to the detectable signals. In general, peroxidases are used as enzyme that react with appropriate substrates such as 2,2′-azinobis [3-ethylbenzothiazoline-6-sulfonic acid] diammonium salt and 3,3′,5,5′-tetramethylbenzidine by changing color. Two types of ELISA techniques are widely used for the detection of analytes, that is, direct ELISA and sandwich ELISA (Fig. 4.2.3). In direct ELISA, analytes are physically adsorbed onto the surface of microplates. The analytes are complexed with enzyme-conjugated antibodies, and then the amount of analyte is quantified by enzymatic reactions. However, the disadvantage of direct ELISA is the nonspecific adsorption of analytes, which is inhibited by the adhesive serum proteins such as albumin and fibrinogen. On the other hand, in sandwich ELISA, analytes are first interacted with primary antibodies attached to the surface of microplates. Then specific antibodies are added to form sandwich-like antibody–analyte–antibody complexes with the analytes bound with the primary antibodies. Finally, the amount of analyte is quantified by the enzyme-conjugated secondary antibodies that bind specifically to the Fc region of antibodies. Although the sandwich ELISA is an expensive and complicated process, it is useful for the detection of minor proteins.

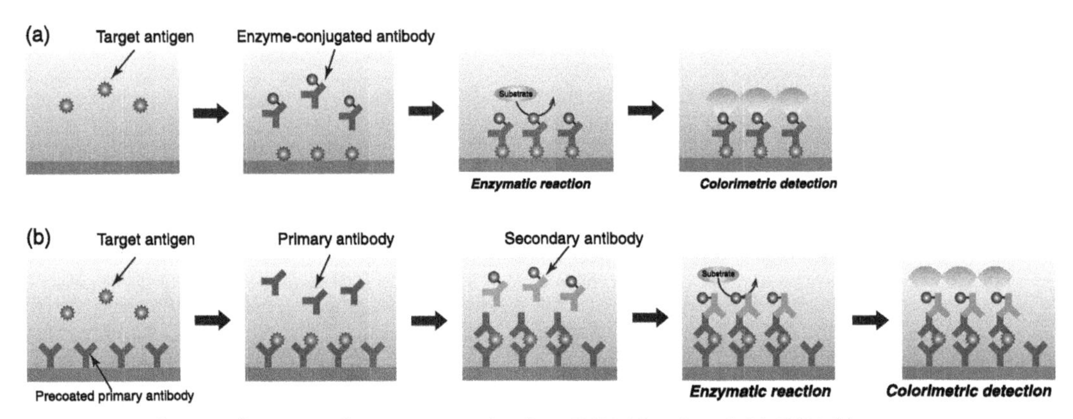

FIGURE 4.2.3 Schematic illustration of protein sensing by direct ELISA (a) and sandwich ELISA (b).

4.2.1.3 Conventional Detection Methods for DNAs and RNAs

Recent advances in genomics have led to the discovery of various kinds of DNAs and RNAs that relate to diseases and prognoses. Measuring the amount of expression of DNAs and RNAs has attracted considerable attention. Quantitative polymerase chain reaction (qPCR) and DNA microarray are modern methods for investigating gene expression. The procedure of qPCR, which is one of the typical methods for the detection and quantification of gene expression, involves the general principle of PCR. During the amplification of the target DNA by the PCR process, a DNA-binding dye such as SYBR Green shows fluorescence caused by the intercalation into the double-stranded DNA. An increase in DNA product during PCR leads to an increase in fluorescence intensity. The amount of target DNA is determined from standard curves obtained using a standard sample. On the other hand, a DNA-based fluorescent reporter probe enables the quantitative qPCR with high specificity even in the presence of nonspecific DNA amplification. The DNA-based fluorescence reporter probe has a fluorescent dye at one end and a quencher of fluorescence at the opposite end. The fluorescence reporter probe was inhibited by the closely arranged quencher molecules. After the probes are hybridized with complementary DNA strands, they are digested by the Taq polymerase that exhibits the 3′ to 5′ exonuclease activity. As a result, the fluorescent dye shows fluorescence because it is released from probes and is separated from the quencher (Fig. 4.2.4).

On the other hand, expression levels of a large number of genes were simultaneously measured with DNA microarray. In the DNA microarray, many types of known DNA fragments are densely attached on several centimeters of a glass slide or plastic resin. The core principle of DNA microarrays is hybridization between target DNA/RNA and DNA fragment for detection on the DNA microarray. In gene expression profiling analysis, mRNAs are extracted from specimens and complementary DNAs (cDNAs) with aminoallyl uracil are obtained from mRNA reverse transcription in the presence of aminoallyl uridine triphosphate. After fluorescence dyes such as Cy3 and Cy5 were conjugated with the cDNAs

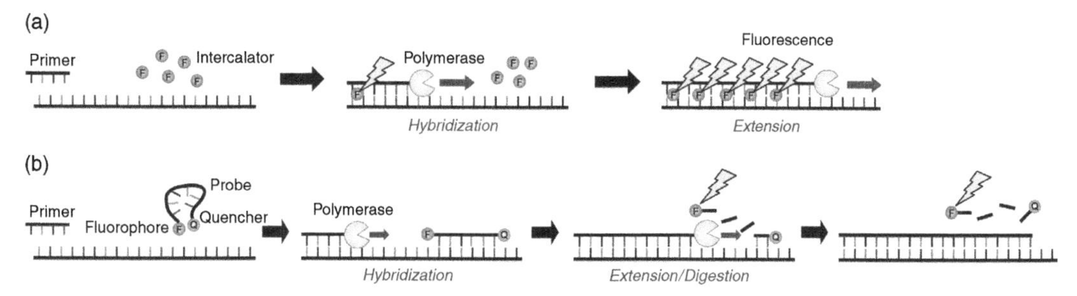

FIGURE 4.2.4 Schematics of the detection of DNA by qPCR. (a) Intercalator method; (b) probe method.

having aminoallyl uracil, the resulting fluorophore-conjugated cDNAs were directly hybridized with DNAs spotted on the DNA microarray. Subsequently, the DNA microarrays are scanned with a microarray scanner to visualize fluorescence. From the fluorescence profiles, upregulated and downregulated genes are identified. However, the disadvantage of this method is poor correlation of data with other experimental methods such as qPCR and a large amount of desired sample. Recently, mRNAs extracted from specimens are generally amplified by combining the reverse transcription and *in vitro* transcription. A small amount of mRNA can be sensitively detected by the use of amplified RNAs with a good correlation with qPCR. Although these detection methods for DNAs and RNAs have a few disadvantages of complicated protocols and high cost, they contribute to advances in molecular biology.

4.2.2 Surface Plasmon Resonance Biosensors

The surface plasmon resonance (SPR) biosensors are most commonly used as sensitive and quantitative tools to monitor binding events and to measure dynamic interactions between biomolecules in biochemical and biomedical fields. The conventional SPR biosensors detect permittivity changes in the region of the gold sensor chip surfaces, which are caused by the formation or dissociation of the bindings of analytes to ligands attached on the surfaces, as resonance angle shifts (Fig. 4.2.5). SPR biosensors are capable of characterizing the binding reactions in real time without labeling.

Basic methods for monitoring the binding of target biomolecules using SPR biosensors have been established, and we can easily obtain the instruments and some functional sensor chips from manufactures of SPR biosensors. Therefore, SPR biosensors are widely used in a variety of fields such as chemistry, biology, medicine, food science, and environmental analysis. Recently, various biomarkers such as proteins, DNAs, and RNAs that are related to the diseases and prognoses have been discovered by progress in proteomics and genomics. To detect minute amounts of such biomarkers, enhancing the sensitivity of SPR sensors is in considerable demand. In addition, preservation stability of SPR sensor chips must be improved for constructing easy-to-handle sensor chips for clinical use. This section describes the recent development of SPR sensor systems.

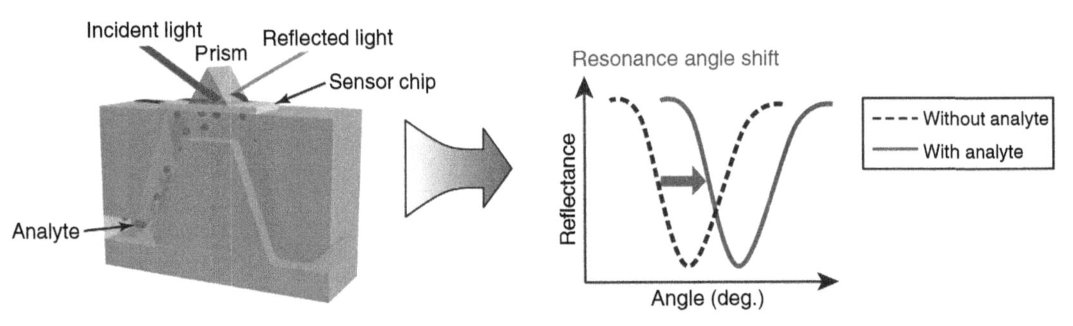

FIGURE 4.2.5 Schematic illustration of SPR sensors.

4.2.2.1 Strategies for Enhancement of SPR Biosensor Sensitivity

SPR biosensors are useful tools for measuring binding constants for biological macromolecules such as antibodies, proteins, DNAs, RNAs, and polysaccharides. However, binding of smaller analytes with a molecular weight of less than 5000 often induces no sufficient change in the refractive index on the SPR sensor chip because responsive resonance angle shift is proportional to the mass of the analyte that binds to the surface [7]. Enhancement of sensor sensitivity for analytes with low molecular weights was achieved by the "labeling" of the analytes with secondary agents with high molecular weights or high refractive indices [8–10]. For example, Lyon et al. reported the amplification of resonance angle shift using AuNPs as a secondary labeling agent (Fig. 4.2.6) [8]. First, antihuman immunoglobulin (anti-*h*IgG) was immobilized onto the SPR gold chip by the standard amino coupling method. After the complexation between AuNPs and human immunoglobulin G (*h*IgG) as an analyte through electrostatic interaction, the resulting *h*IgG–AuNPs complexes were exposed to the anti-*h*IgG-modified SPR sensor chips. A significantly larger shift was observed by the binding of *h*IgG–AuNPs complexes to the anti-*h*IgG-modified SRP sensor chips although the bindings of original *h*IgG resulted in a very small change in resonance angle shift. The approximately 15-fold increase in SPR sensitivity was achieved by the "labeling" using AuNPs. In addition, tremendous signal amplification was observed using the sandwich ELISA-like method. After the target *h*IgG was exposed to the anti-*h*IgG-modified SPR sensor chip, the secondary anti-*h*IgG antibody-conjugated AuNPs were added to the SPR sensor chip. The sandwich ELISA-like amplification in SPR measurements showed the approximately 25-fold increase in SPR sensitivity. The AuNPs-mediated amplification of SPR sensitivity is attributed to the strong optical coupling between the Au film and AuNPs. Furthermore, Mitchell et al. reported that the AuNPs-mediated signal amplification was also applicable for inhibition type analysis [9]. These results indicate that labeling by AuNPs is a useful technique for the amplification of SPR sensitivity. Similarly to the labeling by AuNPs, SPR sensitivity can be improved by the modification of polymer particles such as latex particles [10], and poly(acrylamide) hydrogel microspheres [11,12].

The sensitivity of SPR biosensors was also improved by increasing the amount of ligand biomolecules attached on the SPR sensor chips. As mentioned above, the ligand

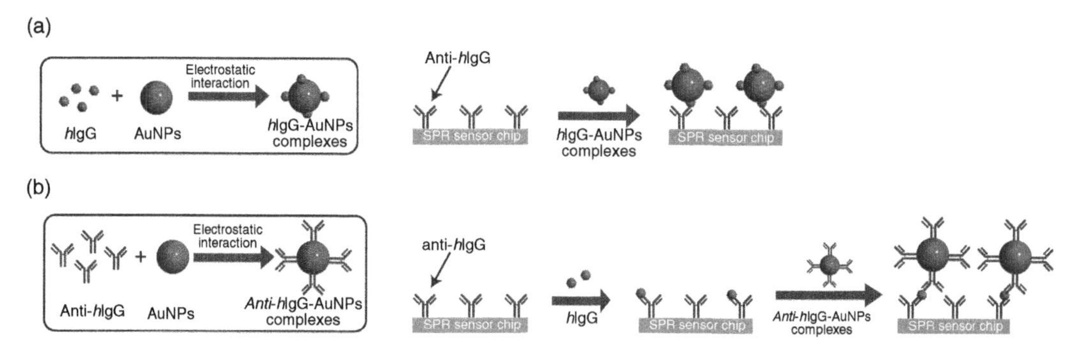

FIGURE 4.2.6 Schematics of AuNPs-mediated signal amplification of SPR measurements. (a) Signal amplification by *h*IgG–AuNPs complexes; (b) sandwich ELISA-like signal amplification.

biomolecules are immobilized onto the surface of SPR sensor chips via the reaction of ligand biomolecules with the activated SPR sensor chip surfaces by standard amine coupling methods. Therefore, the amount of ligands immobilized on the surface of the SPR sensor chips was limited by a two-dimensional space on their surfaces. The detection sensitivity of SPR biosensors was strongly correlated with the amount of the ligands immobilized on the SPR sensor chips. Recently, larger amounts of biomolecular ligands were immobilized by forming polymer brushes or thin hydrogel layers with biomolecule ligands via surface-initiated atom transfer radical polymerization (SI-ATRP) [13]. ATRP is widely utilized as a controlled/living radical polymerization, based on the catalyzed, reversible cleavage of the carbon–halogen bond in the dormant species by a redox process. In ATRP, alkyl halides are used as initiators, and a variety of transition metals and ligands are successfully employed as catalysts. Especially, the catalysts based on copper and N-containing ligands are often used. A wide variety of conjugated monomers such as (meth)acrylic esters, styrene, acrylamide, and acrylonitrile can be precisely polymerized by ATRP. In SI-ATRP, polymerization is directly initiated from the alkyl halides immobilized on the surface of substrates, followed by the formation of polymer brushes. SI-ATPR allows accurate control of the thickness of the polymer brushes formed on the substrate.

By SI-ATRP, antibody-immobilized hydrogel layers were prepared on the surface of SPR sensor chips. The thickness of the antibody-immobilized hydrogel layer on the sensor chip was controlled by the polymerization time. The resonance angle shift of the three-dimensionally antibody-immobilized hydrogel layer chip was larger than that of the directly antibody-immobilized chip prepared by the standard amino coupling method. In addition, the resonance angle shift increased with an increase in thickness of antibody-immobilized hydrogel layer up to 225 nm (Fig. 4.2.7). However, the resonance angle shift of the three-dimensionally antibody-immobilized hydrogel layer chip decreased to a small value similar to that of the directly antibody-immobilized chip when the layer thickness increased above 225 nm. An SPR sensor can detect a change in permittivity in a range of less than 300 nm from top surface of an SPR gold chip [14]. Therefore, a change in permittivity in the vicinity of the gold surface of a too thick hydrogel layer chip becomes small in spite

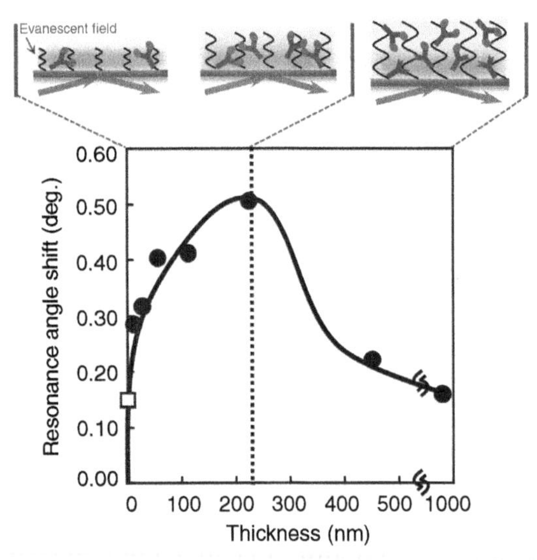

FIGURE 4.2.7 Relationship between gel layer thickness and maximum resonance angle shift of IgG-immobilized gel layer chip in a buffer solution containing rabbit IgG as a target antigen. *Reproduced from Ref. [13], with permission from Chemical Society of Japan, Copyright (2012).*

of a large amount of antibody immobilized within the hydrogel layer. Thus, the sensitivity of SPR sensor chips can be improved by the formation of hydrogel layers with an optimal thickness. Because the recent development of proteomics has led to the great discovery of various minor proteins acting as biomarkers, the successful design of ligand-immobilized hydrogel layer chips with an optimal thickness will contribute to the fabrication of high sensitive diagnostic tools for the detection of these minor proteins.

4.2.2.2 Molecularly Imprinted Layers on SPR Sensor Chips

In the SPR biosensors for detecting relatively large biomolecules as analytes, proteins, saccharides, and DNAs that can interact with target biomolecules are usually utilized as their ligands. However, poor chemical and physical stability of biomolecules sometimes prevents their use in harsh environments such as acidic or basic environments and high temperatures.

Molecular imprinting has attracted considerable attention as a useful technique for creating synthetic hosts having molecular recognition sites [15,16]. In standard molecular imprinting, after polymerizable functional groups as ligands are prearranged around a template molecule by noncovalent interactions, they are copolymerized with a large amount of cross-linker. Molecularly imprinted polymers with molecular recognition sites are then obtained by extraction of the template molecule from the resultant polymer networks to create a complementary molecular cavity (Fig. 4.2.8). Differing from the biomolecular ligands that lose their molecular recognition functions easily by changes in temperature and pH, the molecule recognition sites created by molecular imprinting

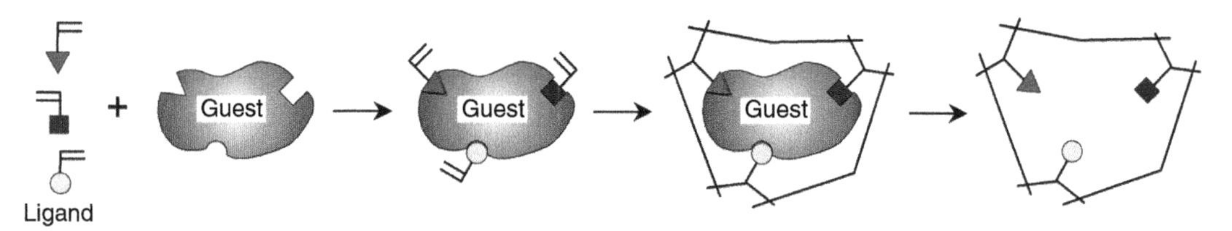

FIGURE 4.2.8 Schematic illustration of molecular imprinting.

are relatively stable. In 1998, pioneering works for the preparation of SPR sensor chips with molecularly imprinted layers were reported by Lai et al. [17]. They synthesized molecularly imprinted polymers by copolymerization of poly(methyl methacrylate) and ethylene glycol dimethacrylate in the presence of theophylline, caffeine, and xanthine as a template. After the removal of the template molecules from the resulting polymer networks, the molecularly imprinted polymer layers were prepared onto the silver thin films by evaporation from polymer solution in acetonitrile–acetic acid (99:1 v/v) spotted on the silver film substrate. The uptake of target molecules such as theophylline, caffeine, and xanthine into the molecularly imprinted polymer layers prepared on the surface of SPR silver chips was measured as a resonance angle shift after the exposure of SPR silver chips to the target molecule solution. The resonance angle shift of the SPR silver chip with molecularly imprinted polymer layer increased with an increase in target molecules and there was good linearity between their concentration and resonance angle shift. On the other hand, cross-recognition studies of the SPR silver chips with theophylline- or caffeine-imprinted polymer layer revealed that no or very slight resonance angel shifts were observed in the presence of molecules having similar structures to theophylline and caffeine. These results indicate that the creation of molecular recognition sites by molecular imprinting with an SPR sensor enables us to fabricate SPR sensor chips without using unstable biomolecular ligands.

In standard molecular imprinting, the resulting polymer networks are highly cross-linked by a large amount of cross-linker to fix the structure of cavities as molecular recognition sites. However, the formation of molecular recognition sites by molecular imprinting using a template protein seems to be difficult because the three-dimensional structure of the protein is denatured under harsh conditions. Molecular imprinting has also been utilized to create molecular recognition sites within swollen hydrogels slightly cross-linked with a minute amount of cross-linker, that is, molecule-imprinted hydrogel. The hydrogels composed of flexible polymer networks with large open spaces can memorize macromolecules with a large size such as proteins in molecular imprinting. For example, α-fetoprotein (AFP)-responsive hydrogels were strategically prepared by molecular imprinting that used lectin and antibody as biomolecular ligands [18,19]. AFP is a tumor-specific marker glycoprotein that is widely used for the diagnosis of hepatocellular carcinoma, germ cell tumors, and metastatic cancers of the liver. In preparing the AFP-responsive hydrogels by molecular imprinting, lectin concanavalin A (ConA) and anti-AFP antibody were utilized as ligands for saccharide and peptide chains of AFP, respectively. First, polymerizable acryloyl groups were conjugated to the ConA and anti-AFP antibody. After synthesis of ConA-conjugated poly(acrylamide) (ConA-PAAm) by copolymerization of acryloyl–ConA with acrylamide, acryloyl anti-AFP antibody was copolymerized with AAm and *N*, *N'*-methylenebisacrylamide (MBAA) with forming ConA–AFP–antibody complexes among ConA-PAAm, template AFP, and acryloyl anti-AFP antibody. AFP-imprinted hydrogel was prepared by the removal of the template AFP from resultant PAAm interpenetrating polymer network hydrogel. The AFP-imprinted hydrogel shrank gradually but nonimprinted hydrogel prepared without template AFP swelled slightly when they were immersed in a phosphate buffer solution with AFP (Fig. 4.2.9). In addition, the swelling ratio of the AFP-imprinted hydrogel decreased with an increase in the AFP concentration of a buffer solution. Molecular imprinting enables lectins and antibodies to be arranged at optimal positions for the simultaneous recognition of saccharide and peptide chains in the AFP molecule. Therefore, AFP-responsive shrinking of the AFP-imprinted hydrogel is attributed to the formation of sandwich-like lectin–AFP–antibody complexes that act as dynamic cross-links. However, as lectins and antibodies in the nonimprinted hydrogel are not arranged at optimal positions for simultaneously recognizing saccharide and peptide moieties of AFP, the cross-linking density of the nonimprinted hydrogel remains unchanged due to the formation of no lectin–AFP–antibody complex. Therefore, a slight swelling of the nonimprinted hydrogel in the presence of AFP was based on a change in osmotic pressure, which was caused by binding of AFP to lectin or antibody.

By combining protein-imprinted hydrogel and SPR sensor, the protein recognition behavior of protein-imprinted hydrogel can be converted to the resonance angle shift. Recently, SPR sensor chips with protein-imprinted hydrogel layers were prepared by SI-ATRP combined with molecular imprinting [20]. For example, recognition sites for a protein in the thin hydrogel layer on the SPR sensor chips were created by molecular imprinting using ConA as a template protein and a monomer with pendant glucose (2-glucosyloxyethyl methacrylate: GEMA) as its ligand. After the complexation of GEMA with ConA with an acryloyl group, the GEMA–ConA complexes were copolymerized with AAm and MBAA by SI-ATRP on SPR sensor chips modified with alkylbromide as an ATRP initiator. The template ConA was removed from the resulting hydrogel network by immersing in an aqueous glucose solution. The thickness of the ConA-imprinted hydrogel layer on the SPR sensor chips increased with an increase in polymerization time of SI-ATRP for layer formation. In the SPR measurements, the resonance angle shift of the ConA-imprinted hydrogel layer chips in response to target ConA was much larger than that of the nonimprinted hydrogel layer chips prepared without using the template ConA (Fig. 4.2.10). In addition, the affinity constant of the ConA-imprinted hydrogel layer chips for ConA was much higher than that of the nonimprinted hydrogel layer chips. The larger resonance angle shift and higher affinity constant of the ConA-imprinted hydrogel layer chip to ConA is attributed to the fact that molecular imprinting with a minute amount of cross-linker enables the arrangement of GEMA ligands at suitable positions for binding target ConA in the imprinted network. In contrast, the nonimprinted hydrogel layer chips had a smaller affinity constant for target

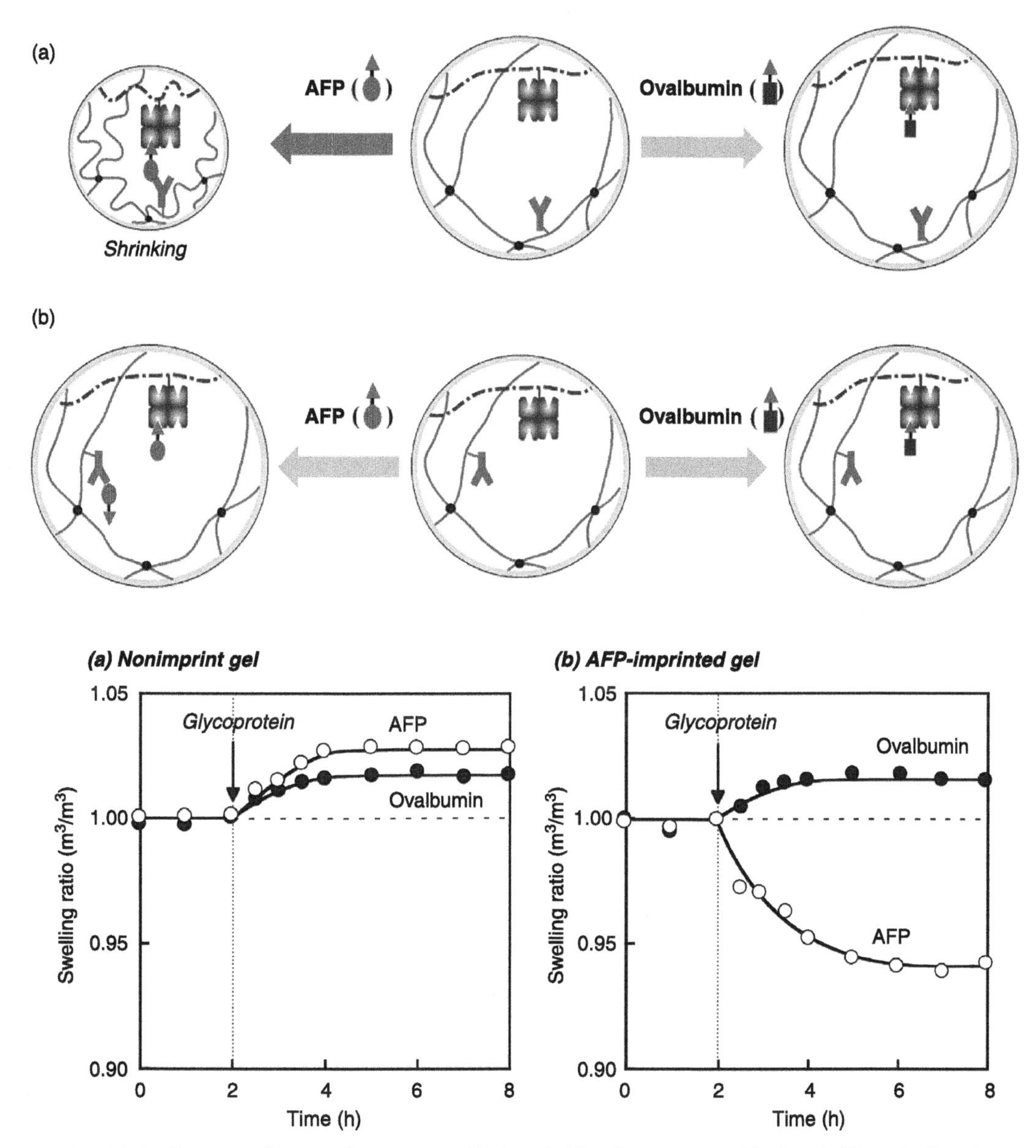

FIGURE 4.2.9 Swelling ratio changes of nonimprinted hydrogels (a) and AFP-imprinted hydrogels (b) in a buffer solution with α-fetoprotein (AFP) (◦) and ovalbumin (•).

ConA because the GEMA ligands were randomly distributed in their network. As a result, the nonimprinted hydrogel layer chips exhibited a smaller change in resonance angle shift in response to target ConA. The SPR sensor chips with biomolecule-imprinted hydrogel layers are likely to be a fundamental system for the highly sensitive and accurate detection of target biomolecules.

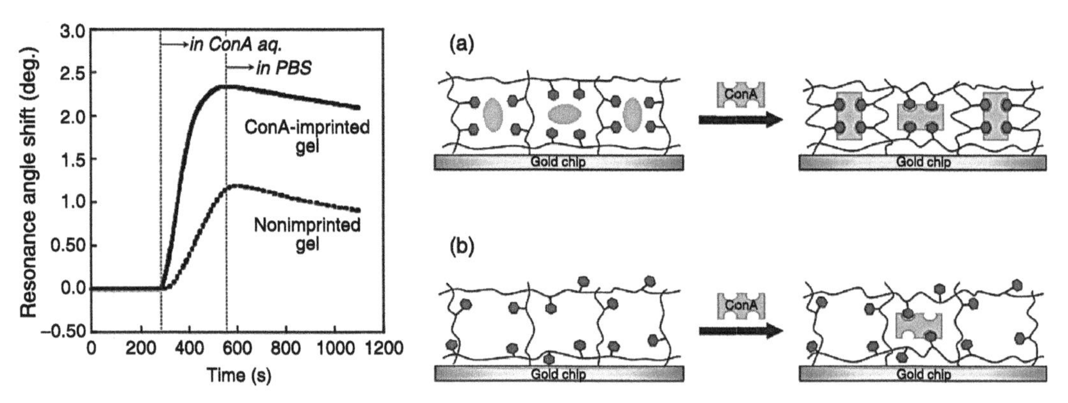

FIGURE 4.2.10 Resonance angle shift of (a) ConA-imprinted hydrogel layer chip (solid line) and (b) nonimprinted hydrogel layer chip (dashed line) in PBS containing 1 μM ConA as an analyte. *Reproduced from Ref. [20], with permission from Chemical Society of Japan, Copyright (2014).*

4.2.3 Field-Effect Transistor-Based Biosensors

Recent developments of nanotechnology provided many essential platforms for the miniaturization and integration of electronic devices. Miniaturization and integration of sensing devices have been extensively studied for the development of biosensors because they enable the diagnosis for point-of-care testing (POCT) with high sensitivity and easy handling. In particular, FETs have attracted considerable attention for fabricating biosensors. FETs consist of *source, drain,* and *gate* electrodes (Fig. 4.2.11). FETs use an electric field to control the conductivity of a source–drain "channel" in a semiconducting material. The conductivity of a source–drain "channel" depended on the changes in electric field potential at the gate electrode. In many different types of FET devices, ion-sensitive FETs (ISFETs) are the most basic and extensively studied for fabricating biosensors. FET-based biosensors are generally prepared by the surface modification of metal gate electrodes with appropriate biological recognition elements such as enzymes, antibodies, and DNAs. When the surface charge density changes by the biomolecular recognition events on the surface of the gate electrode, the corresponding source–drain voltage–current (V_{DS}–I_D) curve is shifted along the voltage axis. The curve shift depends on a concentration of the target biomolecule as an analyte because the carrier density is sensitive to the changes in the electric field in a direction perpendicular to the gate surface [4,21,22]. The most popular FET-based biosensors are the enzymatic reaction-coupled FETs (En-FTEs) in which enzymes are immobilized on the gate surface of ISFET devices. Enzymatic reactions influence the presence of accumulated charge carriers on the gate surface in proportion to the original analyte concentration. Some analytes such as a series of saccharides, urea, penicillin, ethanol, formaldehyde, organophosphorus pesticides, ascorbic acid, acetylcholine, and creatinine were detectable using En-FTE sensing systems.

FETs can monitor the direct binding of target biomolecules onto the surface of a gate electrode because of the changes in charge distribution across the direction perpendicular

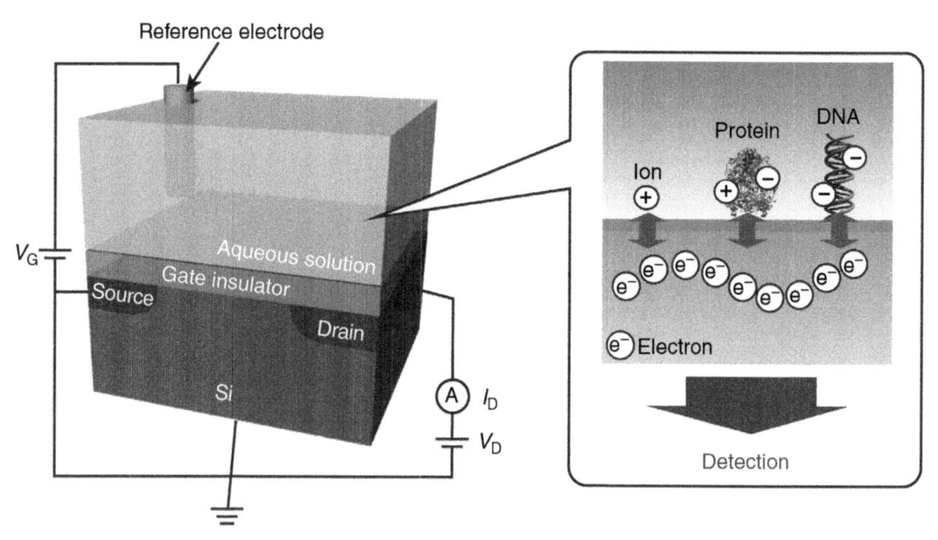

FIGURE 4.2.11 Schematic illustration of structures and principles of FETs.

to the surface of a gate electrode [23]. However, FETs can detect a change in charge within a very short distance corresponding to the Debye length, which is no greater than a few nanometers under physiological ionic strength. The screening effect of counter ions strongly influences the charge detection of FETs, which is severely hampered above the Debye length. To overcome this weakness, dynamic assays involving step-wise addition of target biomolecules and kinetic analysis were applied for the ISFETs. The nonspecific adsorption of proteins was also investigated using ISFETs. Differing from the conventional ISFETs, self-assembled monolayers (SAMs) of alkane thiols with various terminal groups were formed on the surface of a thin gold layer fabricated on the gate electrode. Adsorption of various proteins such as bovine serum albumin, lysozyme, and bovine plasma fibrinogen onto the SAMs was monitored by the gate voltage changes. Although the adsorption of bovine plasma fibrinogen could not be quantitatively detected because of its larger size than the Debye length, highly sensitive and quantitative detection of small proteins was successfully achieved by ISFETs without protein labeling [24].

FETs have attracted much attention as electrochemical devices for monitoring not only proteins but also DNAs and RNAs. Because more and more DNAs and RNAs related to the diseases have been discovered, the development of sensor systems for detecting DNAs and RNAs is in considerable demand. As described in the previous section, the current gold standards for the detection of DNAs and RNAs are real-time PCR and DNA chips. In such standard detection systems, however, fluorescence labeling is needed for the detection of DNAs and RNAs, causing the loss of analytes. In this regard, the FETs offer attractive alternatives as they can detect the negatively charged DNAs and RNAs without labeling. The hybridization of DNAs can be monitored by the shift of the electrical characteristics such as V_{DS}–I_D or the threshold gate voltage (V_T) [25–30]. In addition, FETs enable DNA sequencing by using primer extension reactions [31] (Fig. 4.2.12). For example, after

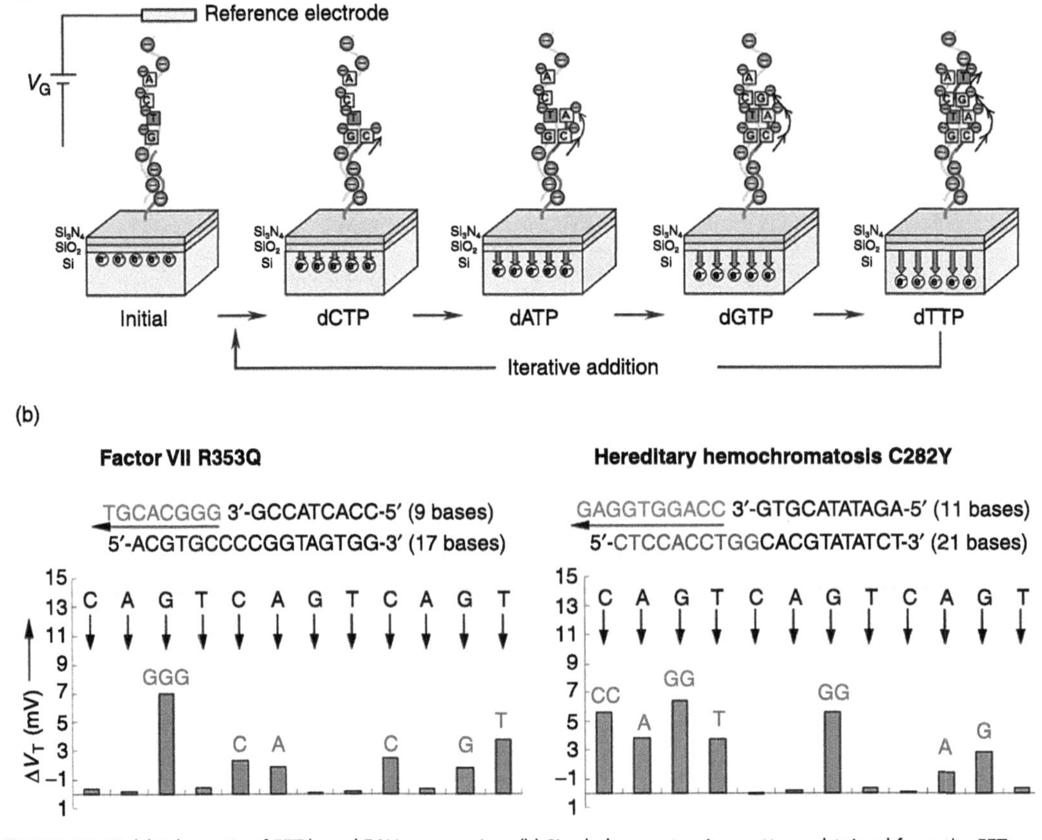

FIGURE 4.2.12 (a) Schematic of FET-based DNA sequencing. (b) Single-base extension pattern obtained from the FET-based DNA sequencing. *Reproduced from Ref. [31], with permission from Wiley-VCH Verlag & Co., Copyright (2006).*

the target DNAs were hybridized with the oligonucleotide probes immobilized on the surface of a FET gate electrode, the DNA polymerase extended the immobilized oligonucleotide probes in a template-dependent manner during sequential addition of each deoxynucleotide. The extension of the template DNAs induced an increase in negative charge, which could be detected as a shift in V_T. This technique enabled the reading of sequence and identification of single nucleotide polymorphisms (SNPs) of target DNAs [32]. Although the readable maximum base number was 40 base or less because of the Debye length effect, the sensing systems using FETs are candidates for fabricating label-free DNA/RNA sensors. In addition, Matsumoto et al. reported the novel strategy for constructing FET-based biosensors with "Debye length-free" molecular recognition functions [33]. They prepared the glucose-responsive hydrogels with phenylboronic acid moieties, which were swollen layers with 50 μm thickness, on the surface of the FET gate electrode. The glucose-responsive hydrogels with phenylboronic acid moieties exhibited swelling in response to glucose because of complex formation between glucose and the phenylboronic acid group, resulting in an increase in negatively charged phenylboronic acid groups [34–37]. The physicochemical changes were initiated from the surface of the hydrogel layers on the gate electrode and geometrically propagated across a macroscopic layer thickness beyond the barrier of "Debye length." The permittivity change of the hydrogel, which was a dominant source of signals, was induced by the volume change of the hydrogel layers. These phase transition-synchronized systems are capable of detecting not only charged molecules but also noncharged molecules such as glucose. These FET-based biosensors have many advantages in constructing biosensing systems because the FETs enable us to monitor target biomolecules without labeling and can be integrated by nanofabrication technologies.

4.2.4 Gold Nanoparticles-Based Optically Detectable Biosensors

Recently, metal nanoparticles have attracted much attention for use in biomedical fields because of their unique physicochemical properties such as catalytic, optical, and magnetic properties. In particular, AuNPs possess distinct physical and chemical properties that are useful as transducer components for fabricating chemical and biological sensors [38]. Unique optical properties of AuNPs are based on SPR resulting from the collective oscillation of the conduction electrons. Monodisperse AuNPs showed a rich red color in solution because SPR phenomena cause absorption of light in the blue-green portion of the spectrum (~450 nm) while red light (~700 nm) is reflected. In addition, the aggregation of AuNPs results in significant red-shifting of SPR absorption maximum and then the color of the AuNP solution changes from red to blue because of the interparticle plasmon coupling at nanomolar concentrations [39]. The changes in color in response to the aggregation of AuNPs provide a practical platform for colorimetric sensors. AuNPs have been successfully applied for colorimetric detection of biomolecules such as proteins, saccharides, and oligonucleotides similarly to latex agglutination assays. The pioneering work of the AuNPs-based colorimetric assays was demonstrated by Mirkin et al. in 1996 [40]. They prepared the AuNPs functionalized with thiolated DNA strands. Two types of thiolated single-strand DNAs (ssDNAs) that are complementary to both ends of a target oligonucleotide were grafted onto the surface of AuNPs. The addition of target ssDNA induced the aggregation of ssDNA-modified AuNPs by hybridization of their DNA strand, leading to a drastic change in color of the solution from red to blue (Fig. 4.2.13). The AuNP aggregates were redispersed by thermal dissociation of double-stranded DNAs (dsDNAs). Furthermore, the AuNPs-based colorimetric DNA sensing systems enabled the differentiation of DNAs with single base pair mismatches by measuring absorbance as a function of temperature [41]. Meanwhile, Maeda et al. reported that the aggregation of DNA-functionalized AuNPs was induced by only hybridization of target DNA without cross-linking between AuNPs [42]. These AuNPs-based DNA sensing systems have several

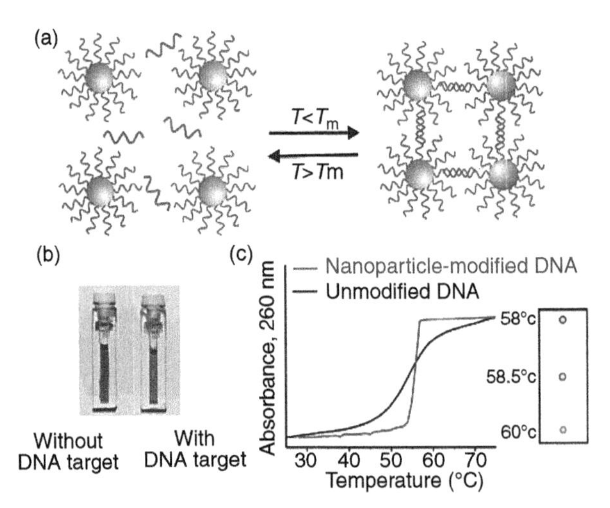

FIGURE 4.2.13 (a) Schematic image of the aggregation of oligonucleotide-modified AuNPs in the presence of complementary target single-strand DNA. (b) Photograph of the oligonucleotide-modified AuNPs without and with target DNA. (c) Thermal dissociation curves for double stranded oligonucleotide-modified AuNPs and double stranded oligonucleotide without AuNPs. *Reproduced from Ref. [38], with permission from American Chemical Society, Copyright (2012).*

advantages over other techniques such as real-time PCR and DNA microarrays probed by fluorescence because they enable "quick and easy" measurements and optical readout with a high degree of discrimination between perfectly matched target oligonucleotides and single base pair mismatches.

AuNPs-based biosensors were fabricated by combining the DNA functions with optical properties of AuNPs because DNAs have unique functions such as target molecular binding and catalytic reactions. For example, aptamer-based AuNP biosensors were strategically designed for colorimetric detection of small molecules. Aptamers are single-stranded oligonucleic acid-based binding molecules that are prepared by the combinatorial method of systematic evolution of ligands by exponential enrichment (SELEX). These functional DNA and RNA structures enable aptamers to bind to a target molecule with high affinity and specificity. Lu et al. prepared the AuNPs-based adenosine sensors by utilizing adenosine aptamers [43]. In the AuNPs-based adenosine sensors, the linker DNA with a certain sequence acted as an adenosine aptamer that was hybridized with ssDNA attached on the surface of AuNPs. When the aptamer on the sensor changed its structure by specific binding to adenosine, the dissociation of AuNP aggregates caused a concomitant blue-to-red color change (Fig. 4.2.14). On the other hand, no change in their color was observed in the presence of other nucleic bases such as cytidine, uridine, and guanosine. The AuNPs-based adenosine sensing systems enabled the selective recognition of adenosine with a dynamic range of 0.3–2 mM. The generality of the sensing system using both aptamers and AuNPs was demonstrated using cocaine [43,44], theophylline [45], Ochratoxin A [46], and platelet-derived growth factors [47] as target molecules.

Numerous carbohydrate-functionalized AuNPs have also been designed for the detection of glucose and lectins. Geddes et al. demonstrated the competitive colorimetric

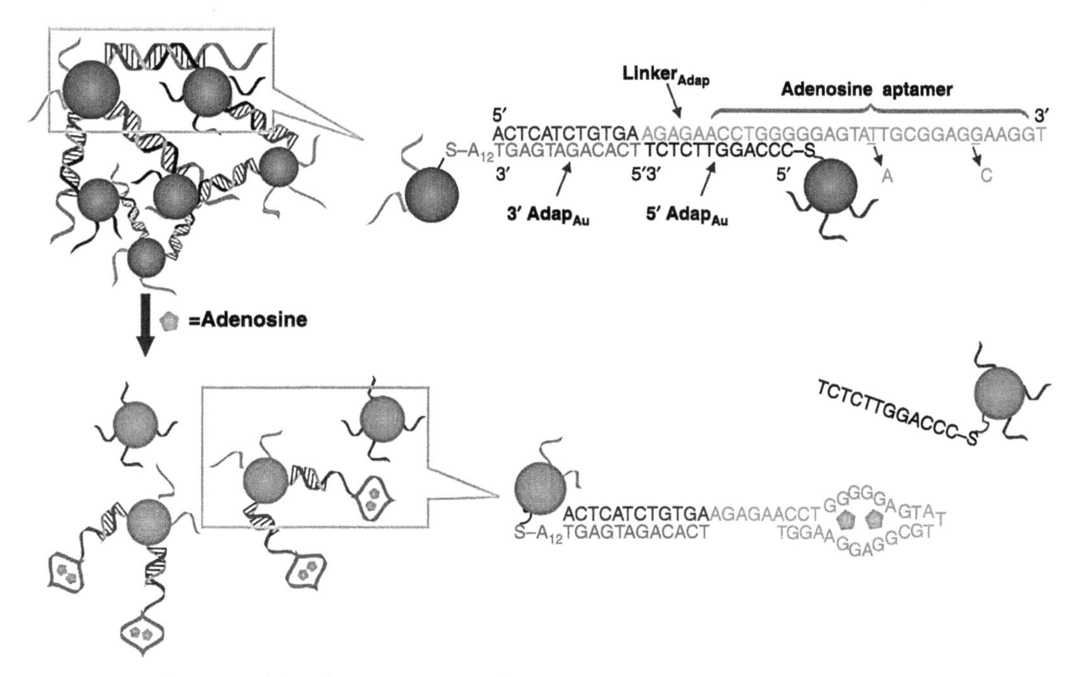

FIGURE 4.2.14 Schematics of the colorimetric sensing of adenosine by aptamer-modified gold nanoparticles (AuNPs). *Reproduced from Ref. [43], with permission from Wiley-VCH Verlag & Co., Copyright (2006).*

glucose assay using dextran-functionalized AuNPs [48,49]. The dextran-functionalized AuNPs were aggregated in the presence of lectin ConA caused by the multivalent complex formation between ConA and dextran. The addition of glucose to the solution containing the AuNP aggregates induced their dissociation because glucose competitively binds to ConA. Using the AuNPs-based glucose sensing system, the glucose concentration with a dynamic range of 1–40 mM was readily monitored by either conventional ultraviolet-visible spectroscopy or wavelength ratiometric resonance light scattering measurement.

There are some reports describing carbohydrate-functionalized AuNPs for the detection of carbohydrate-binding proteins. For example, Otsuka et al. prepared the β-D-lactopyranoside (Lac)-functionalized AuNPs for the detection of *Ricinus communis* agglutinin (RCA_{120}), which is a bivalent lectin specifically recognizing the β-D-galactose residue [50]. They synthesized the heterobifunctional poly(ethylene glycol) (PEG) with both thiol and acetal groups. First, PEG-modified AuNPs were prepared by *in situ* aqueous reduction of chloroauric acid in the presence of heterobifunctional PEG. After the conversion of acetal groups into the aldehyde by gentle acid treatment, the amino-functionalized Lac was conjugated to the aldehyde groups on the surface of PEG-modified AuNPs. The Lac-functionalized AuNPs were aggregated in the presence of RCA_{120}, and the degree of the aggregation was proportional to the RCA_{120} concentration. The Lac-functionalized AuNPs allowed lectin detection with significantly high sensitivity that was nearly the same as that of ELISA. The AuNPs-based biosensors described in this section have some advantages in the detection of target biomolecules because of their easy handling, optical detection, and high sensitivity. They are likely to become important materials for fabricating POCT biosensors.

4.2.5 Summary

Research and development of biosensors is becoming the most extensively studied discipline because the easy, rapid, low-cost, highly sensitive, and highly selective biosensors contribute to advances in next-generation medicines such as individualized medicine and ultrasensitive point-of-care detection of markers for diseases. This chapter overviewed conventional biosensors and biosensing techniques and highlighted the recent advances of important biosensors such as SPR-based biosensors, FET-based biosensors, and AuNPs-based biosensors from the viewpoint of smart biomaterials. The representative works described in this chapter obviously indicate that the biosensor-related researches are literally interdisciplinary. The advances in surface chemistry provide a variety of new methods for designing target molecule recognition systems. Furthermore, the advances in nanofabrication technologies promise not only construction of novel transducers but also miniaturization and integration of biosensors with high throughput. Therefore, interdisciplinary efforts beyond the conventional specialties are required for the development of innovative biosensors. The combination of much interdisciplinary knowledge will accelerate the development of biosensors and contribute to revolutionize the biomedical fields.

References

[1] L.C. Clark, C. Lyons, Electrode systems for continuous monitoring in cardiovascular surgery, Ann. NY Acad. Sci. 102 (1962) 29–45.

[2] J.E. Frew, H.A.O. Hill, Electrochemical biosensors, Anal. Chem. 59 (1987) 933A–944A.

[3] M. Mehrvar, M. Abdi, Recent developments, characteristics, and potential applications of electrochemical biosensors, Anal. Sci. 20 (2004) 1113–1126.

[4] D. Grieshaber, R. MacKenzie, J. Voros, E. Reimhult, Electrochemical biosensors – sensor principles and architectures, Sensors 8 (2008) 1400–1458.

[5] E. Engvall, P. Perlmann, Enzyme-linked immunosorbent assay (ELISA) quantitative assay of immunoglobulin G, Immunochemistry 8 (1971) 871–874.

[6] B.K. Van Weemen, A.H.W.M. Schuurs, Immunoassay using antigen–enzyme conjugates, FEBS Lett. 15 (1971) 232–236.

[7] J. Homola, Surface plasmon resonance sensors for detection of chemical and biological species, Chem. Rev. 108 (2008) 462–493.

[8] L.A. Lyon, M.D. Musick, M.J. Natan, Colloidal Au-enhanced surface plasmon resonance immunosensing, Anal. Chem. 70 (1998) 5177–5183.

[9] J.S. Mitchell, Y. Wu, C.J. Cook, L. Main, Sensitivity enhancement of surface plasmon resonance biosensing of small molecules, Anal. Biochem. 343 (2005) 125–135.

[10] S. Kubitschko, J. Spinke, T. Bruckner, S. Pohl, N. Oranth, Sensitivity enhancement of optical immunosensors with nanoparticles, Anal. Biochem. 253 (1997) 112–122.

[11] Y. Sato, S. Ikegaki, K. Suzuki, H. Kawaguchi, Hydrogel-microsphere-enhanced surface plasmon resonance for the detection of a K-ras point mutation employing peptide nucleic acid, J. Biomater. Sci. – Polym. Ed. 14 (2003) 803–820.

[12] A. Okumura, Y. Sato, M. Kyo, H. Kawaguchi, Point mutation detection with the sandwich method employing hydrogel nanospheres by the surface plasmon resonance imaging technique, Anal. Biochem. 339 (2005) 328–337.

[13] Y. Kuriu, M. Ishikawa, A. Kawamura, T. Uragami, T. Miyata, SPR signals of three-dimensional antibody-immobilized gel layers formed on sensor chips by atom transfer radical polymerization, Chem. Lett. 41 (2012) 1660–1662.

[14] P. Pattnaik, Surface plasmon resonance: applications in understanding receptor–ligand interaction, Appl. Biochem. Biotechnol. 126 (2005) 079–092.

[15] K. Haupt, K. Mosbach, Molecularly imprinted polymers and their use in biomimetic sensors, Chem. Rev. 100 (2000) 2495–2504.

[16] G. Wulff, Enzyme-like catalysis by molecularly imprinted polymers, Chem. Rev. 102 (2002) 1–28.

[17] E.P.C. Lai, A. Fafara, V.A. VanderNoot, M. Kono, B. Polsky, Surface plasmon resonance sensors using molecularly imprinted polymers for sorbent assay of theophylline, caffeine, and xanthine, Can. J. Chem. 76 (1998) 265–273.

[18] T. Miyata, M. Jige, T. Nakaminami, T. Uragami, Tumor marker-responsive behavior of gels prepared by biomolecular imprinting, Proc. Natl. Acad. Sci. USA 103 (2006) 1190–1193.

[19] T. Miyata, T. Hayashi, Y. Kuriu, T. Uragami, Responsive behavior of tumor-marker-imprinted hydrogels using macromolecular cross-linkers, J. Mol. Recog. 25 (2012) 336–343.

[20] Y. Kuriu, A. Kawamura, T. Uragami, T. Miyata, Formation of thin molecularly imprinted hydrogel layers with lectin recognition sites on SPR sensor chips by atom transfer radical polymerization, Chem. Lett. 43 (2014) 825–827.

[21] A. Matsumoto, Y. Miyahara, Current and emerging challenges of field effect transistor based biosensing, Nanoscale 5 (2013) 10702–10718.

[22] P. Bergveld, Thirty years of ISFETOLOGY, Sensors Actuat. B 88 (2003) 1–20.

[23] R.B.M. Schasfoort, R.P.H. Kooyman, P. Bergveld, J. Greve, A new approach to immunoFET operation, Biosens. Bioelectron. 5 (1990) 103–124.

[24] T. Goda, Y. Miyahara, Detection of microenvironmental changes induced by protein adsorption onto self-assembled monolayers using an extended gate-field effect transistor, Anal. Chem. 82 (2010) 1803–1810.

[25] E. Souteyrand, J.P. Cloarec, J.R. Martin, C. Wilson, I. Lawrence, S. Mikkelsen, M.F. Lawrence, Direct detection of the hybridization of synthetic homo-oligomer DNA sequences by field effect, J. Phys. Chem. B 101 (1997) 2980–2985.

[26] J. Fritz, E.B. Cooper, S. Gaudet, P.K. Sorger, S.R. Manalis, Electronic detection of DNA by its intrinsic molecular charge, Proc. Natl. Acad. Sci. USA 99 (2002) 14142–14146.

[27] F. Uslu, S. Ingebrandt, D. Mayer, S. Bocker-Meffert, M. Odenthal, A. Offenhausser, Label-free fully electronic nucleic acid detection system based on a field-effect transistor device, Biosens. Bioelectron. 19 (2004) 1723–1731.

[28] D.S. Kim, Y.T. Jeong, H.J. Park, J.K. Shin, P. Choi, J.H. Lee, G. Lim, An FET-type charge sensor for highly sensitive detection of DNA sequence, Biosens. Bioelectron. 20 (2004) 69–74.

[29] F. Pouthas, C. Gentil, D. Côte, U. Bockelmann, DNA detection on transistor arrays following mutation-specific enzymatic amplification, Appl. Phys. Lett. 84 (2004) 1594.

[30] D.-S. Kim, Y.-T. Jeong, H.-K. Lyu, H.-J. Park, H.S. Kim, J.-K. Shin, P. Choi, J.-H. Lee, G. Lim, M. Ishida, Fabrication and characteristics of a field effect transistor-type charge sensor for detecting deoxyribonucleic acid sequence, Jpn. J. Appl. Phys. 42 (2003) 4111–4115.

[31] T. Sakata, Y. Miyahara, DNA sequencing based on intrinsic molecular charges, Angew. Chem. Int. Ed. Engl. 45 (2006) 2225–2228.

[32] T. Sakata, Y. Miyahara, Potentiometric detection of single nucleotide polymorphism by using a genetic field-effect transistor, ChemBioChem 6 (2005) 703–710.

[33] A. Matsumoto, N. Sato, T. Sakata, R. Yoshida, K. Kataoka, Y. Miyahara, Chemical-to-electrical-signal transduction synchronized with smart gel volume phase transition, Adv. Mater. 21 (2009) 4372–4378.

[34] K. Kataoka, H. Togawa, A. Harada, K. Yasugi, T. Matsumoto, S. Katayose, Spontaneous formation of polyion complex micelles with narrow distribution from antisense oligonucleotide and cationic block copolymer in physiological saline, Macromolecules 29 (1996) 8556–8557.

[35] A. Matsumoto, S. Ikeda, A. Harada, K. Kataoka, Glucose-responsive polymer bearing a novel phenylborate derivative as a glucose-sensing moiety operating at physiological pH conditions, Biomacromolecules 4 (2003) 1410–1416.

[36] A. Matsumoto, T. Ishii, J. Nishida, H. Matsumoto, K. Kataoka, Y. Miyahara, A synthetic approach toward a self-regulated insulin delivery system, Angew. Chem. Int. Ed. Engl. 51 (2012) 2124–2128.

[37] A. Matsumoto, R. Yoshida, K. Kataoka, Glucose-responsive polymer gel bearing phenylborate derivative as a glucose-sensing moiety operating at the physiological pH, Biomacromolecules 5 (2004) 1038–1045.

[38] K. Saha, S.S. Agasti, C. Kim, X. Li, V.M. Rotello, Gold nanoparticles in chemical and biological sensing, Chem. Rev. 112 (2012) 2739–2779.

[39] K.H. Su, Q.H. Wei, X. Zhang, J.J. Mock, D.R. Smith, S. Schultz, Interparticle coupling effects on plasmon resonances of nanogold particles, Nano Lett. 3 (2003) 1087–1090.

[40] C.A. Mirkin, R.L. Letsinger, R.C. Mucic, J.J. Storhoff, A DNA-based method for rationally assembling nanoparticles into macroscopic materials, Nature 382 (1996) 607–609.

[41] R. Elghanian, J.J. Storhoff, R.C. Mucic, R.L. Letsinger, C.A. Mirkin, Selective colorimetric detection of polynucleotides based on the distance-dependent optical properties of gold nanoparticles, Science 277 (1997) 1078–1081.

[42] K. Sato, K. Hosokawa, M. Maeda, Rapid aggregation of gold nanoparticles induced by non-cross-linking DNA hybridization, J. Am. Chem. Soc. 125 (2003) 8102–8103.

[43] J. Liu, Y. Lu, Fast colorimetric sensing of adenosine and cocaine based on a general sensor design involving aptamers and nanoparticles, Angew. Chem. Int. Ed. Engl. 45 (2006) 90–94.

[44] J. Liu, Y. Lu, Smart nanomaterials responsive to multiple chemical stimuli with controllable cooperativity, Adv. Mater. 18 (2006) 1667–1671.

[45] J.L. Chavez, W. Lyon, N. Kelley-Loughnane, M.O. Stone, Theophylline detection using an aptamer and DNA-gold nanoparticle conjugates, Biosens. Bioelectron. 26 (2010) 23–28.

[46] C. Yang, Y. Wang, J.L. Marty, X. Yang, Aptamer-based colorimetric biosensing of Ochratoxin A using unmodified gold nanoparticles indicator, Biosens. Bioelectron. 26 (2011) 2724–2727.

[47] C.C. Huang, Y.F. Huang, Z. Cao, W. Tan, H.T. Chang, Aptamer-modified gold nanoparticles for colorimetric determination of platelet-derived growth factors and their receptors, Anal. Chem. 77 (2005) 5735–5741.

[48] K. Aslan, J.R. Lakowicz, C.D. Geddes, Nanogold-plasmon-resonance-based glucose sensing, Anal. Biochem. 330 (2004) 145–155.

[49] K. Aslan, J.R. Lakowicz, C.D. Geddes, Nanogold plasmon resonance-based glucose sensing. 2. Wavelength-ratiometric resonance light scattering, Anal. Chem. 77 (2005) 2007–2014.

[50] H. Otsuka, Y. Akiyama, Y. Nagasaki, K. Kataoka, Quantitative and reversible lectin-induced association of gold nanoparticles modified with α-lactosyl-ω-mercapto-poly(ethylene glycol), J. Am. Chem. Soc. 123 (2001) 8226–8230.

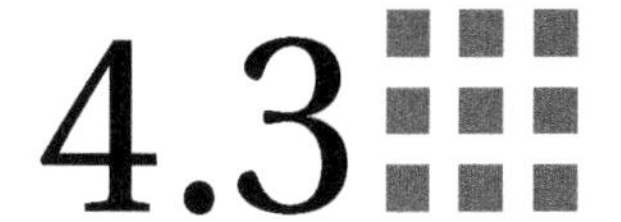

Nanomechanical Sensors

Kota Shiba*, Gaku Imamura*, Genki Yoshikawa**

*INTERNATIONAL CENTER FOR YOUNG SCIENTISTS (ICYS) & INTERNATIONAL CENTER FOR MATERIALS NANOARCHITECTONICS (MANA), NATIONAL INSTITUTE FOR MATERIALS SCIENCE (NIMS), TSUKUBA, JAPAN; **INTERNATIONAL CENTER FOR MATERIALS NANOARCHITECTONICS (MANA), NATIONAL INSTITUTE FOR MATERIALS SCIENCE (NIMS), TSUKUBA, JAPAN

CHAPTER OUTLINE

4.3.1 Introduction

Development of sensing technologies applicable to diverse biological species has been demanded for decades to realize a wide range of applications such as efficient drug screening, point-of-care testing, and early stage/noninvasive diagnostics, etc. To fulfill this demand, various kinds of sensors have been proposed so far. Among such sensors with different working principles, nanomechanical sensors have attracted much attention because of their remarkable features; high sensitivity, wide target range from small molecules to macromolecules, compatibility with industrial technologies, and so on [1]. A number of biological species such as viruses, proteins, bacteria, and cells have been investigated by means of nanomechanical sensors [2].

In this chapter, we will briefly review the basics of nanomechanical sensors, focusing on a microcantilever, which is known as a representative geometry of nanomechanical sensors. In addition to the conventional cantilever, a nanomechanical sensor with a membrane-type geometry will be highlighted as a newly developed sensing platform with various notable features [3–5]. Since affinity of sensors to sensing targets is affected by the type of functional layers, so-called "receptor layers," coated onto the sensor surface, it is important to properly design receptor layers depending on applications. Therefore, we will also discuss a strategy to realize an optimized receptor layer in terms of sensitivity and selectivity. Finally, the biological species measured by nanomechanical sensors will be summarized.

4.3.2 Nanomechanical Sensors

4.3.2.1 General Remarks

A nanomechanical sensor is a mechanical structure that transduces analyte-induced stimuli into a signal via its structural change with nanometer precision. The definition of a nanomechanical sensor can also cover a mechanical transducer with nanometer scale. In either sense, a cantilever sensor is a representative example among various geometries.

The first chemical sensing application using a cantilever sensor was demonstrated by Gimzewski et al. in 1994. They revealed that the static bending of a cantilever can be used as a calorimeter, which can detect the catalytic reaction taking place on the surface of a cantilever [6]. In the same year, Thundat et al. demonstrated a mass detection with picogram resolution using a cantilever. They focused on the shifts in cantilever resonance frequency induced by the exposure of a metal-coated cantilever to humidity or vapors of mercury [7]. Then, the target of cantilever sensors expanded to various phenomena, such as the formation of self-assembled monolayers [8] and the hybridization of DNA [9].

As demonstrated by various groups, nanomechanical sensors are applicable to a wide variety of targets. To take advantage of their attractive feature, it is important to understand the basics of nanomechanical sensors. In the following sections, we will briefly review working principles and readout methods of cantilever sensors [10]. Then, recent developments in the field of nanomechanical sensing will be highlighted.

4.3.2.2 Operation Modes

Cantilever sensors can detect the following two physical parameters: volume and/or mass of target molecules. Since all substances have volume and mass, we can measure almost any kind of substance by using cantilever sensors. To measure volume and mass of target molecules, there are basically two operation modes of cantilever sensors: static mode and dynamic mode (Fig. 4.3.1). Details will be described in the following sections.

4.3.2.2.1 Static Mode

The static mode is known as one of the representative operation modes of cantilever sensors; it measures surface stress, which is not easily measured with other sensing techniques. The major advantage of the static mode is that a cantilever is not affected by damping because the bending motion caused by the analyte-induced surface stress is slow enough, minimizing the damping in most cases. Since the damping of liquid media severely decreases the sensitivity in the dynamic mode, the static mode is a better option for measurements in a liquid environment. It does not require any complicated peripheral devices, such as actuators or high-frequency readout setups, which are usually necessary for dynamic mode measurements.

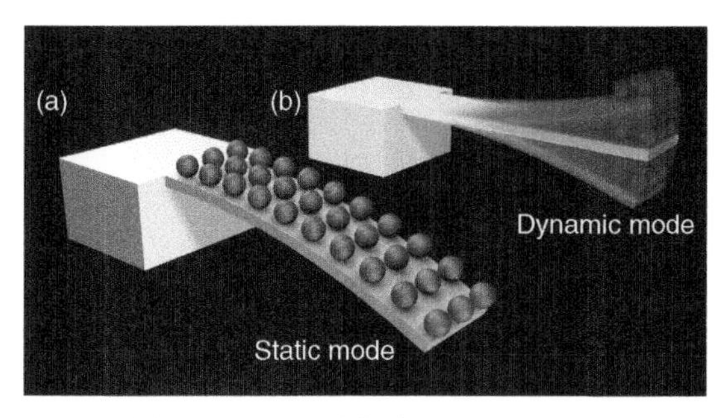

FIGURE 4.3.1 Schematic illustrations of (a) static mode and (b) dynamic mode operations. It is important to note that the bending of a cantilever is caused by the adsorbate-induced surface stress in the case of static mode (the gravity effect is almost negligible). *Reproduced from Ref. [10], with permission from the Royal Society of Chemistry.*

However, there are several issues to be addressed in static mode operation. The long-standing issue is the difficulties in interpreting obtained signals. At present, there is no well-accepted consensus on the origin of surface stress. Although it is roughly regarded as a result of an increase in electrostatic or steric interactions between the adsorbed analytes on the surface of a cantilever, a comprehensive model is still missing. Even for a model system of alkanethiols on a gold (111) surface, several explanations have been reported so far. Thus, the proper calibration should be performed for each application before the actual measurements.

For solid coating layers, a simple analytical model is proposed. It provides general reference values in terms of the strain induced in the coating layer [11,12]. It will help toward analyzing the static behavior of cantilever sensors and various nanomechanical sensors in conjunction with physical properties of coating films as well as optimizing the films for higher sensitivity. The details of the analytical model will be discussed later.

Another difficulty in the interpretation of a signal is the time-dependent complicated behavior, especially in the cases of polymer coatings [13] possibly due to viscoelastic effects [14].

4.3.2.2.2 Dynamic Mode

The concept of dynamic mode operation is same as that for various resonators, such as a quartz crystal microbalance. In this mode, the resonance frequency shift is measured. This shift is due to the change in effective mass induced by the adsorption of analytes on a cantilever. Since signals can be directly correlated to the basic property of adsorbates, that is, mass, the dynamic mode is a useful and powerful technique to derive quantitative information. As the sensitivity generally depends on the resonance frequency determined by the size of a cantilever, a nanometer scale cantilever operated at very high frequency bands (~30~300 MHz) marked several milestones, such as ~7 zeptogram (10^{-21} g) resolution (equivalent to ~30 xenon atoms) in a cryogenically cooled, ultrahigh vacuum (below 10^{-10} torr) apparatus [15], and the mass resolution less than 1 attogram (10^{-18} g) in air at room temperature [16].

The induced mass change (Δm) for a rectangular cantilever with the length of l, thickness of t, width of w, and Young's modulus of E, can be calculated by the following Eq. (4.3.1):

$$\Delta m = \frac{k}{4\pi^2} \times \left(\frac{1}{f_1^2} - \frac{1}{f_0^2} \right) \tag{4.3.1}$$

where $k = Ewt^3/(4l^3)$ is a spring constant of the cantilever, and f_0 and f_1 are the eigenfrequencies before and after the mass change. This equation is derived through pure mechanics, assuming the ideal condition. Thus, in practical situations, several issues still remain. One of the most important issues is the damping effect induced by the surrounding media, as briefly described in the previous section. The damping severely lowers the performance of a cantilever sensor in terms of a low quality factor Q, especially in a liquid environment where Q becomes one-tenth of that in air, resulting in low resolution to track the resonance frequency. Braun and Ghatkesar et al. proposed and demonstrated an elegant way to circumvent the damping effect in a liquid environment using higher flexural modes [17–19]. They succeeded in detecting protein–ligand interactions in a physiological environment at a sensitivity of 2.5 pg/Hz [17], and demonstrated the significant improvement in quality factor of up to ~30 times with the 16th flexural mode [19].

Other factors affecting the signals in the dynamic mode are adsorption-induced effects, such as surface stress and position dependence, which can either stiffen or soften the cantilever, thereby varying the spring constant. The relationship between the surface stress and stiffness of a cantilever has been intensively discussed [20–22]. Lee et al. visually demonstrated the dependence of resonance frequency on a pattern of a gold layer on the surface of a cantilever [23]. In any case, we have to be careful about these effects when we analyze the signals obtained with the dynamic mode.

4.3.2.3 Readout Methods

There are several readout methods to record responses of cantilever sensors [1]. In this section, we will introduce two representative readout methods: optical readout with a laser and electrical readout with a piezoresistor.

4.3.2.3.1 Optical Readout

The most commonly used readout method is the so-called optical readout, which utilizes laser light emitted from, for example, a vertical cavity surface emitting laser (VCSEL). The laser is reflected on the surface of a cantilever and then the position is measured by a position-sensitive detector (PSD) (Fig. 4.3.2). It gives high sensitivity in terms of signal-to-noise ratio because of its relatively low noise. Another practical advantage of this method is that there is no requirement for wiring on a cantilever array sensor chip because both the source and detector of laser light are placed at remote positions.

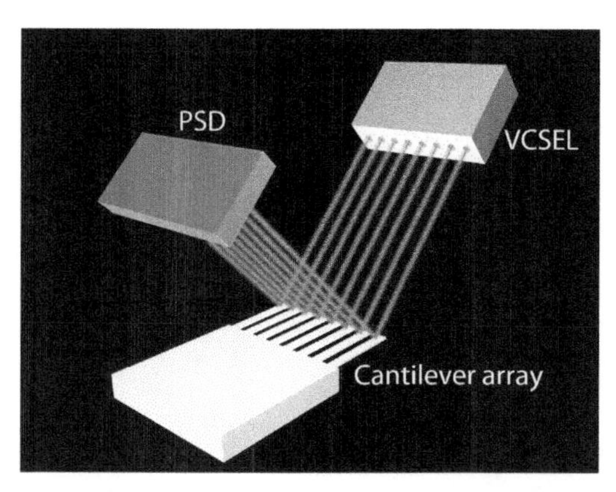

FIGURE 4.3.2 Typical setup for the optical (laser) readout system. VCSEL is usually used as a source of multiple laser light. Each laser light reflected on the surface of each cantilever is measured by a PSD. *Reproduced from Ref. [10], with permission from the Royal Society of Chemistry.*

However, optical readout has several drawbacks when we consider actual applications. First of all, laser-related peripherals are bulky and expensive in most cases. For multiple cantilevers such as a cantilever array, the same number of laser sources must be prepared. While highly integrated VCSEL or multiple optical fiber systems might be able to solve this problem, each laser light should be always aligned on each cantilever precisely. Thus, optical readout is not suitable for large one- or two-dimensional arrays. Another critical problem is the difficulty in measurements in opaque liquids, such as blood. In such a liquid, the optical signal is significantly attenuated owing to low transmission or refractive index change.

4.3.2.3.2 Piezoresistive Readout

Piezoresistive readout can be utilized by using a piezoresistive cantilever, in which a sensing element (piezoresistor) is embedded at the clamped end; thereby it is sometimes called a "self-sensing" cantilever (Fig. 4.3.3). In contrast to the optical readout method, no bulky and complex peripherals are required because a piezoresistive readout electrically measures the change in resistance of a piezoresistor with a simple circuit (Fig. 4.3.4). By means of the piezoresistive readout, it is also possible to perform measurements even in

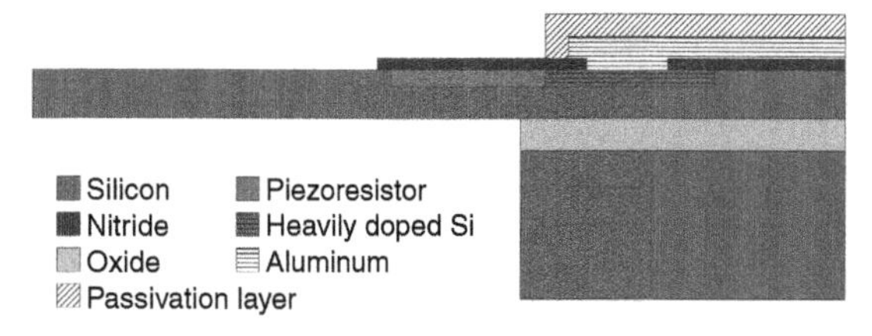

FIGURE 4.3.3 An example of the cross-section of a piezoresistive cantilever. It is important to cover the piezoresistor with a passivation layer, such as silicon nitride, to prevent leakage of current, especially in the case of measurements in a liquid environment. *Reprinted from Ref. [24], with permission from Elsevier B.V.*

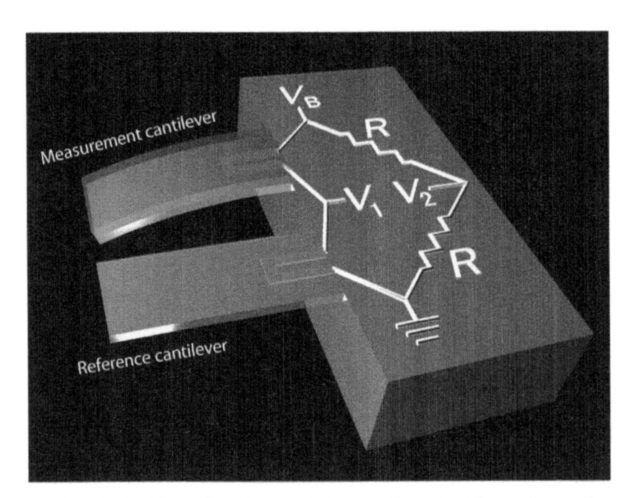

FIGURE 4.3.4 An example of electrical wiring of a piezoresistive readout. In this configuration, the differential signal is given as an output of the Wheatstone bridge, while it is also possible to place measurement and reference cantilevers in individual Wheatstone bridges and obtain differential signals by subtracting the output of the reference lever bridge from that of measurement lever bridge. *Reproduced from Ref. [10], with permission from the Royal Society of Chemistry.*

opaque liquids. In addition, because of its complementary metal-oxide semiconductor compatibility, the whole sensor unit including readout parts can be integrated into common semiconductor devices, such as mobile phones. It is also technically feasible by mass production to produce inexpensive disposal chips, which are important for various applications, especially for medical diagnosis. Thus, the piezoresistive readout has been regarded as one of the most promising approaches to overcome the problems arising from the optical readout. In spite of these inherent advantages, piezoresistive cantilevers have not been widely utilized for sensing applications because of their critically low sensitivity. In other words, they will open the door to the applications of nanomechanical sensors if the sensitivity of a piezoresistive cantilever can be significantly improved. Therefore, various trials have been made for more than a decade to improve the sensitivity of a piezoresistive cantilever toward practical uses. However, significant improvement in sensitivity has not been achieved to make piezoresistive detection comparable to the optical approach.

4.3.2.4 Structural Optimization of Nanomechanical Sensors for Improved Sensitivity

Various strategies have been proposed to improve the sensitivity of a piezoresistive cantilever by structural modification, such as making a through-hole [25,26], patterning of the cantilever surface [27], or variation of geometrical parameters (e.g., length, width, and overall shapes) [28,29]. Although these approaches gained some improvements in sensitivity (typically, a few tens of a percent, while up to ~5 times in some cases [29]), significant enhancement has not been achieved.

To realize the appropriate scheme for the enhanced sensitivity, it is important to note the basic properties of a piezoresistive cantilever for surface stress sensing [3]. One notable parameter is piezocoefficient. P-type piezoresistors created by boron diffusion onto a single-crystal silicon (100) surface can be effectively utilized because of its high piezocoefficient [30–32]. Plain stress (i.e., $\sigma_z = 0$) is assumed because of the intrinsically two-dimensional feature of surface stress. In this case, relative resistance change can be described as follows [32,33]:

$$\frac{\Delta R}{R} \approx \frac{1}{2}\pi_{44}(\sigma_x - \sigma_y) \tag{4.3.2}$$

where $\pi_{44}(\sim 138.1 \times 10^{-11}\ \mathrm{Pa}^{-1})$ is one of the fundamental piezoresistance coefficients of the silicon crystal. σ_x, σ_y, and σ_z are stresses induced on the piezoresistor in the [110], [1-10], and [001] directions of the crystal, respectively. Based on this equation, both enhancement of σ_x (σ_y) and suppression of σ_y (σ_x) are required to yield a substantial amount of $\Delta R/R$. However, in the case of surface stress sensing, the stress is basically isotropic. In other words, σ_x is almost equal to σ_y, resulting in $\Delta R/R \sim 0$. Therefore, the resultant signal is virtually zero on the whole surface. Because of this intrinsic material property, it is difficult to significantly improve sensitivity as long as we consider simple cantilever-type structures.

Through a detailed structural investigation, a new geometry with high sensitivity was developed. This structure is called a membrane-type surface stress sensor (MSS, Fig. 4.3.5a) [3]. In addition to the geometry, MSS was also optimized in terms of electric circuit. For p-type silicon (100), the relative resistance change with a current flow in the x-direction is given by Eq. (4.3.2). In case all four resistors ($R_1 \sim R_4$) are practically equal and that the relative resistance changes are small with $\Delta R_i/R_i << 1$ ($i = 1 \sim 4$), the total output signal V_{out} of the Wheatstone bridge can be approximated by:

$$V_{out} = \frac{V_B}{4}\left(\frac{\Delta R_1}{R_1} - \frac{\Delta R_2}{R_2} + \frac{\Delta R_3}{R_3} - \frac{\Delta R_4}{R_4}\right) \tag{4.3.3}$$

where V_B is a bias voltage of the Wheatstone bridge. Thus, if the sign of the resistance changes ΔR_1 and ΔR_3 are opposite to those of ΔR_2 and ΔR_4, the full Wheatstone bridge yields an amplification of another factor of 4. If we configure the MSS structure (i.e., membrane-type structure), this condition is fulfilled since the dominant stresses induced on the membrane are σ_x in R_1, R_3, and σ_y in R_2, R_4, resulting in opposite signs for the relative resistance changes in each set of resistors. Therefore, the whole induced surface stress is efficiently utilized, and thus MSS realizes the following properties: high sensitivity, self-compensating low-drift operation with full Wheatstone bridge, and stable operation without a free end.

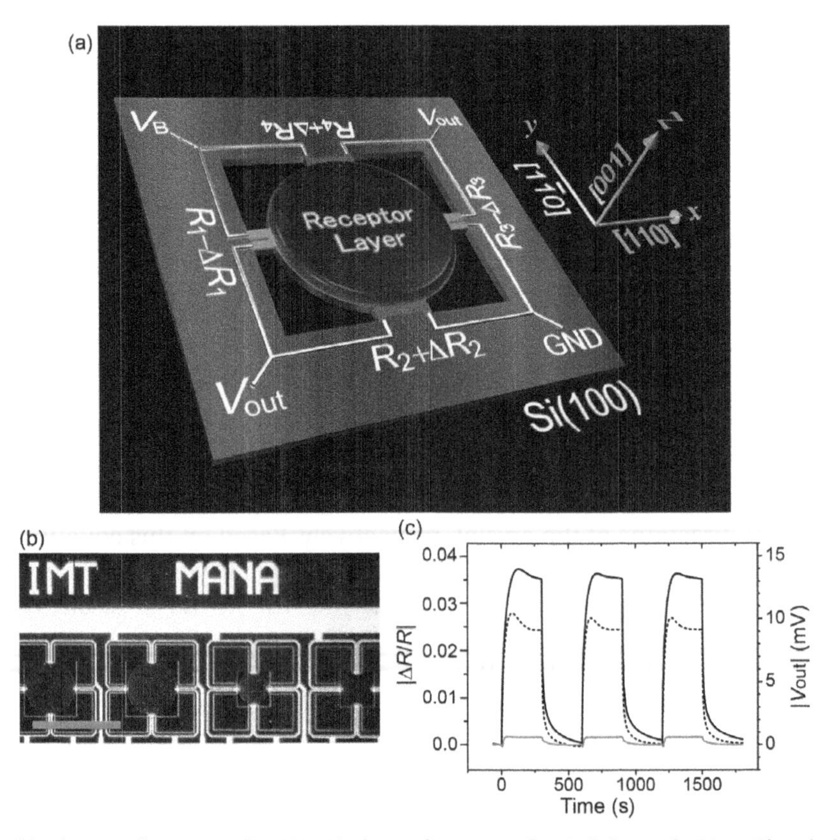

FIGURE 4.3.5 (a) Schematic illustration of a MSS with the configuration of typical electrical wirings. The whole surface stress induced on the round center membrane is efficiently detected by piezoresistors embedded in the constricted beams. (b) Photo of membranes aligned in a fabricated MSS chip. Scale bar corresponds to 1 mm. Membranes with diameters of 500 and 300 μm are fabricated in the same chip to examine the size dependence under the same condition. (c) Output signals (V_{out}) and corresponding values of $|\Delta R/R|$ obtained by the MSS having a diameters of 500 μm (solid line) and 300 μm (dashed line), and by a standard piezoresistive cantilever (gray line). Significant enhancement in sensitivity is confirmed in addition to the size dependence of MSS. *Reproduced from Ref. [10], with permission from the Royal Society of Chemistry.*

4.3.3 Functionalization of Nanomechanical Sensors

In this section, we focus on the fabrication of receptor layers. Nanomechanical sensors are usually coated with various kinds of materials, so-called "receptor layers," where analytes are captured. The adsorbed/absorbed analytes then cause surface stress, which results in the deflection of nanomechanical sensing units. Therefore, the sensing features depend on the quality of the coating (i.e., surface roughness, a coffee ring, etc.) as well as physical/chemical properties of receptor layers. A major factor that affects the quality of the coating is a coating method. Thus, we briefly review common coating techniques for the functionalization of nanomechanical sensors. Effects of the coating quality will be discussed using

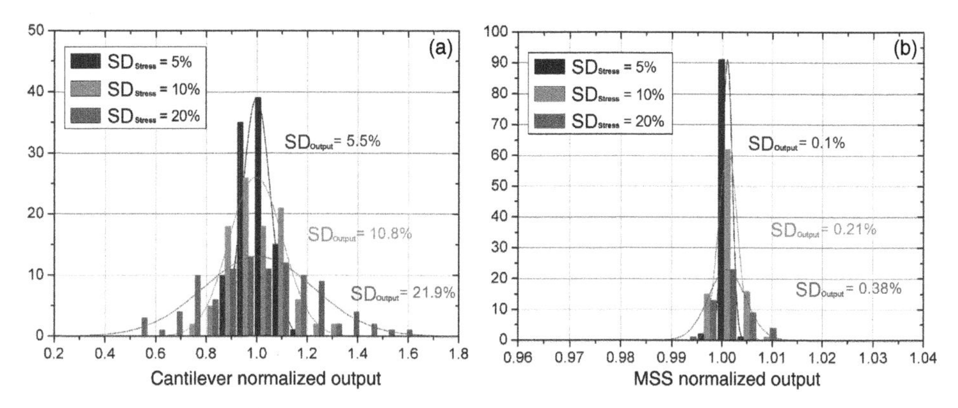

FIGURE 4.3.6 Sensor output distributions of 100 simulated cantilevers (a) and a MSS (b) while a randomly distributed surface stress is applied on their surfaces. *Reprinted from Ref. [34], with permission from Elsevier B.V.*

a cantilever and MSS, focusing on reproducibility of measurements. We also show guidelines to design receptor layers; the structural optimization strategy for high sensitivity.

4.3.3.1 Coating of Receptor Layers

4.3.3.1.1 Reproducibility

Constant sensing performance is a crucial factor for the manufacture of sensors. Loizeau et al. investigated the reproducibility of MSS comparing with a typical cantilever-based sensor [34]. For the practical coating methods such as inkjet spotting and spray coating, the coated receptor layer has a certain amount of roughness in thickness. Such roughness causes inhomogeneous surface stress on the sensors. The stability of the sensing signals for such inhomogeneous surface stress is investigated by means of finite element analysis (FEA), and the results are also confirmed experimentally [34].

The surface stress simulation was conducted for both the cantilever-based sensor and MSS. The surface stress of 0.2 N/m was nonuniformly applied to the sensors with the standard deviation of 5, 10, and 20%. One hundred cases were simulated for each sensor. Figure 4.3.6 shows the distribution of the output signals. In the case of the cantilever-based sensor, the distribution of the output signals had almost the same standard deviations as the surface stress. On the other hand, the standard deviations of the output signals dramatically decreased for the MSS; approximately 50 times smaller than the standard deviations of the surface stress. These results indicate that the MSS has a higher stability for the inhomogeneous surface stress compared to a cantilever-based sensor. As the inhomogeneous surface stress is mainly caused by the roughness of the receptor layers, these results suggest that the MSS is less influenced by the quality of the coatings, leading to the higher uniformity of the sensing performance. The results of the FEA simulations were also confirmed experimentally (Fig. 4.3.7). On the basis of the FEA simulation and the experimental results, the higher reproducibility of the MSS compared to a cantilever-based sensor was demonstrated; the output signal of the MSS is less influenced by the

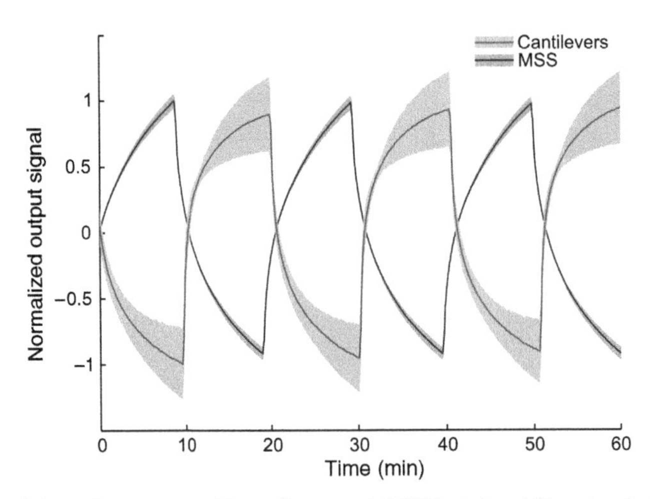

FIGURE 4.3.7 Normalized dynamic responses of 8 cantilevers and 15 MSSs to humidity pulses between 0% and 5%. Solid lines represent average curves and shaded zones highlight standard deviations. Note that the opposite signs of output signals of cantilevers and MSS are due to the opposite directions of stresses on the piezoresistors. *Reprinted from Ref. [34] with permission from Elsevier B.V.*

roughness of the receptor layer. This enhanced sensor-to-sensor repeatability leads not only to accurate and reliable data acquisition in research, but also to the mass production of nanomechanical sensors.

4.3.3.1.2 Double-Side Coating

One of the important challenges of nanomechanical sensors is how to prepare receptor layers in a reproducible manner without any complicated apparatus. Drop casting and dip-coating are examples of fast and convenient coating methods. These methods, however, lead to coatings on both sides. In the case of a cantilever-based sensor with the optical (laser) readout method, the double-side coating does not work because the cantilever does not have measurable vertical deformation as shown in Fig. 4.3.8b. In contrast to the optical readout case, signals are obtained with a double-side-coated piezoresistive cantilever sensor [35,36]. An in-plane elongation caused by the surface stresses on both sides can be detected by the piezoresistor embedded at the clamped end (Fig. 4.3.8d). However, only a local stress induced at the surface where the piezoresistor is embedded can be detected, leading to low sensitivity. Taking account of the conventional cantilever-type geometry and the material property of silicon, it is difficult to realize high sensitivity with the double-side coating.

The MSS geometry is an effective solution to overcome this issue [5]. The in-plane stress induced in the membrane can be detected at the four beams. Figures 4.3.8g and h are the results of FEA simulations on the MSS structure. A surface stress of −3.0 N/m is uniformly applied only on the top surface (Fig. 4.3.8g) or both sides (Fig. 4.3.8h). The distribution of the relative resistance change ($\Delta R/R$) is presented by light and shade. Large relative resistance changes can be observed for the single-side-coated MSS [3]. Although the signal is not as large as the single-side-coated MSS, the

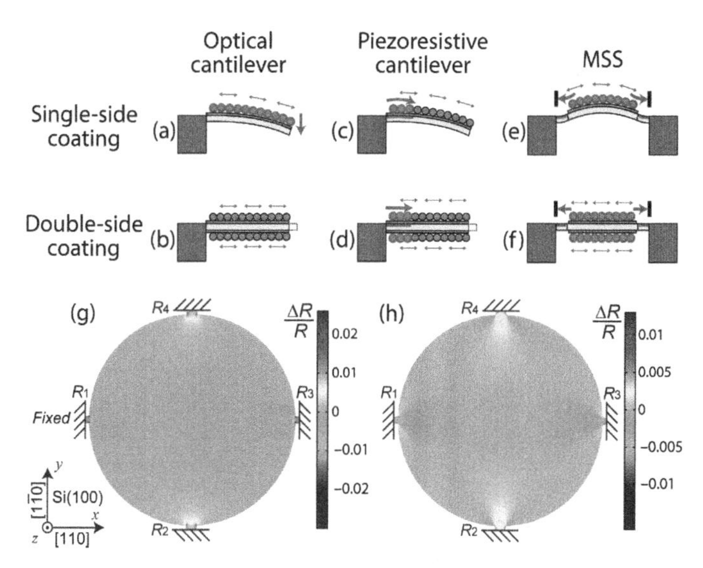

FIGURE 4.3.8 Schematic side views of (a, b) optical and (c, d) piezoresistive cantilevers and (e, f) a MSS with single- and double-side coatings, respectively. FEA of the distribution of $\Delta R/R$ in the middle plane (150 nm below the top surface) of the piezoresistors. A surface stress of −3.0 N/m is applied uniformly on (g) the top surface and (h) on both the top and bottom surfaces of the center circular membranes. *Reprinted from Ref. [5], with permission from the American Chemical Society.*

double-side-coated MSS also exhibits notable relative resistance changes. The double-side-coated MSS yields approximately 37% of the relative resistance change observed with the single-side-coated MSS.

To demonstrate the feasibility of the double-side coating method, the MSS membrane was functionalized by simply dipping it into an aqueous solution containing polyvinylpyrrolidone (PVP). Figure 4.3.9a shows a photograph of a simple hand-operated dipping process. An MSS chip was dipped into the PVP aqueous solution, and then dried in air. The coated MSS was used to measure water vapor. Fig. 4.3.9b shows the results of the measurements. Sufficient signal outputs are obtained with a good reproducibility. Such consistent signals from different channels would compensate the decreased sensitivity compared to the single-side-coated MSS because consistent signals from N channels improve the signal-to-noise ratio by a factor of $N^{1/2}$.

4.3.3.2 Guideline to the Design of Receptor Layers

4.3.3.2.1 Thickness

According to a recent study [11], deflection (signal intensity) of a nanomechanical sensor strongly depends on the thickness of a receptor layer. In this section, we focus on the analytical model that describes the relationship between deflection of a cantilever and various physical parameters of a cantilever itself and receptor layer on it. This analysis provides a practical guideline to optimize the thickness of a receptor layer.

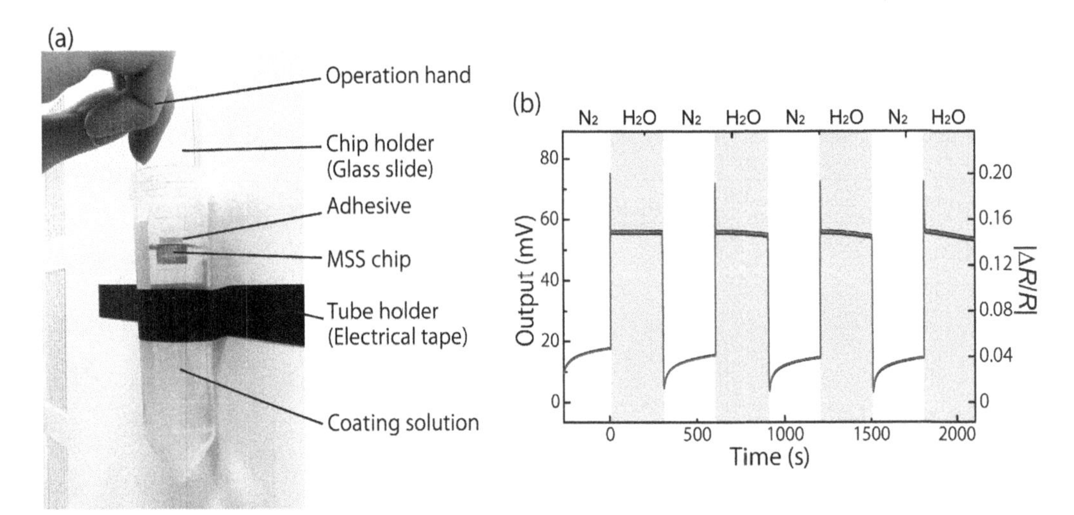

FIGURE 4.3.9 (a) Photograph of the hand-operated dip coating setup for creating double-sided coatings for the MSS chip. (b) Obtained output signals (V_{out}) for three MSS membranes on the same double-side-coated chip. This MSS chip was coated with PVP using hand-operated dip coating. *Reprinted from Ref. [5], with permission from the American Chemical Society.*

The Stoney's equation is widely used to estimate the deflection of a cantilever [37]. According to the Stoney's equation, the deflection of a cantilever (Δz) caused by surface stress (σ_{surf}) is written as:

$$\Delta z = \frac{3(1-\nu_c)l_c^2}{E_c t_c^2}\sigma_{surf} \tag{4.3.4}$$

where E_c and ν_c are the Young's modulus and Poisson's ratio, and l_c and t_c correspond to the length and thickness of a cantilever, respectively. Although this equation has been widely used, no parameters relating to a receptor layer are included. It leads to a large discrepancy for a cantilever with a relatively thick receptor layer.

To consider the effect of a receptor layer, Timoshenko beam theory, which was originally developed to analyze a bimetal strip, can be used [38]. Based on the Timoshenko beam theory, an analytical model for the static deflection of a cantilever sensor coated with a solid layer was derived. In a simple cantilever coated with a solid receptor layer as shown in Fig. 4.3.10, the deflection of the cantilever is described as:

$$\Delta z = \frac{3l^2(t_f + t_c)}{(A+4)t_f^2 + (A^{-1}+4)t_c^2 + 6t_f t_c}\varepsilon_f \tag{4.3.5}$$

$$A = \frac{E_f w_f t_f (1-\nu_c)}{E_c w_c t_c (1-\nu_f)}, \tag{4.3.6}$$

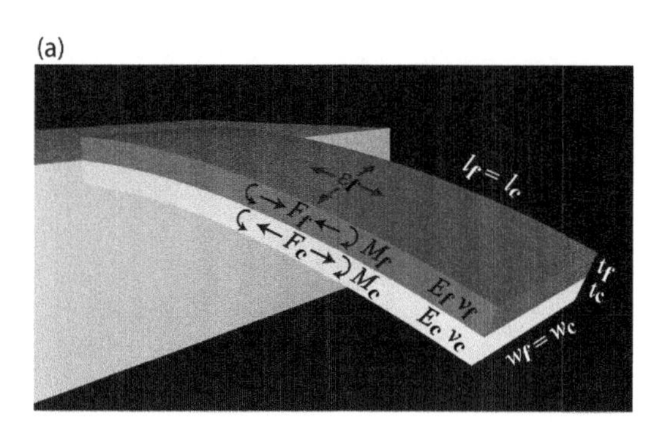

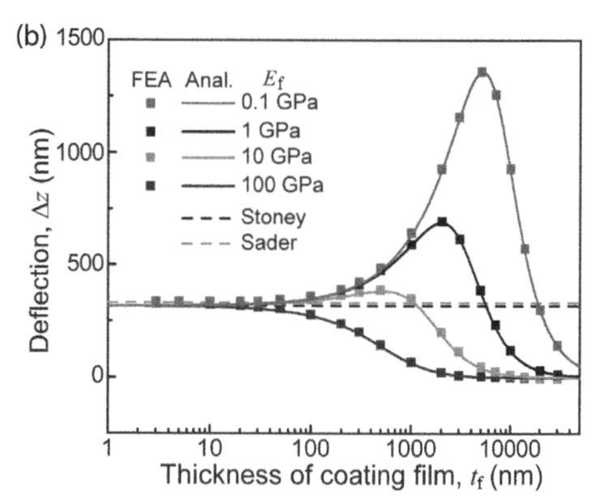

FIGURE 4.3.10 (a) Schematic illustration of a cantilever covered by a coating film with isotropic internal strain. (b) Dependence of cantilever deflection on the thickness of coating films with various Young's moduli from 0.1 GPa to 100 GPa. The values calculated by FEA are represented with filled squares. Black and gray dashed lines correspond to the cantilever deflection calculated by the Stoney's equation and Sader's model, respectively. l = 500 μm, $w_c = w_f$ = 100 μm, t_c = 1 μm, E_c = 170 GPa, ν_c = 0.28, ν_f = 0.30, and σ_{surf} = 0.1 N/m. *Reprinted from Ref. [11], with permission from the American Institute of Physics.*

where E_f, ν_f, and t_f are the Young's modulus, the Poisson's ratio, and the thickness of a receptor layer, and w_c and w_f are the width of a cantilever and a receptor layer, respectively. By replacing the strain of a coating film (ε_f) using the relations $\varepsilon_f = \sigma_f(1 - \nu_f)/E_f$ or $\sigma_f = \sigma_{surf}/t_f$, the deflection of a cantilever (Δz) can be described as a function of internal stress in the receptor layer (σ_f) or surface stress (σ_{surf}). In the case of $t_c \gg t_f$ and $w_c = w_f$, Eq. (4.3.5) reduces to the Stoney's equation.

To verify this analytical result, FEA simulation was also performed for a cantilever with the same geometry. The results are shown in Fig. 4.3.10b. The values obtained from the FEA simulation show a good agreement with the analytically derived curves. The Stoney's model and Sader's model are also drawn in Fig. 4.3.10b, both of which show significant deviations from the FEA analysis [39].

The thickness of a receptor layer can be optimized based on Eq. (4.3.5). The deflection reaches maximum at $t_{t\text{-op}}$, at which $d\Delta z/dt$ becomes zero. In the case of $w_c = w_f$, $t_{t\text{-op}}$ can be written as:

$$t_{t\text{-op}} = \frac{t_c}{2}\left(X^{1/3} + X^{-1/3} - 1\right) \tag{4.3.7}$$

$$X = \frac{2U_c - U_f - 2\sqrt{U_c(U_c - U_f)}}{U_f} \tag{4.3.8}$$

where $U_c = E_c(1 - \nu_f)$ and $U_f = E_f(1 - \nu_c)$. Thus, one can easily find the optimum thickness of a receptor layer by using Eqs. (4.3.7) and (4.3.8).

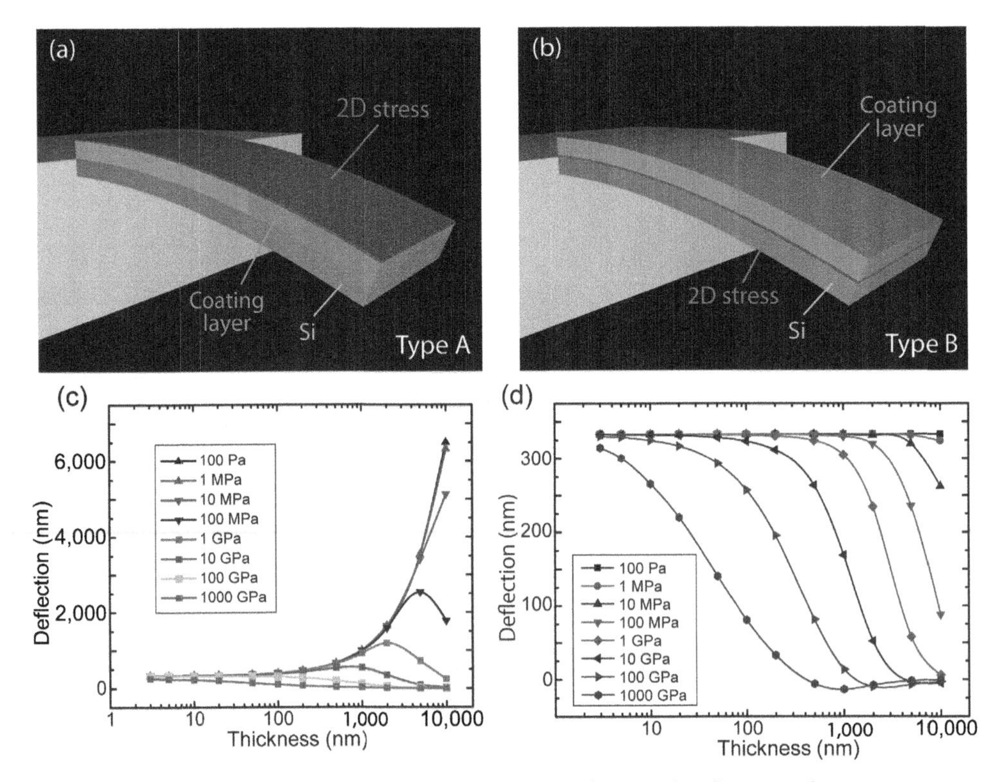

FIGURE 4.3.11 (a) Visualization of the two systems of two-dimensional stress induced on a cantilever-type nanomechanical sensor. (a) Type A system in which the stress is induced on the top surface of the coating layer. (b) Type B system in which the stress is induced at the interface between the silicon cantilever and the coating layer. Note that the dimensions and deflections of the cantilever and the coating layer are exaggerated. Thickness dependence on the deflection of the cantilever in the case of (c) Type A and (d) Type B. Poisson's ratio of coating layers is 0.30 for all plots. *Reprinted from Ref. [12], with permission from the American Scientific Publishers.*

4.3.3.2.2 Configuration

Analytes adsorbed/absorbed on a cantilever sensor can induce two-dimensional stress on the surface of the receptor layer (type A) or on the interface between the receptor layer and the cantilever (type B) as depicted in Fig. 4.3.11. The type A stress is induced when the surface of a cantilever is modified by functional groups including self-assembled monolayers. Analytes that induce charge distribution at the interface by dipole interactions can cause the type B stress. Here, we focus on these two cases [12].

The deflection of a cantilever sensor is investigated by FEA simulation. The length, width, and thickness of the cantilever are set at 500, 100, and 1 μm, respectively. The results are depicted in Fig. 4.3.11c and d. The deflection is plotted as a function of thickness. As we have seen in the previous section, the deflection increases by decreasing the Young's modulus for the type A stress. There is an optimal thickness $t_{t\text{-}op}$ written as Eq. (4.3.7). The type B stress gives rise to even lower deflections compared to the type A stress. In contrast to the type A, the deflection monotonically decreases with increasing thickness regardless of Young's modulus.

4.3.4 Nanomechanical Sensing of Biomolecules

Detection of biomolecules is an important issue in various fields. For example, detection of biomarkers for cancer in an early stage could significantly reduce the mortality of the patients. Detection of glucose in blood enables us to monitor the blood sugar level, which is essential for diagnosis of diabetes. Biosensors that can detect infectious viruses in real time with high sensitivity are highly required with regard to the control of epidemics. In fundamental science, detection of physical forces generated by a single cell or a number of cells, which are known to show collective motion, is a major challenge to investigate various stimuli-responsive behaviors of cells. Here, we focus on the sensing techniques for biomolecules using nanomechanical sensors. First, we give an overview of previous nanomechanical sensing studies related to the detection of biomolecules. Then, we describe the nanomechanical approach to detect cellular forces.

4.3.4.1 General

Many biomolecules and microorganisms have been detected by means of nanomechanical sensors. Table 4.3.1 summarizes the reported studies [40]. Molecular recognition techniques play an important role in biosensing applications. Antigen–antibody interaction is one of the most powerful tools to detect biomolecules, making it possible to detect targets with high sensitivity and selectivity. Not only peptides including antigens and antibodies themselves, but also microorganisms such as viruses and fungi can be detected by antigen–antibody binding. Another promising technique to detect biomolecules is enzyme reactions. Enzyme reactions can be applied to detect smaller biomolecules such as hydrogen peroxide and glucose.

4.3.4.2 Cells

Mechanobiology is a discipline at the interface of biology and engineering [88]. It focuses on how cells or tissues respond to mechanical stimuli. Since some diseases are known to closely correlate with mechanical changes in cellular systems, advances in mechanobiology lead to the development of mechanical therapies. Moreover, it is reported that biomechanical forces trigger stem cell differentiation, implying its possible control [89]. Thus, mechanobiology has a great potential for the discovery of fundamental biological concepts as well as the development of mechanical therapies.

To investigate the mechanics in cellular systems, measuring the mechanical properties of living cells such as Young's modulus, surface tension, and force distribution is an important

Table 4.3.1 Reported Studies of the Many Biomolecules and Microorganisms that have been Detected by Means of Nanomechanical Sensors [40]

Analytes	References
Glucose	[41–44]
Fructose	[45]
Hydrogen peroxide	[46–48]
α-Amino acid and peptides	[49,50]
Acetylcholine	[47]
Lipid bilayer	[51]
Myoglobin	[52,53]
C-reactive protein	[54–56]
Bovine serum albumin	[57]
Human serum albumin	[58,59]
Human growth hormone	[60]
Protein kinase	[61]
Prostate-specific antigen	[62–64]
Single-chain Fv	[65]
Cytokine	[66]
Human estrogen receptor protein	[67]
Low density lipoproteins	[68]
Cyclin-dependent protein kinase	[69]
Human epidermal growth factor receptor 2	[70]
Immunoglobulin G	[57,71]
Alpha-fetoprotein	[72
Human immunodeficiency virus	[72]
Vaccinia virus	[74]
Bacterial virus T5	[75]
Severe acute respiratory syndrome associated coronavirus	[76]
A. niger	[77]
Bacillus anthracis	[78–80]
Enterohemorrhagic *Escherichia coli* serotype	[81–84]
Salmonella typhimurium	[85]
Tularemia	[86]
Cryptosporidium	[87]

challenge [90]. Nanomechanical sensors have a distinct advantage over measuring the mechanical properties of cellular systems as the principle of nanomechanical sensors is based on the detection of strain/stress and the resultant deflection. Maloney et al. reported the monitoring of single *Aspergillus niger* spore growth by means of functionalized cantilevers [91]. They detected the growth of single spores as changes in resonant frequency. It has been reported by Bischofs et al. that cell migration causes surface tension of ~2 mN/m, which is larger than the detection limit of the nanomechanical sensors with high sensitivity, such as optical readout cantilevers (typically 0.15–0.90 mN/m) and MSS (<0.1 mN/m) [3]. Thus, nanomechanical sensors would provide new grounds for exploring the mechanical properties of living cells.

4.3.5 Conclusions and Future Trends

In this chapter, we briefly overviewed the basics of nanomechanical sensing, focusing on the working principles and representative readout methods. Then, we reviewed a recently developed nanomechanical sensing platform; MSS, which has various practical advantages over conventional nanomechanical sensors. The analytical approach to designing a receptor layer with optimized sensitivity was explained. Since they can detect volume and/or mass of analytes, nanomechanical sensors are promising devices for the measurements of diverse biomaterials, ranging from small molecules (e.g., volatile organic compounds, amino acid) to microorganisms (e.g., viruses, cells) as summarized in this chapter. In addition, application of nanomechanical sensors to mechanobiology, an emerging field of science, would provide new biological concepts; clarifying the mechanics in cellular systems and mechanical basis of tissue regulation.

References

[1] N.V. Lavrik, M.J. Sepaniak, P.G. Datskos, Rev. Sci. Instrum. 75 (2004) 2229.

[2] K.R. Buchapudi, X. Huang, X. Yang, H.-F. Ji, T. Thundat, Analyst 136 (2011) 1539.

[3] G. Yoshikawa, T. Akiyama, S. Gautsch, P. Vettiger, H. Rohrer, Nano Lett. 11 (2011) 1044.

[4] G. Yoshikawa, T. Akiyama, F. Loizeau, K. Shiba, S. Gautsch, T. Nakayama, P. Vettiger, N.F. de Rooij, M. Aono, Sensors 12 (2012) 15873.

[5] G. Yoshikawa, F. Loizeau, C.J.Y. Lee, T. Akiyama, K. Shiba, S. Gautsch, T. Nakayama, P. Vettiger, N.F. de Rooij, M. Aono, Langmuir 29 (2013) 7551.

[6] J.K. Gimzewski, C. Gerber, E. Meyer, R.R. Schlittler, Chem. Phys. Lett. 217 (1994) 589.

[7] T. Thundat, R.J. Warmack, G.Y. Chen, D.P. Allison, Appl. Phys. Lett. 64 (1994) 2894.

[8] R. Berger, E. Delamarche, H.P. Lang, C. Gerber, J.K. Gimzewski, E. Meyer, H.J. Guntherodt, Science 276 (1997) 2021.

[9] J. Fritz, M.K. Baller, H.P. Lang, H. Rothuizen, P. Vettiger, E. Meyer, H.J. Guntherodt, C. Gerber, J.K. Gimzewski, Science 288 (2000) 316.

[10] G. Yoshikawa, Nanomechanical sensors and membrane-type surface stress sensor (MSS) for medical, security and environmental applications, Manipulation of Nanoscale Materials: An Introduction to Nanoarchitectonics, The Royal Society of Chemistry, Burlington House, London, UK, (2012) pp. 428.

[11] G. Yoshikawa, Appl. Phys. Lett. 98 (2011) 173502.

[12] G. Yoshikawa, C.J.Y. Lee, K. Shiba, J. Nanosci. Nanotechnol. 14 (2014) 2908.

[13] A. Bietsch, J.Y. Zhang, M. Hegner, H.P. Lang, C. Gerber, Nanotechnology 15 (2004) 873.

[14] S.M. Heinrich, M.J. Wenzel, F. Josse, I. Dufour, J. Appl. Phys. 105 (2009) 124903.

[15] Y.T. Yang, C. Callegari, X.L. Feng, K.L. Ekinci, M.L. Roukes, Nano Lett. 6 (2006) 583.

[16] M. Li, H.X. Tang, M.L. Roukes, Nat. Nanotechnol. 2 (2007) 114.

[17] T. Braun, V. Barwich, M.K. Ghatkesar, A.H. Bredekamp, C. Gerber, M. Hegner, H.P. Lang, Phys. Rev. E 72 (2005) 031907.

[18] M.K. Ghatkesar, V. Barwich, T. Braun, J.P. Ramseyer, C. Gerber, M. Hegner, H.P. Lang, U. Drechsler, M. Despont, Nanotechnology 18 (2007) 445502.

[19] M.K. Ghatkesar, T. Braun, V. Barwich, J.P. Ramseyer, C. Gerber, M. Hegner, H.P. Lang, Appl. Phys. Lett. 92 (2008).

[20] A.W. McFarland, M.A. Poggi, M.J. Doyle, L.A. Bottomley, J.S. Colton, Appl. Phys. Lett. 87 (2005) 053505.

[21] M.J. Lachut, J.E. Sader, Phys. Rev. Lett. 99 (2007) 206102.

[22] M.J. Lachut, J.E. Sader, Appl. Phys. Lett. 95 (2009) 193505.

[23] D. Lee, S. Kim, N. Jung, T. Thundat, S. Jeon, J. Appl. Phys. 106 (2009) 024310.

[24] L. Aeschimann, A. Meister, T. Akiyama, B.W. Chui, P. Niedermann, H. Heinzelmann, N.F. De Rooij, U. Staufer, P. Vettiger, Microelectron. Eng. 83 (2006) 1698.

[25] J.H. He, Y.F. Li, J. Phys. 34 (2006) 429.

[26] X.M. Yu, Y.Q. Tang, H.T. Zhang, T. Li, W. Wang, IEEE Sens. J. 7 (2007) 489.

[27] N.L. Privorotskaya, W.P. King, Microsyst. Technol. 15 (2008) 333.

[28] F.T. Goericke, W.P. King, IEEE Sens. J. 8 (2008) 1404.

[29] A. Loui, F.T. Goericke, T.V. Ratto, J. Lee, B.R. Hart, W.P. King, Sensors Actuat. A. 147 (2008) 516.

[30] Y. Kanda, IEEE Trans. Electron. Devices 29 (1982) 64.

[31] W.G. Pfann, R.N. Thurston, J. Appl. Phys. 32 (1961) 2008.

[32] Y. Kanda, Sensors Actuat. A 28 (1991) 83.

[33] P.A. Rasmussen, O. Hansen, A. Boisen, Appl. Phys. Lett. 86 (2005) 203502.

[34] F. Loizeau, T. Akiyama, S. Gautsch, P. Vettiger, G. Yoshikawa, N.F. de Rooij, Sensors Actuat. A 228 (2015) 9.

[35] P.A. Rasmussen, A.V. Grigorov, A. Boisen, J. Micromech. Microeng. 15 (2005) 1088.

[36] A. Choudhury, P.J. Hesketh, T.G. Thundat, H. Zhiyu, R. Vujanic, Design and testing of single and double sided cantilevers for chemical sensing, Sensors, 2007 IEEE 1–3 (2007) 1432.

[37] G.G. Stoney, Proc. R. Soc. Lond. Ser. A 82 (1909) 172.

[38] S. Timoshenko, J. Opt. Soc. Am. 11 (1925) 233.

[39] J.E. Sader, J. Appl. Phys. 89 (2001) 2911.

[40] K.R. Buchapudi, X. Huang, X. Yang, H.F. Ji, T. Thundat, Analyst. 136 (2011) 1539.

[41] A. Subramanian, P.I. Oden, S.J. Kennel, K.B. Jacobson, R.J. Warmack, T. Thundat, M.J. Doktycz, Appl. Phys. Lett. 81 (2002) 385.

[42] J. Pei, F. Tian, T. Thundat, Anal. Chem. 76 (2004) 292.

[43] T. Chen, D.P. Chang, T. Liu, R. Desikan, R. Datar, T. Thundat, R. Berger, S. Zauscher, J. Mater. Chem. 20 (2010) 3391.

[44] X. Huang, S. Li, J.S. Schultz, Q. Wang, Q. Lin, Sensors Actuat. B 140 (2009) 603.

[45] G.A. Baker, R. Desikan, T. Thundat, Anal. Chem. 80 (2008) 4860.

[46] X.D. Yan, X.L. Shi, K. Hill, H.F. Ji, Anal. Sci. 22 (2006) 205.

[47] H. Gao, K.R. Buchapudi, A. Harms-Smyth, M.K. Schulte, X. Xu, H.-F. Ji, Langmuir 24 (2008) 345.

[48] J.P. Lock, E. Geraghty, L.C. Kagumba, K.K. Mahmud, Thin Solid Films 517 (2009) 3584.

[49] P. Dutta, C.A. Tipple, N.V. Lavrik, P.G. Datskos, H. Hofstetter, O. Hofstetter, M.J. Sepaniak, Anal. Chem. 75 (2003) 2342.

[50] B.H. Kim, O. Mader, U. Weimar, R. Brock, D.P. Kern, J. Vac. Sci. Technol. B 21 (2003) 1472.

[51] I. Pera, J. Fritz, Langmuir 23 (2007) 1543.

[52] Y. Arntz, J.D. Seelig, H.P. Lang, J. Zhang, P. Hunziker, J.P. Ramseyer, E. Meyer, M. Hegner, C. Gerber, Nanotechnology 14 (2003) 86.

[53] G.Y. Kang, G.Y. Han, J.Y. Kang, I.-H. Cho, H.-H. Park, S.-H. Paek, T.S. Kim, Sensors Actuat. B 117 (2006) 332.

[54] J.H. Lee, K.H. Yoon, K.S. Hwang, J. Park, S. Ahn, T.S. Kim, Biosens. Bioelectron. 20 (2004) 269.

[55] T.Y. Kwon, K. Eom, J.H. Park, D.S. Yoon, T.S. Kim, H.L. Lee, Appl. Phys. Lett. 90 (2007) 223903.

[56] K.W. Wee, G.Y. Kang, J. Park, J.Y. Kang, D.S. Yoon, J.H. Park, T.S. Kim, Biosens. Bioelectron. 20 (2005) 1932.

[57] A.M. Moulin, S.J. O'Shea, R.A. Badley, P. Doyle, M.E. Welland, Langmuir 15 (1999) 8776.

[58] S. Stolyarova, S. Cherian, R. Raiteri, J. Zeravik, P. Skladal, Y. Nemirovsky, Sensors Actuat. B 131 (2008) 509.

[59] G.A. Campbell, R. Mutharasan, Anal. Chem. 78 (2006) 2328.

[60] M. Calleja, J. Tamayo, M. Nordström, A. Boisen, Appl. Phys. Lett. 88 (2006) 113901.

[61] H.-S. Kwon, K.-C. Han, K.S. Hwang, J.H. Lee, T.S. Kim, D.S. Yoon, E.G. Yang, Anal. Chim. Acta 585 (2007) 344.

[62] G.H. Wu, R.H. Datar, K.M. Hansen, T. Thundat, R.J. Cote, A. Majumdar, Nat. Biotechnol. 19 (2001) 856.

[63] C. Vancˇura, Y. Li, J. Lichtenberg, K.-U. Kirstein, A. Hierlemann, F. Josse, Anal. Chem. 79 (2007) 1646.

[64] S.M. Lee, K.S. Hwang, H.J. Yoon, D.S. Yoon, S.K. Kim, Y.S. Lee, T.S. Kim, Lab Chip 9 (2009) 2683.

[65] N. Backmann, C. Zahnd, F. Huber, A. Bietsch, A. Pluckthun, H.P. Lang, H.J. Güntherodt, M. Hegner, C. Gerber, Proc. Natl. Acad. Sci. USA 102 (2005) 14587.

[66] P. Dutta, J. Sanseverino, P.G. Datskos, M.J. Sepaniak, Nanobiotechnology 1 (2005) 237.

[67] R. Mukhopadhyay, V.V. Sumbayev, M. Lorentzen, J. Kjems, P.A. Andreasen, F. Besenbacher, Nano Lett. 5 (2005) 2385.

[68] A.M. Moulin, S.J. O'Shea, M.E. Welland, Ultramicroscopy 82 (2000) 23.

[69] W. Tan, Y. Huang, T. Nan, C. Xue, Z. Li, Q. Zhang, B. Wang, Anal. Chem. 82 (2010) 615.

[70] J.A. Capobianco, W.Y. Shih, Q.-A. Yuan, G.P. Adams, W.-H. Shih, Rev. Sci. Instrum. 79 (2008) 076101.

[71] T. Kwon, J. Park, J. Yang, D.S. Yoon, S. Na, C.-W. Kim, J.-S. Suh, Y.-M. Huh, S. Haam, K. Eom, PLoS One 4 (2009) e6248.

[72] Y.J. Liu, X.X. Li, Z.X. Zhang, G.M. Zuo, Z.X. Cheng, H.T. Yu, Biomed. Microdevices 11 (2009) 183.

[73] Y. Lam, N.I. Abu-Lail, M.S. Alam, S. Zauscher, Nanomed. Nanotechnol. Biol. Med. 2 (2006) 222.

[74] R.L. Gunter, W.G. Delinger, K. Manygoats, A. Kooser, T.L. Porter, Sensors Actuat. A 107 (2003) 219.

[75] T. Braun, M.K. Ghatkesar, N. Backmann, W. Grange, P. Boulanger, L. Letellier, H.-P. Lang, A. Bietsch, C. Gerber, M. Hegner, Nat. Nano. 4 (2009) 179.

[76] V. Sreepriya, J. Hai-Feng, Meas. Sci. Technol. 17 (2006) 2964.

[77] N. Nugaeva, K.Y. Gfeller, N. Backmann, M. Duggelin, H.P. Lang, H.J. Guntherodt, M. Hegner, Microsc. Microanal. 13 (2007) 13.

[78] A.P. Davila, J. Jang, A.K. Gupta, T. Walter, A. Aronson, R. Bashir, Biosens. Bioelectron. 22 (2007) 3028.

[79] J.-P. McGovern, W.Y. Shih, R. Rest, M. Purohit, Y. Pandya, W.-H. Shih, Analyst 133 (2008) 649.

[80] L. Fu, S. Li, K. Zhang, Z.-Y. Cheng, MRS Online Proc. Library 951 (2006) E05 04.

[81] J. Zhang, H.F. Ji, Anal. Sci. 20 (2004) 585.

[82] K.Y. Gfeller, N. Nugaeva, M. Hegner, Appl. Environ. Microbiol. 71 (2005) 2626.

[83] J.A. Capobianco, W.Y. Shih, W.-H. Shih, Rev. Sci. Instrum. 77 (2006) 125105.

[84] L. Fu, K. Zhang, S. Li, Y. Wang, T.-S. Huang, A. Zhang, Z.Y. Cheng, Sensors Actuat. B 150 (2010) 220.

[85] Q. Zhu, W.Y. Shih, W.-H. Shih, Biosens. Bioelectron. 22 (2007) 3132.

[86] H.F. Ji, X. Yang, J. Zhang, T. Thundat, Expert Rev. Mol. Diagn. 4 (2004) 859.
[87] G.A. Campbell, R. Mutharasan, Biosens. Bioelectron. 23 (2008) 1039.
[88] T. Mammoto, A. Mammoto, D.E. Ingber, Annu. Rev. Cell Dev. Biol. 29 (2013) 27.
[89] D.A. Lee, M.M. Knight, J.J. Campbell, D.L. Bader, J. Cell. Biochem. 112 (2011) 1.
[90] Z. Xiaoyu Rayne, Z. Xin, J. Micromech. Microeng. 21 (2011) 054003.
[91] N. Maloney, G. Lukacs, J. Jensen, M. Hegner, Nanoscale 6 (2014) 8242.

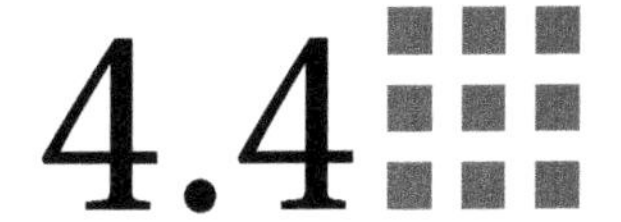

Theranostics

Rajendrakumar Santhosh Kalash*, Vinoth Kumar Lakshmanan*, Chong-Su Cho**, In-Kyu Park*

*DEPARTMENT OF BIOMEDICAL SCIENCES, BK21 PLUS CENTER FOR CREATIVE BIOMEDICAL SCIENTISTS AT CHONNAM NATIONAL UNIVERSITY, RESEARCH INSTITUTE OF MEDICAL SCIENCES, CHONNAM NATIONAL UNIVERSITY MEDICAL SCHOOL, GWANGJU, SOUTH KOREA; **DEPARTMENT OF AGRICULTURAL BIOTECHNOLOGY AND RESEARCH INSTITUTE FOR AGRICULTURE AND LIFE SCIENCES, SEOUL NATIONAL UNIVERSITY, SEOUL, SOUTH KOREA

CHAPTER OUTLINE

4.4.1 Introduction

In clinical trials, there is quite a demand for overcoming variations in drug response due to genetic variability in large patient populations. Thus, individualized treatment is the current strategy chosen for overcoming this problem [1]. According to the National Academy of Sciences, personalized medicine (PM) or precision medicine is defined as "the use of genomic, epigenetics, exposure and other data to define individual patterns of disease, potentially leading to better individual treatment" [2]. For the past few decades, clinician practice habits shifted toward PM and PM has been considered to offer promising benefits for improving the health care system.

One of the major challenges in personalized treatment is pharmacokinetic variability of drugs in patients. Real-time pharmacokinetic monitoring in patients will provide information for planning or designing further treatment plans and may also decrease the occurrence of drug-related adverse events. For the past few decades, the combination

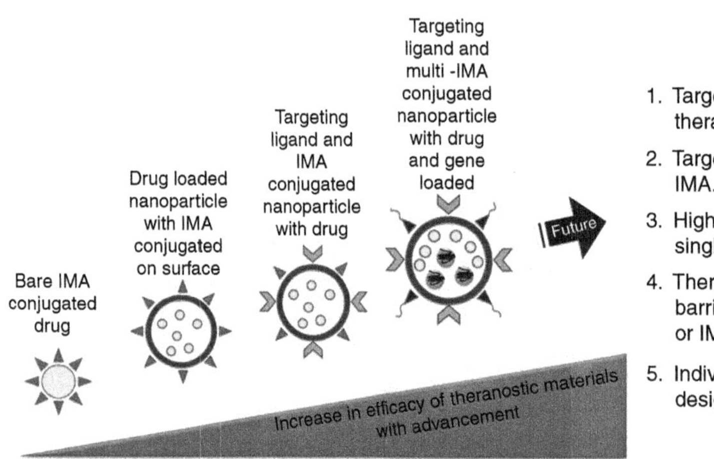

FIGURE 4.4.1 Schematic illustration of advancements in the field of nanotheranostics. IMA, Imaging agent.

of therapy with an imaging modality has been achieved through the development of nanomedicine and this image-guided therapeutic system is commonly referred as "nano-theranostics" [3].

In 2002, "theranostics" was coined by Funkhouser and is defined as the integration of two modalities, that is, therapy and medical imaging into a single "package" material for overcoming the undesirable variations in biodistribution and therapeutic efficacy [4–6]. Theranostic materials will provide a window for monitoring the pharmacokinetics and pharmacodynamics of the drug injected into the body. The concept was largely focused on cancer therapy, but later was expanded for other diseases like inflammatory diseases, autoimmune disorders like type 1 diabetes, cardiovascular diseases and neurological disorders [7–10]. The integration is achieved through the development of various nanoplatforms that have the ability to carry or act as both a therapeutic and an imaging agent along with the targeting moiety for specific delivery to the site of interest.

With engineered multifunctional theranostic nanomaterials, treatment and diagnosis can be done simultaneously and the progress of treatment can be viewed using diagnostics tools such as magnetic resonance imaging (MRI), computed tomography/positron emission tomography (CT/PET) scan, or fluorescent imaging [11]. Figure 4.4.1 shows that nanosystems can be used for tailor-made treatment for a specific patient and to improve their survival rate. The theranostic efficacy of nanomaterials will gradually increase with the use of "smart and novel" biomaterials. Theranostic nanomaterials can be made in response to the biological microenvironment such as temperature, pH, enzyme, or specific targeting moiety, which provides system-specific drug release and reduces toxicity to healthy tissues [12]. In this chapter, nanomaterials in the field of theranostics will be discussed in detail and also future prospects of theranostics in PM will be emphasized further in each topic.

4.4.2 Concept of Nanotheranostics

In the ever-growing field of PM, nanotechnology plays a vital role by integrating diagnostics and therapeutic function in a single system termed "nanotheranostics" [13]. With help of nanomaterials, proper diagnosis and therapeutic intervention by simultaneously targeting diseased cells after systemic circulation, evading the immune system, and imaging the pathological sites can be achieved [14]. For theranostics, many inorganic materials and carbon-based and polymer-based nanomaterials have been studied and also have been shown to act efficiently as an imaging agent or carrier/delivery agent. The following topics will describe the therapeutic and imaging strategies used in the field of theranostics.

4.4.2.1 Nanotheranostics in Therapy

4.4.2.1.1 Photodynamic Therapy

Around 3500 years ago, the Egyptians treated vitiligo, a chronic skin disease, by feeding patients a plant extract from *Ammi majus* L. and then exposing them to sunlight [15]. Also around that time, Indian healers used the seeds of the Bavachee plant (*Psoralea corylifolia*) in combination with sunlight for the treatment of leucoderma [15]. In the modern era, phototherapy was popularized by the Danish physician and Nobel laureate Niels Finsen who developed a focusable carbon-arc torch used for treating lupus vulgaris. Later on, gradually the development of the phototherapy approach toward other major diseases like cancer started to progress [16].

The therapies designed by the ancient Egyptians and Indians for skin diseases were based on the principles of photochemotherapy, where the exogenous photosensitizing agent (plant extract) absorbs the photons and reacts with neighboring biomolecules for therapeutic effect. For the past few decades, photodynamic therapy (PDT) has been used as an alternative treatment for many cancerous and noncancerous diseases. In PDT, a photosensitizing agent absorbs light of a particular wavelength and produces singlet oxygen ($^1O_2$) by converting molecular oxygen ($^3O_2$) in the cytoplasm of cells resulting in either apoptosis or necrosis of the cells [17].

According to the illustration of Jablonski (Fig. 4.4.2), the photochemical reaction can take place in two steps: (1) after absorbing incident light, the electrons in the photosensitizer excite from the ground state to the excited state, and (2) instead of decaying from singlet state to ground state, the electrons have intersystem crossing and therefore transfer the energy to either other photosensitizer molecules to form harmful intermediates such as hydrogen peroxides or superoxide (absence of oxygen), or transfer to the ground triplet dioxygen molecules to produce singlet oxygen (presence of oxygen) [18]. Either way it brings selective destruction to diseased cells by damaging the cellular organelles such as the mitochondria or nucleus (DNA) and leads to cell apoptosis or necrosis.

The photosensitizing agent or photosensitizer is a chemical entity that modulates the chemical changes inside the cells by absorbing light [19], and in preclinical studies, they have been shown to have potentially useful characteristics for PDT [20]. Phorphine,

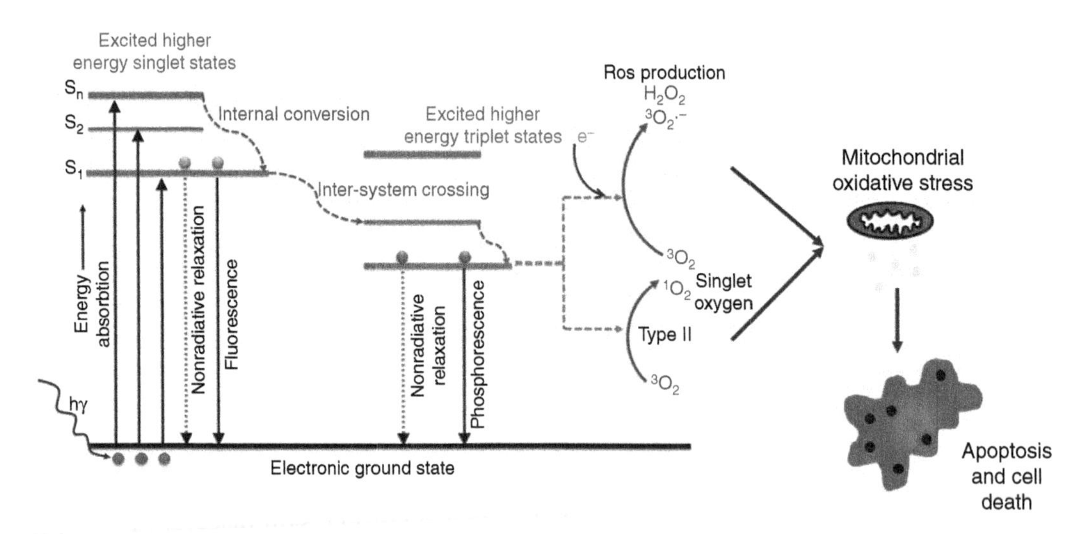

FIGURE 4.4.2 Schematic illustration of a Jablonski diagram explaining light-induced ROS production by photosensitizers and their role in causing apoptosis in cancer cells.

chlorins, and phthalocyanine derivatives were commonly used PDT photosensitizers for various clinical and preclinical cancer treatments [21]. For effective PDT, photosensitizers are either conjugated or loaded in various polymers, metallic or nonmetallic and carbon-based nanoparticles. In clinical applications, PDT has been mostly applied for various cancerous diseases like brain, head, and neck cancer, but it is also used in dermatological diseases, ophthalmic diseases, cardiovascular diseases, and urological diseases [22].

The major drawback of PDT is that after treatment, the long-term presence of photosensitizers in the blood stream of the patient makes them sensitive to light [23]. Hence, after treatment, the patients have to be kept in a dark room to prevent any further phototoxicity. But PDT with a nanotheranostics platform can be made safe and effective by specifically targeting only diseased cells.

4.4.2.1.2 Photothermal Therapy

Heat is one of the most efficient weapons to destroy tumor cells. But to induce a moderate heat of 41–47°C for a short duration (5–10 min) in the body without affecting normal tissue is quite difficult. Some of the commonly used heating sources to induce localized hyperthermia in the body are radiofrequency (RF), microwaves, ultrasound, magnetic field, and light [24].

In photothermal therapy (PTT), after near-infrared irradiation (NIR), PTT agents in cancer cells will absorb light/energy and at the subatomic level electrons will excite from the ground state to the excited state. Then, upon returning to the ground state through nonradiative decay channels, kinetic energy is emitted, which leads to the production of heat energy in the local tumor environment. The generated heat energy (1) disrupts the cell membrane and (2) degrades the cellular proteins and other molecules (Fig. 4.4.3). The

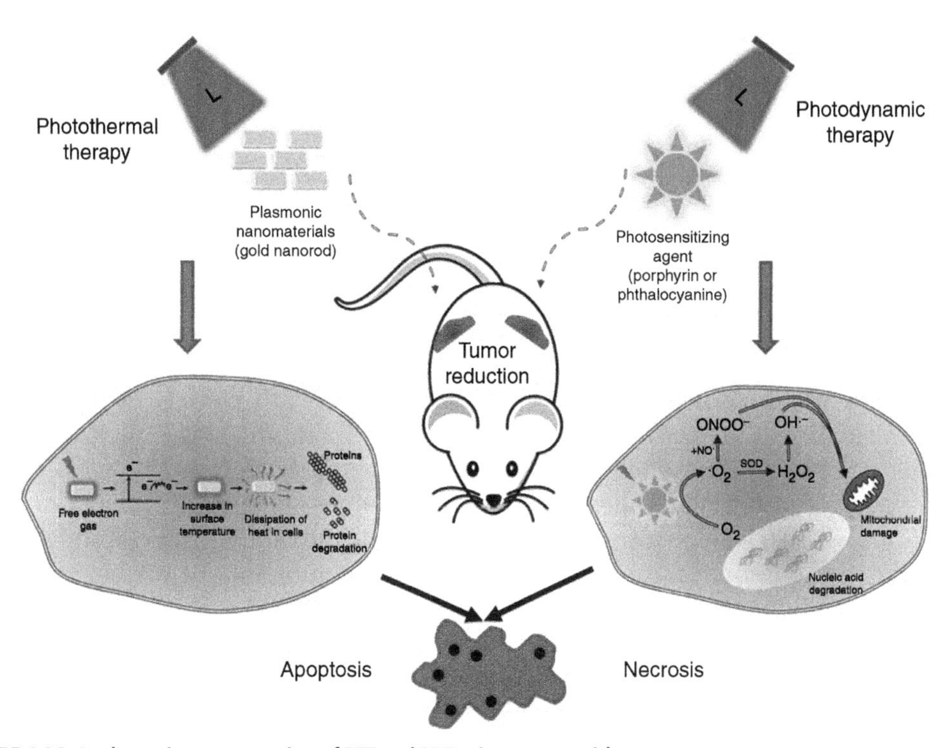

FIGURE 4.4.3 A schematic representation of PTT and PDT using nanoparticles.

reason behind the high thermal production in only the tumor region compared to normal tissues is due to the poor vasculature in tumor tissue and therefore heat dissipation is quite reduced [25]. Hence, the heat produced does not affect the normal tissue and causes thermal ablation in tumor tissue only. For PTT, nanomaterials of both organic and inorganic forms that have the ability to excite upon induction of light result in the production of heat. Noble metals such as gold and silver and carbon-based nanomaterials such as graphene oxide (GO) or carbon nanotube (CNT) have been used for cancer photothermal ablation. Currently this technique has been applied mostly in cancer treatment; however, application has also focused on other diseases such as Alzheimer's disease [26].

In image-guided PTT, plasmonic gold nanoparticles are kept in the spotlight because of the unique surface plasmon resonance (SPR) properties, which confines photons and enhances all radiative and nonradiative properties of the particle [27]. Gold nanoparticles of different shapes such as nanorod, nanosphere, nanocage, and nanostar are used for PTT and by varying the size and shell thickness, they can be tuned to absorb incident light in the NIR range. Therefore, in the NIR range, light can penetrate through the tissue and be absorbed by the nanoparticles, which then can heat up and destroy the nearby cancer cells. The currently emerging nanoparticles for PTT are carbon-based nanoparticles such as GO and CNT, which are under intense study. With proper fine tuning and implementation of certain functionalization strategies in GO and CNT, they can be used for PTT, apart from drug delivery. Robinson et al. developed nanosized, PEGylated reduced GO sheets for PTT and the NIR absorbance capacity is >sixfold. However, since GO is hydrophobic, it is necessary to coat it with an amphiphilic surfactant [28].

4.4.2.1.3 Hyperthermia Treatment

In cancer treatment, minimal treatment strategy limits surgery to diagnostic puncture procedures, such as core biopsy or fine needle biopsy to yield acceptable rates of local control. In order to achieve this, with the aid of MRI or CT scan detection, malignant tumors can be ablated using minimal invasive techniques like laser thermotherapy [29]. During this process, the laser is focused toward the tumor site and generates heat energy that leads to the death of cancer cells. Thus, such therapy is popularly known as hyperthermia. Here, the cancer cells are killed by exposure to high temperature (45°C) and healthy cells are protected by specifically exposing only tumor tissues to the heat.

In hyperthermia, the killing effect is achieved at a temperature range between 40°C and 45°C, during which the following events take place inside the cancer cells: (1) proteins start denaturing, (2) apoptotic factors induce apoptosis, (3) inhibition of DNA repair mechanism, and (4) inhibition of heat shock protein synthesis [30]. Apart from these cellular events, the tumor microenvironment makes the cells more sensitive to heat. Importantly, the nervous system has to be taken into consideration while applying this technique because nerve cells are sensitive to heat and may be irreversibly damaged. Thus, exposure time and temperature have to be maintained and focused on the region of interest [31,32].

Based on source type, the materials can vary upon their characteristic properties, for example, magnetic nanoparticles (MNP) with enhanced magnetic properties produce heat when a magnetic field is applied [33] or gold nanoparticles with high absorbance produce heat when a laser is applied (photothermal).

MNP-based hyperthermia is the most prominent method to conduct this noninvasive technique, without affecting healthy tissues. In an alternating magnetic field (AMF), MNPs vibrate and produce heat energy and their efficiency to produce heat is measured in terms of specific absorption rate (SAR) [34]. MNPs are good candidates since they have high MR T2 relaxivity and SAR and MRI-guided thermal ablation for cancer can be achieved [35].

4.4.2.2 Nanotheranostics for Imaging

4.4.2.2.1 Optical Imaging

Optical imaging has been a powerful modality for studying molecular recognition and molecular imaging in a noninvasive, sensitive, and real-time manner. Optical imaging is cost-effective, convenient, and safe due to nonionization. Also, optical imaging has the capacity to be combined with other imaging modalities such as PET, single-photon emission computed tomography (SPECT), and MRI. For *in vivo* applications, bioluminescence and fluorescence imaging are the most widely used techniques for image-guided surgery (IGS) and tumor diagnosis. IGS is the current technique used for excising tumors that are small in nature, such as gastric polypoid lesions or breast cancer tumors [36]. In this manner, removal of healthy tissues or cancer metastasis can be prevented and further treatment plans can be made if necessary.

The combination of optical imaging techniques with cancer-specific imaging agents provides a barrier to hinder cancer recurrence caused by the presence of tumor margins. Specificity of the imaging agents toward cancer cells can be achieved by conjugating the imaging dye with biomolecules such as an antibody, cell penetrating peptides, cyclic RGD or drug molecules that specifically bind to cancer cells [37–39].

The bioluminescence technique is applied for quantitative measurement of tumor burden, treatment response, immune cell trafficking, and detection of gene transfer [40]. The luminescence property depends on adenosine triphosphate and oxygen-dependent enzymatic conversion of exogenous luciferin to oxyluciferin by luciferase within living cells. An emission spectrum is produced with a peak of approximately 560 nm, which can be detected by a highly sensitive charge coupled device camera at 10–15 min after injection of luciferin and lasts for 60 min in mice [41].

Infrared dyes for fluorescent imaging have been used because background noise can be avoided while imaging a target tissue. At 650–900 nm range, autofluorescence from blood, water, and lipids is reduced and clear images of the target tissue can be visualized and therefore diagnosis for a particular disease can be easily achieved [42]. Hence, NIR dyes are widely used for tracking drug molecules as well as drug accumulation in organs.

In theranostics, anticancer therapy with fluorescent imaging can be also achieved with metal nanoparticles. It has been reported that silver nanoparticles with high metal enhanced fluorescence can be used for cell imaging [43].

4.4.2.2.2 MRI Imaging

Magnetic resonance imaging (MRI) is widely used for diagnosing solid tumors and brain tumors, and it is considered to be the most efficient and noninvasive imaging system due to its high spatial resolution as well as its high sensitivity. MRI basically reveals a detailed map of the anatomical structure, detecting lesions for diagnosis, and also provides information about the functional aspects within the body. In MRI, RF radiation is applied in the presence of a controlled magnetic field to produce high-quality cross-sectional images of the body in any plane. When the magnetic field is applied, all of the hydrogen atoms align along the external field and become excited after RF is applied. The excited atoms release energy, which will be received by the wire coils in the MRI unit and MR mapping is done using a computer. From MRI, two images are obtained: (1) T_1-weighted image and (2) T_2-weighted image; these images solely depend on the property of MRI contrast agents used. In T_2-weighted images, the contrast agents have a very large transverse relaxivity (r_2) of 100–200 s^{-1} mM^{-1} and produce darker images whereas in the T_1-weighted image, contrast agents possessing a longitudinal relaxivity r_1 of 3–5 s^{-1} mM^{-1} produce brighter images [44]. The T_1 and T_2 relaxation times are generally correlated with the water content, tissue structure, and contrast agent uptake [45]. The available MRI contrast agents are paramagnetic such as gadolinium (Gd^{3+}) or manganese (Mn^{2+}), which have a permanent magnetic moment, and superparamagnetic agents such as iron oxide core or an Fe/Mn composite metal core covered in a polymer matrix, which have a larger magnetic moment compared to the paramagnetic agents [46]. Even though MRI allows high spatial resolution (0.2–1 mm), it lacks sensitivity (10^{-3}–10^{-5} mol/L). Therefore, to improve the imaging quality and visualization of tissue morphology and function, MRI is combined with other imaging modalities such as CT, PET, SPECT, or ultrasound [47,48].

4.4.2.2.3 Ultrasound Imaging

When high-frequency sound waves are sent to interact with the living tissues, the echoes from the sound waves will be captured and an image of the moving tissue, primarily blood, abnormal masses of tissue, and tissue size, is produced. This ultrasound imaging technique is well established, noninvasive, versatile, and widely used as a diagnostic tool in humans. In the ultrasound imaging technique, no contrast agents are used and vascular information derived from color or power Doppler is generally sufficient for correct diagnosis. In order to image inflammatory sites or thromboses, it is necessary to diagnose with contrast ultrasound imaging. The trend of contrast ultrasound imaging started with microbubbles (MBs), and has been shown to be quite a promising technique for theranostics [49]. The MBs are free gas bubbles in solution over bubbles stabilized by surfactants with a shell made from phospholipids, proteins, or polymers, which is several micrometers in size. These MBs reflect the ultrasound waves, which are quite different from the tissues. Thus, it gives an insight about the vasculature through which the blood and MBs are traveling [50].

These MBs can be attached to a targeting antibody, peptide, or ligand for targeted imaging in the body. Also, they can be used for transporting drugs and genes to specific cells such as cancer cells.

MB application in drug delivery to the brain by crossing the blood–brain barrier (BBB) was shown by Fan et al., where vascular endothelial growth factor-targeted drug-loaded MBs were used for targeting brain glioma tumors in rats, and using ultrasound, drug release was achieved with a burst of MBs making the focused ultrasound BBB open. During the short opening, drug molecules reached the tumor site and promoted tumor killing [51].

Recently, ultrasound imaging has been intensified using a single nanoparticle with double scattering/reflection properties. Zhang et al. developed a rattle-type mesoporous silica nanostructure with two contributing interfaces, that is, incident ultrasound will be scattered and reflected twice between these two interfaces in the nanoparticle [52].

4.4.3 Metallic Nanomaterials for Theranostics

For centuries, metallic nanoparticles have been widely used by clinicians and researchers from all around the world and they have been studied greatly in the field of nanobiotechnology. They have been positioned in various aspects of medical applications such as diagnosis, drug delivery, gene delivery, and noninvasive therapy including hyperthermia and PTT. With proper surface functionalization using ligands or polymers, they can also be applied in cancer theranostics.

4.4.3.1 Superparamagnetic Iron Oxide Nanoparticles (SPIONs)

In the field of biomedical sciences, SPIONs are used widely for various applications such as magnetic separation, temperature-mediated drug delivery, cancer therapy, and MRI contrast agents [53,54]. SPIONs consisting of an iron oxide core have excellent superparamagnetic properties and with proper surface functionalization they can be used for drug or gene delivery, which is guided by an external magnetic field [55]. They have great potential to improve the following aspects: (1) MRI contrast imaging, (2) enhanced drug or gene delivery, and (3) hyperthermia [56]. With smaller size and proper surface modification, SPIONs have significant binding kinetics toward various biomolecules [57].

In clinical MRI, SPIONs will shorten the T_2 proton relaxation times, thus leading to dark negative contrast areas in T_2-weighted MR images [58]. For stabilization and biocompatibility, SPIONs are coated with biopolymers such as dextran or carboxyl dextran. However, studies have shown that dextran coating of SPIONs resulted in immune-related adverse effects in patients, enhanced renal clearance, and endocytosis by macrophages [59–62]. Therefore, to avoid detection by the immune system, masking the foreignness of SPIONs is necessary for long-term immune evasion as well as *in vivo* longevity. Wang et al. have successfully masked immune reactivity and improved the long-term circulation of SPION nanoworms with high R_2 relativity by cross-linking dextran with epichlorohydrin in the presence of NaOH [63].

In magnetic hyperthermia, heat is generated when SPIONs are stimulated by an external high-frequency AMF. The local heat generated is sufficient for killing cancerous cells, although the main challenge of this will be tuning the nanoparticle property in order to generate sufficient heat at the clinical-allowed magnetic field conditions. However, compared to iron oxide nanoparticles (IONPs), SPIONs can generate significantly higher heat in intracellular magnetic hyperthermia. The reason behind this was explained by Soukup et al.: IONPs generate less heat due to immobilization inside the cells. In detail, IONPs follow the Brownian mechanism for the magnetization relaxation process, which is drastically reduced inside the cells leading to a significant reduction in heat generation, whereas SPIONs relax by thermal processes (Neel relaxation), which is not affected by cellular immobilization and heat generation occurs at minimal AMF [64]. Another insight given by this study was that, IONs or SPIONs are released after cell lysis in their original state and they can be taken up by viable cells again for additional hyperthermia.

For long-term circulation and targeted delivery, formulation of drug and biotherapeutics such as nucleic acids, proteins, and cells with SPIONs were used as an alternative treatment for various nontreatable diseases [65]. In drug delivery to the brain, SPIONs can replace invasive methods, such as intraneoplastic injection or drug-loaded wafers implanted in the resection cavity during brain surgery, by delivering the drug specifically to the site in the brain guided by a targeting ligand [66–71]. SPIONs are not only an efficient drug carrier, but also have been investigated for effective gene delivery [72]. Using cationic lipids or polymers, the surface of SPIONs can be modified for efficient binding of negatively charged nucleic acids such as plasmids, siRNA, and miRNA.

Lo et al. coated SPIONs with chondritin sulfate–polyethylenimine copolymer for the efficient delivery of a microRNA-128 encoding plasmid *in vitro* and in a U87-xenograft nude mouse model [73].

SPIONs can be produced as multifunctional nanoparticles by following various strategies to fabricate theranostic iron oxide nanoparticles such as (1) drug-conjugated/loaded polymeric micelles loaded with SPIONs, (2) SPIONs coated with drug, and (3) PTT or PDT agent with SPIONs.

Nanocomposite micelles were formed by SPIONs stabilized by poly(styrene)-*b*-poly(acrylic acid) block copolymer (PS-*b*-PAA), with peripheral surfacing folic acid and loaded with doxorubicin (DOX) drug. These nanocomposite micelles have pH-controlled release of drug, real-time monitoring of particle distribution by MRI, and a tumor-specific sensing property [74]. Similarly, SPION can also be coated with drug and then functionalized with hydrophilic polymers. Kaaki et al. demonstrated DOX attached to SPIONs and buried under the poly(ethylene glycol) (PEG) layer conjugated with folic acid for cancer targeting [75].

With the PDT/PTT agent, employing SPIONs facilitates obtaining visual information of the target site (MRI), efficient drug delivery, and NIR hyperthermia. Urries et al. studied hybrid double shell nanoparticles prepared with gold (Au) and SPIONs for MRI, PTT, and drug delivery. The hybrid nanoshell was achieved by growing a silica shell over SPIONs and then coating with Au. After PEGylation, the silica is slowly etched using NaOH and buffered with hydrofluoric acid [76].

4.4.3.2 Gold Nanoparticles

SPR is a unique property of plasmonic or noble metal nanoparticles such as gold nanoparticles. This unique property offers multimodalities for medical applications due to photon confinement to a small particle size and enhancing all radiative and nonradiative properties of the nanoparticles [77].

When an oscillating electromagnetic radiation falls over a plasmonic metal surface, it induces collective coherent oscillation of the free electron gas on the surface. This creates a charge separation with respect to the ionic lattice, forming a dipole oscillation along the direction of the electric field of the light. The amplitude of the oscillation in SPR reaches a maximum at a specific frequency and induces strong absorption and scattering of the incident light. Based on size, absorption, and scattering ratio, gold nanoparticles produce intense colors [27]. Therefore, for imaging, larger nanoparticles are preferred because of the higher scattering efficiency, that is, more intense color, whereas smaller nanoparticles are preferred for PTT because the high light absorption is required for heat conversion [27].

For cancer-based gene therapy, gold nanoparticles are used for the safe, specific, and effective delivery of siRNA. The gold surface has affinity toward thiol and amine groups. Therefore, thiolated nucleic acids can be linked via an Au–thiol linkage. It has been reported that cross-linking of multimerized siRNA by gold nanoparticles is achieved by immobilizing gold nanoparticles with single-stranded antisense siRNA and then assembled by complementary hybridization with AuNPs having the other single-stranded sense siRNA [78].

Gold nanoparticles as a drug carrier are possible through proper functionalization of the metal surface where the drug does not directly interact with gold unless a linker is added. Zhang et al. developed a strategy to increase the solubility and efficacy of the hydrophobic drug paclitaxel (PTX) by conjugating the drug with polyvalent DNA and then later coating over the gold surface via the thiol linkage. The DNA linker labeled with fluorophore provided a visual image of drug delivery in the cells [79].

For PTT, the absorption of NIR light by gold nanoparticles provides better conversion of light to heat and can also be designed in such a way that light is absorbed at a higher wavelength, that is, the NIR region [80]. Recently, it was shown that hollow gold nanoparticles could be loaded with drugs like DOX and irradiated with NIR light thus triggering release of the drug and inducing thermal ablation with enhanced radio sensitization of the tumor [81].

Theranostic nanoparticles with gold can be made with other metallic nanoparticles such as SPIONs, for providing multi-imaging modality and dual therapeutic outcomes. A recent study showed that gold and SPIONs loaded in an amphiphilic diblock copolymer PEG-*b*-PCL had selective tumor accumulation, enabling MRI of the tumor margins and improved survival rate of tumor-bearing mice after NIR irradiation [82].

4.4.4 Carbon-Based Nanomaterials for Theranostics

In biomedical research, carbon nanomaterials (CNMs) are considered to be the most attractive materials since they possess distinctive physical and chemical properties such as excellent mechanical strength, electrical and thermal conductivity, and optical properties [83]. Much effort is being taken to utilize these properties for developing various biomedical applications.

CNMs have emerged as an efficient carrier for genes and drugs as well as an imaging agent. In drug delivery, hydrophobic drugs are loaded to the CNMs via π–π interaction [84]. Even though CNMs have a large surface area that provides higher loading of drug, this comes with certain limitations such as toxicity, renal clearance issues, and low solubility, which can be overcome by surface modification via oxygen containing functionality of carbon structures [85].

4.4.4.1 Graphene Oxide (GO)

GO is obtained by treating graphite material with strong oxidizers such as potassium chlorate and fuming nitric acid. By this method, tightly stacked graphite layers are loosened by the introduction of oxygen atoms to the carbon. Dimiev et al. have explained the step-by-step formation of GO from solid graphite: (1) graphite is converted to graphite intercalation compound (GIC), (2) then GIC is converted to oxidized graphite as pristine graphene oxide (PGO), and finally (3) exposing the PGO to water gives conventional GO, where it undergoes hydrolysis of covalent sulfates and loss of all interlayer registry.

GO possesses a single layered two-dimensional sp^2 hybrid structure with sufficient hydrophilic surface groups and therefore forms stable colloids in water. But under physiological buffers, GO aggregates due to the presence of salts, which has a charge screening effect [84].

Both reduced graphene oxide (rGO) and GO have the ability to absorb NIR, visible, and UV light and fluoresce at a particular wavelength. But mechanisms responsible for the fluorescence are still unclear [86]. According to a study by Shang et al., three different kinds of functional groups, C–O, C═O, O═C–OH, on GO were found to be involved in GO fluorescence [87].

GO exhibits a higher NIR light absorption property, making it a potent photothermal agent. Compared to ultrasmall GO, rGO prepared by PEGylation showed a >6-fold increase in NIR absorbance and irradiation with an 808 nm laser resulting in a temperature rise up to 55°C in 8 min along with an increase in concentration [86].

By taking advantage of this property, many studies have shown that GO can be used for combinatorial therapy where it can be tagged with any ligand such as folic acid [88] or chlorotoxin [89] and loaded with DOX for specific cancer chemotherapy and PTT.

The presence of functional groups on the basal plane and edges of GO facilitates the bioconjugation of various biomolecules such as proteins or peptides. For gene delivery, GO needs to be functionalized with cationic polymers or peptides in order to bind the negatively charged DNA. GO functionalized with octaarginine has been shown to be an efficient gene carrier and less cytotoxic compared to the cationic polymer such as a branched polyethylenimine [90].

Hydrophobic drugs such as DOX or camptothecin can be loaded over the surface of GO through noncovalent conjugation via π–π interaction. As PTX has no π structure to interact with larger aromatic rings, it can be conjugated to GO via a cleavable ester bond [91].

4.4.4.2 Carbon Nanotube (CNT)

CNTs with their cylindrical carbon structure possess a wide range of electrical and optical properties, which have been explored for use in biomedical applications. Due to their mechanical strength and optical properties, CNTs have been used as tissue scaffolds, drug delivery, and imaging. Similar to GO, CNTs also have optical transition in the NIR region, which makes them a potent imaging agent for NIR fluorescence microscopy and optical coherence tomography.

The limitations of CNTs are (1) insolubility, (2) toxicity, (3) agglomeration, and (4) they induce inflammation. These limitations can be overcome by functionalizing the surface of CNTs with PEG, or other biomolecules such as DNA, protein, or carbohydrate.

For theranostic application, CNTs must have the following: (1) the ability to deliver drugs or genes, (2) PTT properties, and (3) sensitivity toward Raman scattering. CNTs are highly sensitive to Raman scattering because of their extensive symmetric carbon bonds and thus by using different Raman spectrum signatures of CNTs, selective PTT can be achieved in tumor cells [92].

CNTs have frequently proven to be an efficient carrier of drugs and genes. In gene delivery, very few metallic and polymeric nanoparticles have been employed, since they provide better protection from enzymatic degradation and interference from DNA binding proteins. But apart from protection, CNTs have shown higher transfection efficiency in hard-to-transfect cells such as bone marrow mesenchymal stem cells and other primary cells [93]. CNTs in combination with metal nanoparticles such as gold, silver, or SPIONs can be employed for theranostic applications [94]. Recently, SPIONs-decorated multiwalled CNTs (MWCNTs) radiolabeled with technetium-99m was used as a dual MRI and SPECT contrast agent. In this construct, the MWCNTs were functionalized with bisphosphonate (dipicolylamine-alendronate) for radiolabeling and then coated with SPIONs. Overall, the hybrid nanoparticles were shown to be stable and capable for MRI and SPECT imaging [95]. Similarly, single-stranded DNA/polymer functionalized single-walled CNTs can be coated with gold nanoparticles for surface enhanced Raman scattering imaging and PTT [96].

4.4.5 Polymer-Based Theranostics Nanomaterials

In theranostic applications, both synthetic and natural polymers have been used for delivering drugs, genes, and imaging agents. For sustained release of therapeutic agents over a period of time, synthetic polymers have been found to be more advantageous compared to natural polymers [97]. With other nanoplatforms such as GO, SPIONs, or gold nanoparticles, biodegradable polymers were employed because solubility and biocompatibility were improved and also provided a site for biomolecule conjugation [98].

4.4.5.1 Polymeric Liposome

Similar to living cells, liposomes composed of phospholipids and cholesterol are spherical vesicles with a unilamellar or multivesicular lipid bilayer structure. Due to this bilayer structure, both lipophilic and hydrophilic drug or gene molecules can be accommodated together, thus making them multifunctional nanoparticles with biocompatible, nontoxic, and biodegradable properties. They can accumulate passively into the tumor either through an enhanced permeability and retention effect effect or by specific targeting toward the cancer cells.

This versatile modifiable property allows liposomes to encapsulate functional molecules in the interior, inserted in the bilayer or attached on the bilayer membrane surface. Hence, they have been considered for application in multifunctional platforms, that is, therapy and imaging. They protect the amphiphilic, hydrophobic, and hydrophilic therapeutic agents against various threats that lead to their immediate dilution and degradation.

Liposomes are limited by their instability, drug leakiness, and slow release kinetics in the tumor and hence PEG is coated on the surface to form stealth liposomes that are not

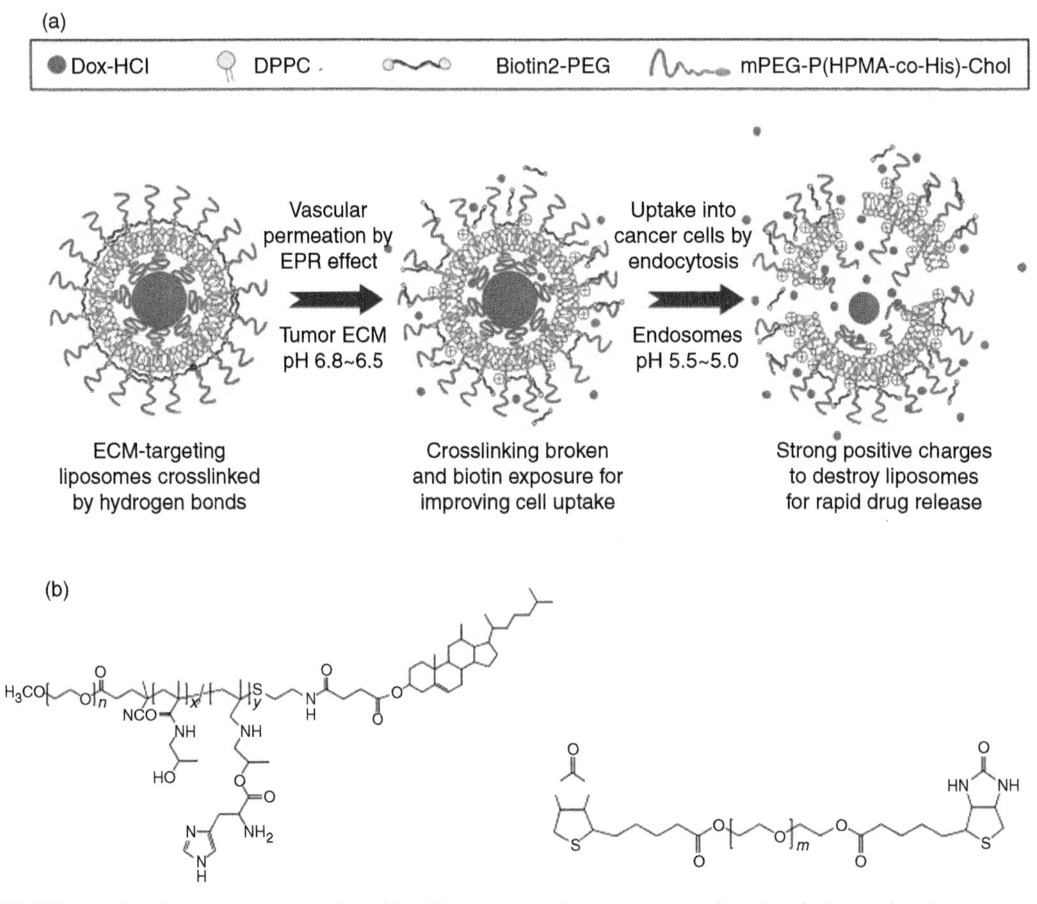

FIGURE 4.4.4 (a) Schematic representation of the ECM-targeting liposome concept based on hydrogen bond cross-linking, targeting ability, and drug release after tumor accumulation. (b) Chemical structures of mPEG-P(HPMA-co-His)-Chol copolymer and biotin2-PEG cross-linker [103].

recognized by the reticuloendothelial system that prolongs the blood circulation time [99–101]. Even though stealth liposomes are slow to release drug due to their compact structure [102], this problem can be overcome by using various methods such as: (1) highly pH-sensitive polymers for polymeric liposome, (2) cancer-associated enzyme-sensitive probes, or (3) cancer targeting polymers such as hyaluronic acid (HA), which can internalize and enhance drug release.

Polymeric liposomes are composed of liposomes functionalized with biodegradable polymers used for drug and gene delivery. In Fig. 4.4.4, Chiang et al. developed a stable and ECM, target-specific, pH-sensitive polymeric liposome to overcome slow drug release for anticancer therapy. The polymeric liposome showed an increase in antitumor activity and lower toxicity due to prevention of drug leakage, protein absorption, exposing biotin for cancer cell uptake by breaking the hydrogen bond in the cross-linker, and an increase in particle accumulation in the tumor [103].

Natural polymers such as chitosan and HA were grafted over liposomes for stability and biocompatibility. HA also aided in CD44-based cancer cell targeting and was also used as a backbone for many polymeric micelles and liposome formulations. Grafting HA with PEG of different molecular weights to liposomes, PEG–HA–liposome was found to have similar tumor accumulation to that of PEG–liposome in solid tumors, although cellular internalization was higher in the former compared to the latter [104]. Also, to facilitate MRI contrast agent accumulation in the target site, Smith et al. used chitosan to conjugate with the hydrophobic octadecyl chain (C18) and diethylenetriaminepentaacetic acid for gadolinium binding. The hydrophobic chain facilitated the binding of chitosan to the liposome, thus functionalizing them rapidly [105].

4.4.5.2 Polymeric Micelle Nanoparticles

Lipid molecules with an amphipathic nature form spherical particles such as micelles in aqueous medium. Polymeric micelles have a polymer backbone conjugated to a hydrophobic unit and the hydrophobic core formed accommodates hydrophobic drugs, dye molecules, or SPIONs, which can be used for simultaneous imaging and drug/gene delivery. It is an ideal carrier system for delivering hydrophobic drugs or dye molecules that are insoluble in water. Polymeric micelles have prolonged circulation kinetics necessary for drug accumulation in tumor target sites and also improve the solubility of drugs.

But the critical problem for current polymeric micelle-based drug delivery is that low stability and fast release of drug make it unsuitable for systemic drug delivery. However, Shi et al. overcame this problem and reported that π–π interaction between PTX and the aromatic ring of methoxy poly(ethylene glycol)-*b*-(N-[2-benzoyloxypropyl] methacrylamide) (mPEGb-*p*[HPMAm-Bz]) polymeric chains in the core increased drug loading capacity and showed strong drug retention [106].

In therapeutic gene and anticancer drug delivery, self-assembled polymeric micelles prepared from amphiphilic block copolymers represent one of the potential nanodelivery systems [107]. Xiong et al. developed a multifunctional polymeric micelle system that can deliver both DOX and siRNA to intracellular targets. The micellar formulation showed that 6% (wt ratio of DOX/polymer) DOX loading content and spermine-conjugated copolymer facilitated siRNA binding. As a whole, the polymeric micelle has shown to be efficient in protecting and delivering siRNA to target sites and also obtained proper pH-sensitive DOX release in MDA-MB-435/LCC6MDR1-resistant tumor murine models [108].

In order to monitor drug action toward solid tumors, Cho et al. administered micelles containing three different drugs and an NIR optical imaging agent in sequential manner. Here the poorly water-soluble drugs such as PTX, 17-allylamino-17-demethoxygeldanamycin and rapamycin were loaded in poly(ethylene glycol)-block-poly(D,L-lactic acid) and was given as a single intravenous injection in an LS180 human colon xenograft model. After 48 h of first intravenous injection, poly(ethylene glycol)-block-poly(ε-caprolactone) loaded with carbocyanine dye was given as a second intravenous injection. In the first case, there was a 1.6fold reduction in tumor volume and in the second case, the NIR optical signal was 2.1-fold higher in the excised solid tumors compared to the negative control. Thus, this system can be used as a promising multimodal strategy for theranostic application [109].

4.4.6 Conclusion and Future Prospects

Currently, clinicians and researchers in the field of biomedical sciences have the motivation to progress toward PM. Due to genetic differences between patient groups, therapeutic drugs that have shown significant efficacy in preclinical stages have failed in clinical trials. Even the pharmaceutical and diagnostic industries have diverted attention to develop a platform for PM for individual or small patient populations. Since the application of nanomedicine has started to progress from bench to bedside, nanomedicine is no longer considered futuristic medicine. Theranostics is an emerging field that is progressing rapidly although it is still naïve for clinical applications. Currently, there are numerous studies employing nanoparticle-based systems for fusing both therapies such as PTT and/or PDT and diagnostic imaging modalities such as MRI, and optical and ultrasound imaging. For preclinical studies, it is necessary to understand the behavior of nanoparticles in cellular and *in vivo* systems. Therefore, labeling agents such as quantum dots or dye have been used to track the nanoparticles after being injected. Theranostics is currently focused on cancer therapy although application to other chronic diseases such as autoimmune diseases and neurological disorders such as Alzheimer's disease is currently in progress. In this chapter, the overall role and application of nanomaterials in the field of theranostics was explained in detail. In the future, nanotheranostics will have significant potential to move from the bench toward the bedside.

References

[1] T. Tursz, R. Bernards, Mol. Oncol. 9 (2015) 935.

[2] National Research Council CommitteeToward Precision Medicine: Building a Knowledge Network for Biomedical Research and a New Taxonomy of Disease, National Academies Press, Washington DC, (2011).

[3] T. Lammers, L.Y. Rizzo, G. Storm, F. Kiessling, Clin. Cancer Res. 18 (2012) 4889.

[4] H. Ding, F. Wu, Theranostics 2 (2012) 1040.

[5] L.S. Wang, M.C. Chuang, J.A. Ho, Int. J. Nanomed. 7 (2012) 4679.

[6] S.S. Kelkar, T.M. Reineke, Bioconjug. Chem. 22 (2011) 1879.

[7] P. Wang, A. Moore, Quant. Imag. Med. Surg. 2 (2012) 151.

[8] S.K. Patel, J.M. Janjic, Theranostics 5 (2015) 150.

[9] B. Sriramoju, R. Kanwar, R.N. Veedu, J.R. Kanwar, Curr. Top. Med. Chem. 15 (2015) 1115.

[10] D. Wang, B. Lin, H. Ai, Pharm. Res. 31 (2014) 1390.

[11] S.M. Janib, A.S. Moses, J.A. MacKay, Adv. Drug Deliv. Rev. 62 (2010) 1052.

[12] M.E. Caldorera-Moore, W.B. Liechty, N.A. Peppas, Acc. Chem. Res. 44 (2011) 1061.

[13] T.H. Kim, S. Lee, X. Chen, Expert Rev. Mol. Diagn. 13 (2013) 257.
[14] M.S. Muthu, D.T. Leong, L. Mei, S.S. Feng, Theranostics 4 (2014) 660.
[15] H. Honigsmann, Photochem. Photobiol. Sci. 12 (2013) 16.
[16] M.D. Daniell, J.S. Hill, Aust. N. Z. J. Surg. 61 (1991) 340.
[17] E. Paszko, C. Ehrhardt, M.O. Senge, D.P. Kelleher, et al., Photodiagnosis Photodyn. Ther. 8 (2011) 14.
[18] P.G. Calzavara-Pinton, M. Venturini, R. Sala, J. Eur. Acad. Dermatol. Venereol. 21 (2007) 293.
[19] K. Berg, P.K. Selbo, A. Weyergang, A. Dietze, et al., J. Microsc. 218 (2005) 133.
[20] J.G. Levy, Semin. Oncol. 21 (1994) 4.
[21] R.R. Allison, G.H. Downie, R. Cuenca, X.H. Hu, et al., Photodiagnosis Photodyn. Ther. 1 (2004) 27.
[22] Z. Huang, Technol. Cancer Res. Treat. 4 (2005) 283.
[23] B. Zhao, Y.Y. He, Expert Rev. Anticancer Ther. 10 (2010) 1797.
[24] P. Wust, B. Hildebrandt, G. Sreenivasa, B. Rau, et al., Lancet Oncol. 3 (2002) 487.
[25] C.W. Song, Cancer Res. 44 (1984) 4721s.
[26] M. Li, X. Yang, J. Ren, K. Qu, et al., Adv. Mater. 24 (2012) 1722.
[27] X. Huang, P.K. Jain, I.H. El-Sayed, M.A. El-Sayed, Nanomed. (Lond.) 2 (2007) 681.
[28] J.T. Robinson, S.M. Tabakman, Y. Liang, H. Wang, et al., J. Am. Chem. Soc. 133 (2011) 6825.
[29] A.B. Akimov, V.E. Seregin, K.V. Rusanov, E.G. Tyurina, et al., Lasers Surg. Med. 22 (1998) 257.
[30] B. Hildebrandt, P. Wust, O. Ahlers, A. Dieing, et al., Crit. Rev. Oncol. Hematol. 43 (2002) 33.
[31] J. van der Zee, Ann. Oncol. 13 (2002) 1173.
[32] T.J. Vogl, P. Farshid, N.N. Naguib, A. Darvishi, et al., Radiol. Med. 119 (2014) 451.
[33] M. Banobre-Lopez, A. Teijeiro, J. Rivas, Rep. Pract. Oncol. Radiother. 18 (2013) 397.
[34] R.R. Shah, T.P. Davis, A.L. Glover, D.E. Nikles, et al., J. Magn. Magn. Mater. 387 (2015) 96.
[35] C.S. Kumar, F. Mohammad, Adv. Drug Deliv. Rev. 63 (2011) 789.
[36] E. de Boer, N.J. Harlaar, A. Taruttis, W.B. Nagengast, et al., Br. J. Surg. 102 (2015) e56.
[37] J.E. Bugaj, S. Achilefu, R.B. Dorshow, R. Rajagopalan, J. Biomed. Opt. 6 (2001) 122.
[38] S. Achilefu, H.N. Jimenez, R.B. Dorshow, J.E. Bugaj, et al., J. Med. Chem. 45 (2002) 2003.
[39] Y. Ye, X. Chen, Theranostics 1 (2011) 102.
[40] T.J. Sweeney, V. Mailander, A.A. Tucker, A.B. Olomu, et al., Proc. Natl. Acad. Sci. USA 96 (1999) 12044.
[41] F. Togel, Y. Yang, P. Zhang, Z. Hu, et al., Am. J. Physiol. Renal. Physiol. 295 (2008) F315.
[42] X. Yi, F. Wang, W. Qin, X. Yang, et al., Int. J. Nanomed. 9 (2014) 1347.
[43] H. Li, H. Hu, Y. Zhao, X. Chen, et al., Anal. Chem. 87 (2015) 3736.
[44] W. Xu, K. Kattel, J.Y. Park, Y. Chang, et al., Phys. Chem. Chem. Phys. 14 (2012) 12687.
[45] D. Galanaud, F. Nicoli, Y. Le Fur, M. Guye, et al., Biochimie 85 (2003) 905.
[46] H. Shokrollahi, Mater. Sci. Eng. C 33 (2013) 4485.
[47] O. Keunen, T. Taxt, R. Gruner, M. Lund-Johansen, et al., Adv. Drug Deliv. Rev. 76 (2014) 98.
[48] K.M. Bennett, J. Jo, H. Cabral, R. Bakalova, et al., Adv. Drug Deliv. Rev. 74 (2014) 75.
[49] C.Z. Behm, J.R. Lindner, Ultrasound Q. 22 (2006) 67.
[50] T.V. Bartolotta, A. Taibbi, M. Midiri, R. Lagalla, Abdom. Imag. 34 (2009) 193.
[51] B. Sivakumar, R.G. Aswathy, Y. Nagaoka, M. Suzuki, et al., Langmuir 29 (2013) 3453.

[52] K. Zhang, H. Chen, X. Guo, D. Zhang, et al., Sci. Rep. 5 (2015) 8766.

[53] I. Giouroudi, J. Kosel, Recent Pat. Nanotechnol. 4 (2010) 111.

[54] E. Zhang, M.F. Kircher, M. Koch, L. Eliasson, et al., ACS Nano 8 (2014) 3192.

[55] M. Mahmoudi, S. Sant, B. Wang, S. Laurent, et al., Adv. Drug Deliv. Rev. 63 (2011) 24.

[56] M.M. Lin, K. Kim do, A.J. El Haj, J. Dobson, IEEE Trans. Nanobiosci. 7 (2008) 298.

[57] P.B. Santhosh, N.P. Ulrih, Cancer Lett. 336 (2013) 8.

[58] A.K. Gupta, M. Gupta, Biomaterials 26 (2005) 3995.

[59] A. Moore, R. Weissleder, A. Bogdanov Jr., J. Magn. Reson. Imag. 7 (1997) 1140.

[60] J.W. Bulte, D.L. Kraitchman, NMR Biomed. 17 (2004) 484.

[61] D. Simberg, J.H. Park, P.P. Karmali, W.M. Zhang, et al., Biomaterials 30 (2009) 3926.

[62] I. Raynal, P. Prigent, S. Peyramaure, A. Najid, et al., Invest. Radiol. 39 (2004) 56.

[63] G. Wang, S. Inturi, N.J. Serkova, S. Merkulov, et al., ACS Nano 8 (2014) 12437.

[64] D. Soukup, S. Moise, E. Cespedes, J. Dobson, et al., ACS Nano 9 (2015) 231.

[65] O. Veiseh, J.W. Gunn, M. Zhang, Adv. Drug Deliv. Rev. 62 (2010) 284.

[66] E. Allard, C. Passirani, J.P. Benoit, Biomaterials 30 (2009) 2302.

[67] R. Saito, M.T. Krauze, C.O. Noble, M. Tamas, et al., J. Neurosci. Methods 154 (2006) 225.

[68] Z.R. Stephen, F.M. Kievit, O. Veiseh, P.A. Chiarelli, et al., ACS Nano 8 (2014) 10383.

[69] D. Allhenn, M.A. Boushehri, A. Lamprecht, Int. J. Pharm. 436 (2012) 299.

[70] P.P. Wang, J. Frazier, H. Brem, Adv. Drug Deliv. Rev. 54 (2002) 987.

[71] A. Boiardi, M. Eoli, A. Salmaggi, E. Lamperti, et al., Neurol. Sci. 26 (Suppl. 1) (2005) S37.

[72] H. Mok, M. Zhang, Expert Opin. Drug Deliv. 10 (2013) 73.

[73] Y.L. Lo, H.L. Chou, Z.X. Liao, S.J. Huang, et al., Nanoscale 7 (2015) 8554.

[74] H.K. Patra, N. Ul Khaliq, T. Romu, E. Wiechec, et al., Adv. Healthc. Mater. 3 (2014) 526.

[75] K. Kaaki, K. Herve-Aubert, M. Chiper, A. Shkilnyy, et al., Langmuir 28 (2012) 1496.

[76] I. Urries, C. Munoz, L. Gomez, C. Marquina, et al., Nanoscale 6 (2014) 9230.

[77] R. Shukla, V. Bansal, M. Chaudhary, A. Basu, et al., Langmuir 21 (2005) 10644.

[78] W.H. Kong, K.H. Bae, C.A. Hong, Y. Lee, et al., Bioconjug. Chem. 22 (2011) 1962.

[79] X.Q. Zhang, X. Xu, R. Lam, D. Giljohann, et al., ACS Nano 5 (2011) 6962.

[80] A.M. Gobin, M.H. Lee, N.J. Halas, W.D. James, et al., Nano Lett. 7 (2007) 1929.

[81] J. Park, E.J. Ju, S.S. Park, J. Choi, et al., J. Control. Release 207 (2015) 77.

[82] C. McQuade, A. Al Zaki, Y. Desai, M. Vido, et al., Small 11 (2015) 834.

[83] C. Cha, S.R. Shin, N. Annabi, M.R. Dokmeci, et al., ACS Nano 7 (2013) 2891.

[84] J. Liu, L. Cui, D. Losic, Acta Biomater. 9 (2013) 9243.

[85] E.K. Lim, T. Kim, S. Paik, S. Haam, et al., Chem. Rev. 115 (2015) 327.

[86] K.P. Loh, Q. Bao, G. Eda, M. Chhowalla, Nat. Chem. 2 (2010) 1015.

[87] J. Shang, L. Ma, J. Li, W. Ai, et al., Sci. Rep. 2 (2012) 792.

[88] X.C. Qin, Z.Y. Guo, Z.M. Liu, W. Zhang, et al., J. Photochem. Photobiol. B 120 (2013) 156.

[89] H. Wang, W. Gu, N. Xiao, L. Ye, et al., Int. J. Nanomedicine 9 (2014) 1433.

[90] R. Imani, S.H. Emami, S. Faghihi, Phys. Chem. Chem. Phys. 17 (2015) 6328.

[91] H. Xu, M. Fan, A.M. Elhissi, Z. Zhang, et al., Nanomedicine (Lond.) 10 (2015) 1247.
[92] A.A. Bhirde, G. Liu, A. Jin, R. Iglesias-Bartolome, et al., Theranostics 1 (2011) 310.
[93] H. Moradian, H. Fasehee, H. Keshvari, S. Faghihi, Colloids Surf. B 122 (2014) 115.
[94] G. Modugno, C. Menard-Moyon, M. Prato, A. Bianco, Br. J. Pharmacol. 172 (2015) 975.
[95] J.T.W. Wang, L. Cabana, M. Bourgognon, H. Kafa, et al., Adv. Funct. Mater. 24 (2014) 1880.
[96] X. Wang, C. Wang, L. Cheng, S.T. Lee, et al., J. Am. Chem. Soc. 134 (2012) 7414.
[97] S. Parveen, S.K. Sahoo, J. Drug Target. 16 (2008) 108.
[98] T. Krasia-Christoforou, T.K. Georgiou, J. Mater. Chem. B 1 (2013) 3002.
[99] D.C. Drummond, O. Meyer, K. Hong, D.B. Kirpotin, et al., Pharmacol. Rev. 51 (1999) 691.
[100] D. Papahadjopoulos, T.M. Allen, A. Gabizon, E. Mayhew, et al., Proc. Natl. Acad. Sci. USA 88 (1991) 11460.
[101] G. Molineux, Cancer Treat. Rev. 28 (Suppl. A) (2002) 13.
[102] M.B. Yatvin, W. Kreutz, B.A. Horwitz, M. Shinitzky, Science 210 (1980) 1253.
[103] Y.T. Chiang, C.L. Lo, Biomaterials 35 (2014) 5414.
[104] H.S. Qhattal, T. Hye, A. Alali, X. Liu, ACS Nano 8 (2014) 5423.
[105] C.E. Smith, A. Shkumatov, S.G. Withers, B. Yang, et al., ACS Nano 7 (2013) 9599.
[106] Y. Shi, R. van der Meel, B. Theek, E. Oude Blenke, et al., ACS Nano 9 (2015) 3740.
[107] C. Zhu, S. Jung, S. Luo, F. Meng, et al., Biomaterials 31 (2010) 2408.
[108] X.B. Xiong, A. Lavasanifar, ACS Nano 5 (2011) 5202.
[109] H. Cho, G.S. Kwon, ACS Nano 5 (2011) 8721.

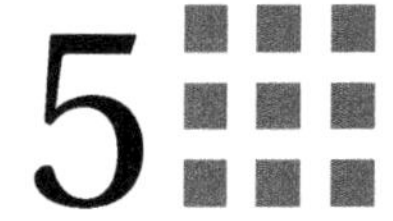

Next Generation Technologies

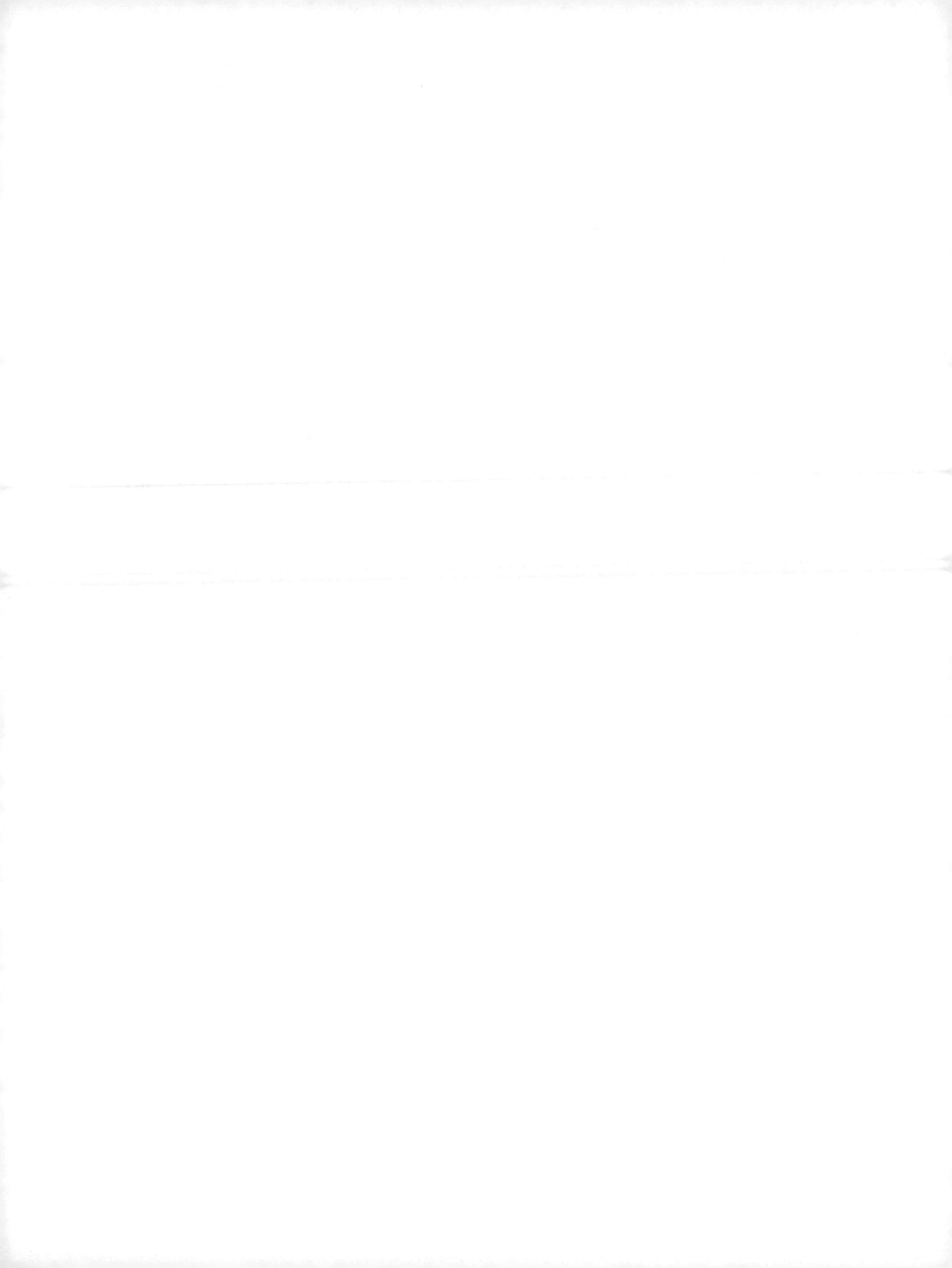

5.1

Self-Oscillating Polymer Materials

Tsukuru Masuda, Aya Mizutani Akimoto, Ryo Yoshida

DEPARTMENT OF MATERIALS ENGINEERING, SCHOOL OF ENGINEERING, THE UNIVERSITY OF TOKYO, TOKYO, JAPAN

CHAPTER OUTLINE

5.1.1 Introduction

Polymer gels are defined widely as cross-linked polymer networks that are swollen in solvents. The gels have attracted much attention because of their unique physiochemical properties. In 1978, T. Tanaka discovered that polymer gels change volume discontinuously and reversibly in response to external environmental changes such as pH, temperature, and solvent composition ("volume-phase transition" phenomena of the polymer gels) [1]. Since the discovery of the phenomena as a turning point, the study of polymer gels for functional soft materials has progressed rapidly. To date, these gels have been proposed as various applications including soft actuators (artificial muscle), drug delivery systems, purification or separation systems, regenerative medicine, biosensors, shape memory materials, molecular recognition systems, etc. [2–9]. Furthermore, with the advances in polymer synthesis technologies including supramolecular chemistry, the polymer network structures have been precisely designed in nanoscale to show unique properties or functions such as rapid response [10,11], self-healing properties [12], and high mechanical strength [13–16].

In these ways, stimuli-responsive gels and their applications have been widely studied. One of the most important strategies of designing the polymer gels as functional materials is mimicking living systems. Among the characteristics of the living systems, autonomous oscillation, that is, spontaneous changes with temporal periodicity (called "temporal structure"), such as heartbeat, brain waves, pulsatile secretion of hormones, cell cycles, and biorhythms, are important behaviors. The stimuli-responding behavior of the gels is a temporary action toward an equilibrium state, and the on/off switching of the external stimuli is necessary to induce the action of the gels. If autonomously oscillating gel systems can be constructed by using artificially designed materials, unprecedented biomimetic materials are expected. Based on this concept, we have developed "self-oscillating" gels as a novel biomimetic material.

In order to construct cyclic gel systems, coupling stimuli-responsive gels and chemical reactions have been attempted. For instance, Siegel et al. demonstrated an oscillatory release hormone system by using a pH-responsive gel membrane coupled with enzyme reaction [17]. On the other hand, we designed a coupling system of pH-responsive gels and pH oscillating reaction [18] (the $H_2O_2/HSO_3^-/Fe(CN)_6^{4-}$ system, etc.) in a continuously stirred tank reactor (CSTR). In these systems, periodic swelling–deswelling of the gel under constant conditions without external on/off switching was achieved [19,20]. However, the swelling–deswelling oscillation of the gel passively followed the oscillating outer conditions, which were created by membrane permeation cells or CSTR. Therefore, we further attempted to develop a novel gel that provides mechanical oscillation without external control in a complete closed system. Eventually, we succeeded in developing "self-oscillating" polymer gels by incorporating an oscillating chemical reaction in a polymer network, that is, by constructing a built-in circuit of an energy conversion cycle system that produced mechanical oscillation within the polymer network itself (Fig. 5.1.1) [21]. In contrast to conventional stimuli-responsive gels, the "self-oscillating" polymer gel exhibits an autonomous mechanical swelling–deswelling oscillation without any on/off switching of external stimuli. Since the first report in 1996 [21], we have systematically studied the self-oscillating polymer gels as well as their application to biomimetic smart materials (Fig. 5.1.2) [22,23]. Herein, development of the self-oscillating polymer gels and our recent progress are summarized.

5.1.2 Design of Self-Oscillating Polymer Gels

5.1.2.1 Oscillating Chemical Reaction

For the design of the autonomous polymer systems, we focused on the Belousov–Zhabotinsky (BZ) reaction [24–27], a well-known chemical oscillating reaction with temporal rhythm and spatial pattern formation. The overall process of the BZ reaction is the oxidization of an organic substrate (malonic acid [MA], citric acid, etc.) by an oxidizing agent (typically bromate ion) in the presence of a metal catalyst under acidic conditions. For the catalysts of the BZ reaction, metal ions or metal complexes with high redox potentials, such as cerium ion, ferroin, and ruthenium *tris*(2,2′-bipyridine) ($Ru(bpy)_3$) are widely used. In the course of the reaction, the catalyst undergoes spontaneous redox oscillation. Thus, the BZ reaction shows periodic color changes in the homogeneously stirred solution. When the solution is placed in stationary conditions, wave patterns appear in the solution. The

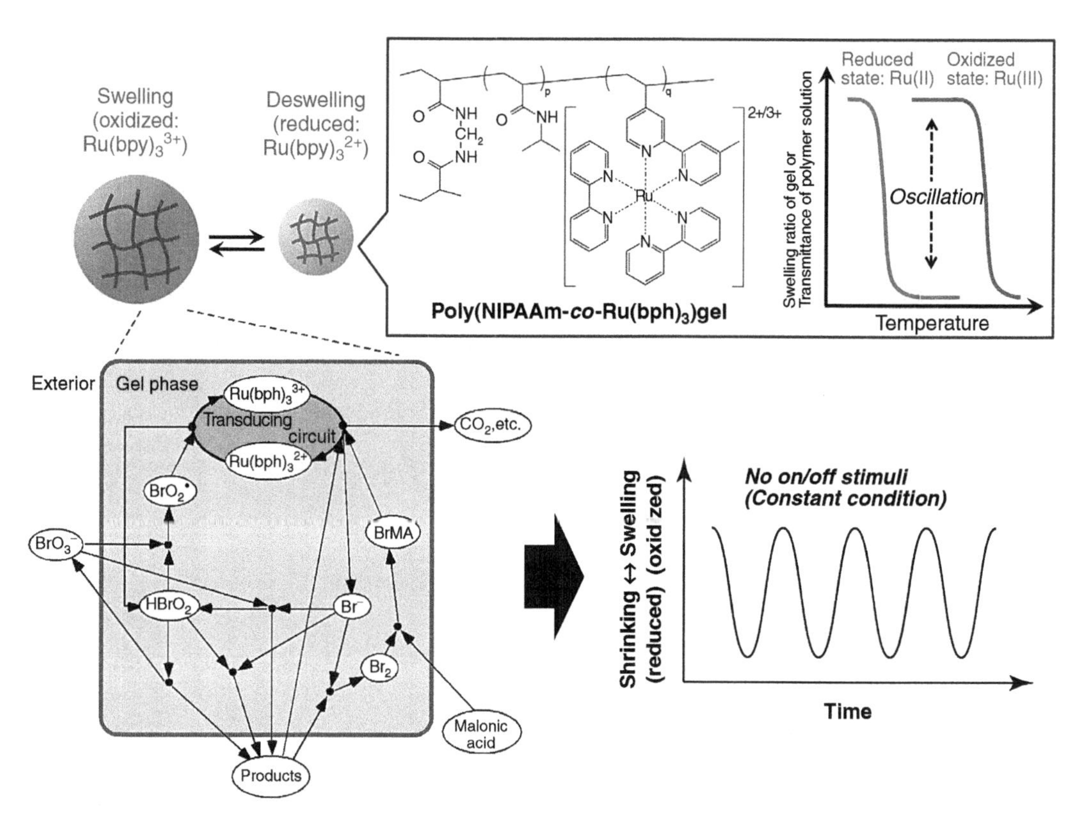

FIGURE 5.1.1 Design concept of self-oscillating gel using the Belousov-Zhanotinsky (BZ) reaction.

wave of the oxidized state propagating in the medium is called a "chemical wave." The BZ reaction is often analogized with a tricarboxylic acid cycle, a key metabolic process in the living body, which is also recognized as a chemical model for understanding several autonomous phenomena in biological systems such as glycolytic oscillations or biorhythms, cardiac fibrillation, self-organization of ameba cells, pattern formation on animal skin, etc.

5.1.2.2 Mechanism of Self-Oscillating Gels

We attempted to convert the chemical oscillation of the BZ reaction into the mechanical changes of the gels and to generate autonomous swelling–deswelling oscillation under nonoscillatory outer conditions. For this purpose, we designed a copolymer gel containing *N*-isopropylacrylamide (NIPAAm) and $Ru(bpy)_3$ (i.e., poly(NIPAAm-*co*-$Ru(bpy)_3$) gel) (Fig. 5.1.1). PNIPAAm, which is a well-known thermoresponsive polymer, has a lower critical solution temperature (LCST) around 32°C. The homopolymer gels of NIPAAm undergo an abrupt volume collapse (volume phase transition) when heated above the transition temperature. Redox changes of the polymerized $Ru(bpy)_3$ moiety change the volume phase transition temperature (VPTT) of the poly(NIPAAm-*co*-$Ru(bpy)_3$) gels as well as the swelling ratio because the hydrophilicity of the polymer chain changes with an alternation

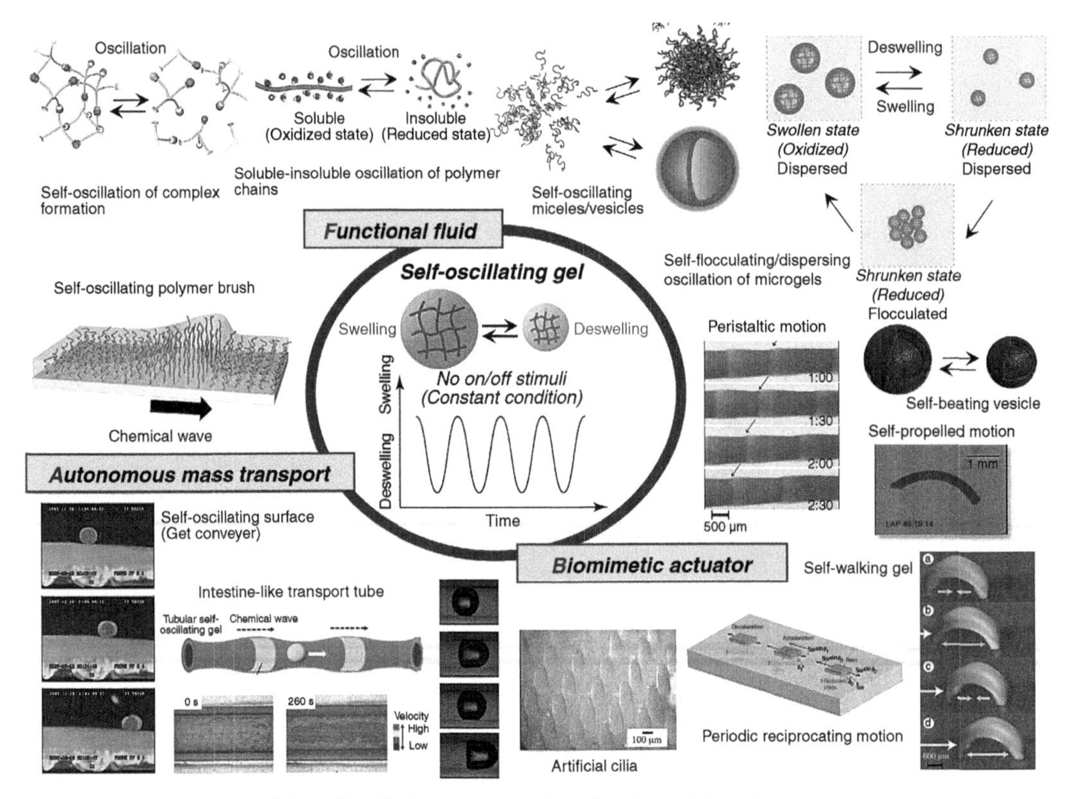

FIGURE 5.1.2 Development of the self-oscillating polymer as functional materials systems.

of the valency of Ru(bpy)$_3$ and the VPTT shifts to higher temperature in the oxidized state. When the poly(NIPAAm-*co*-Ru(bpy)$_3$) gel is immersed in an aqueous solution containing all the substrates of the BZ reaction except for the metal catalyst (i.e., MA, $NaBrO_3$, and nitric acid), the oscillating reaction occurs in the gel phase by the catalytic function of the polymerized Ru(bpy)$_3$. As a result, the gel undergoes spontaneous and cyclic swelling–deswelling changes synchronized with the redox changes of Ru(bpy)$_3$ in the closed solution under constant conditions.

5.1.2.3 Self-Oscillating Behaviors on Several Scales

Self-oscillation can be induced on several scales, from the order of polymer chains to bulk gels (Fig. 5.1.3). In the case of an uncross-linked linear polymer, the polymer chain undergoes periodic soluble–insoluble changes, and the optical transmittance or the viscosity of the polymer solution oscillates autonomously. When the gel size is much smaller than the chemical wavelength, redox changes occur homogeneously in the gel without pattern formation [28]. In that case, the swelling–deswelling of the gel becomes isotropic. In contrast, when the gel size is larger than the chemical wavelength, the chemical wave propagates autonomously in the gel by coupling with diffusion of the intermediates [29–31]. Then,

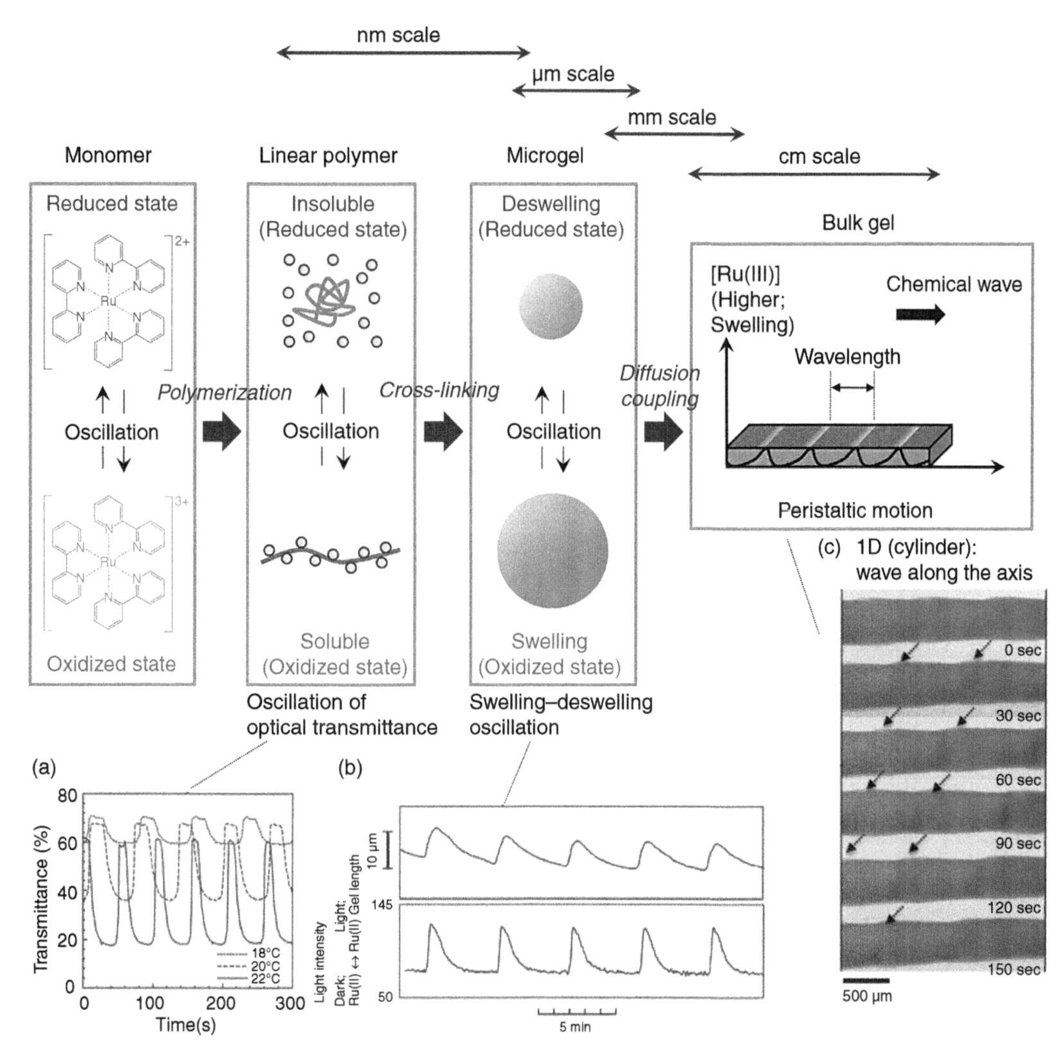

FIGURE 5.1.3 Self-oscillation on several scales. (a) Self-oscillating profiles of optical transmittance for poly(NIPAAm-*co*-Ru(bpy)$_3$) solution. (b) Periodic redox changes of the miniature poly(NIPAAm-*co*-Ru(bpy)$_3$) gel (lower) and the swelling–deswelling oscillation (upper) at 20°C. (c) Time course of peristaltic motion of poly(NIPAAm-*co*-AMPS-*co*-Ru(bpy)$_3$) gel in a catalyst-free BZ reaction solution.

the peristaltic motion of the gel is created. Figure 5.1.3c shows the time course of the peristaltic motion of the cylindrical gel in a catalyst-free BZ reaction solution [29]. The green and orange colors correspond to the oxidized Ru(III) state and the reduced Ru(II) state of the Ru(bpy)$_3$ moiety in the gel, respectively. The chemical waves propagate in the gel at a constant speed in the direction of the gel length. Considering that the orange (Ru(II)) and green (Ru(III)) zones represent simply the shrunken and swollen parts, respectively, the locally swollen and shrunken parts move with the chemical wave, as in the peristaltic motion of living worms or intestines.

5.1.2.4 Control of Self-Oscillating Chemomechanical Behaviors

The oscillating profile of the BZ reaction changes depending on the concentration of the substrates and temperature as characteristics of the chemical reaction. Typically, the oscillation period becomes shorter with increase in the initial concentration of the substrates. The oscillation frequency (the reciprocal of the period) of the BZ reaction increases as the temperature increases, in accordance with the Arrhenius equation. The swelling–deswelling amplitude of the gel increases with an increase in the oscillation period and amplitude of the redox potential changes [28]. Thus, the amplitude and period of swelling–deswelling of the self-oscillating gels can be controlled by changing the initial concentration of the substrates and temperature.

For controlling the chemomechanical behavior of the self-oscillating gels, the polymer architecture is also important. We have already shown several strategies to improve the dynamic properties of the self-oscillating gels such as microgel-aggregated structure [32] and comb-type self-oscillating gels [33]. Furthermore, self-oscillation at higher temperature and physiological body temperature while maintaining larger amplitude was investigated considering the potential application for biomaterials. We prepared a self-oscillating gel composed of a thermosensitive *N,N'*-ethylmethylacrylamide (EMAAm) polymer which exhibits a higher LCST than that of PNIPAAm, and the poly(EMAAm-*co*-Ru(bpy)$_3$) gel exhibited swelling–deswelling oscillation with a large amplitude and higher frequency around physiological temperature [34]. Recently, the ternary self-oscillating gel, poly(NIPAAm-*co*-NAPMAm-*co*-Ru(bpy)$_3$NAPMAm) gel was newly designed by using the postmodification method [35]. It was demonstrated that swelling–deswelling behaviors of the self-oscillating gels can be controlled by changing the composition ratio of the free amino group and the conjugated Ru(bpy)$_3$ moieties. The swelling–deswelling oscillation with a comparable amplitude around physiological temperature was also achieved. Recently, it was found for the first time that the BZ reaction occurred in certain hydrated protic ionic liquids (PILs) without adding strong acid such as nitric acid. Further, a stable and long-lasting self-oscillation under milder conditions than the typical BZ reaction can be achieved when the component concentrations of the BZ medium are optimized [36]. A systematic study of the correlation between the chemical structure of PILs, the characteristics of the BZ reaction, and the application to the self-oscillating polymer materials has been also in progress [37].

5.1.3 Design of Biomimetic Soft Actuators

We have been investigating novel biomimetic soft actuators by exploiting the macroscopic swelling–deswelling oscillation of the gels. For example, ciliary motion actuators (artificial cilia) were prepared by using microfabrication techniques [38,39]. Furthermore, we successfully developed a novel biomimetic walking gel actuator (self-walking gel) [40]. The self-oscillating gel having gradient distribution in the polymer network was prepared to generate asymmetrical swelling–deswelling motion. By putting the gel on the ratchet base, the gel repeatedly bends and stretches autonomously, resulting in the self-walking motion. Recently, it was also found that the self-oscillating gel undergoes reciprocating motion on the BZ reaction substrate solution, the driving force of which is the contact angles around the gel [41].

The theoretical simulation of the self-oscillating gel will be helpful in understanding the chemomechanical behavior of the self-oscillating gels and applying the self-oscillating gels as soft actuators. In the case of the self-oscillating gels, the chemical reaction and the mechanical motion affect each other with feedback control, and the oscillating behavior of the self-oscillating gels becomes more complicated compared with the swelling–deswelling behavior of conventional stimuli-responsive gels. Balazs et al. developed a mathematical model for simulating the chemomechanical behaviors of the self-oscillating gels [42–45]. Since the first report in 2006 [42], Balazs et al. have demonstrated several aspects of the self-oscillating behavior of the gels by theoretical simulation. Many interesting phenomena and possible actuating behaviors have been demonstrated theoretically, some of which have been realized experimentally. Using both experiments and computer simulations, control of the motion of the gel by preparing a composite gel made of self-oscillating gel and poly(acrylamide) (PAAm) gel as a nonactive gel was attempted [43]. The disk-shaped self-oscillating gels were arranged around the corners of a polygonal sheet of PAAm gel. Wave propagation was controlled by changing the patch size, the catalyst concentration of the BZ gel, and the spacing between the patches. The oscillating profile and the synchronization mechanism of this heterogeneous self-oscillating gel were also revealed by computational studies.

5.1.4 Design of Autonomous Mass Transport Systems

5.1.4.1 Self-Oscillating Gel Conveyers: Autonomous Mass Transport Surface Using Peristaltic Motion of the Gels

To realize a self-driven gel conveyer as a novel autonomous mass transport system, we attempted to transport an object by utilizing the peristaltic motion of the self-oscillating gel [46–49]. A model object, such as a cylindrical or spherical PAAm gel, was put on the surface of the self-oscillating gel sheet. It was observed that the object was transported on the gel surface with the propagation of the chemical wave as it rolled. The velocity and the indication angle of the propagating wave were changed by altering the concentration of the outer solution. The ability of the cylindrical gel to be transported was estimated for controlled chemical waves with several inclination angles (0–10°) and velocities (1–5 mm/min^{-1}). The cylindrical PAAm gel was not transported when the inclination angle was less than approximately 3°. The mass transportability did not depend on the velocity of the chemical wave, but on the diameter of the cylindrical PAAm gel and the inclination angle of the wave front. To analyze this result, we proposed a model to describe these mass transport phenomena based on the Hertz contact theory, and the relationship between the transportability and the peristaltic motion was investigated. Calculation using the theoretical equation indicated that the minimum inclination angle was 3°, the same as the angle determined from the experiment. The model supported the idea that the sheer wave front of the peristaltic motion was necessary to transport the cylindrical gels. Further, in order to fabricate a more versatile self-driven gel conveyer, the surface figure capable of transporting microparticles was designed as the self-oscillating gel having a grooved surface. For a wider use including biomedical applications, the influence of the physical interaction between the self-oscillating gel surface and the loaded cargo was also investigated.

5.1.4.2 Autonomous Intense-Like Motion of a Tubular Self-Oscillating Gel

To construct an autonomous mechanical pumping system such as intestines, we fabricated a self-oscillating gel in a tubular shape by photopolymerization (Fig. 5.1.4) [50]. Several types of tubular self-oscillating gels that exhibit autonomous peristaltic motion were

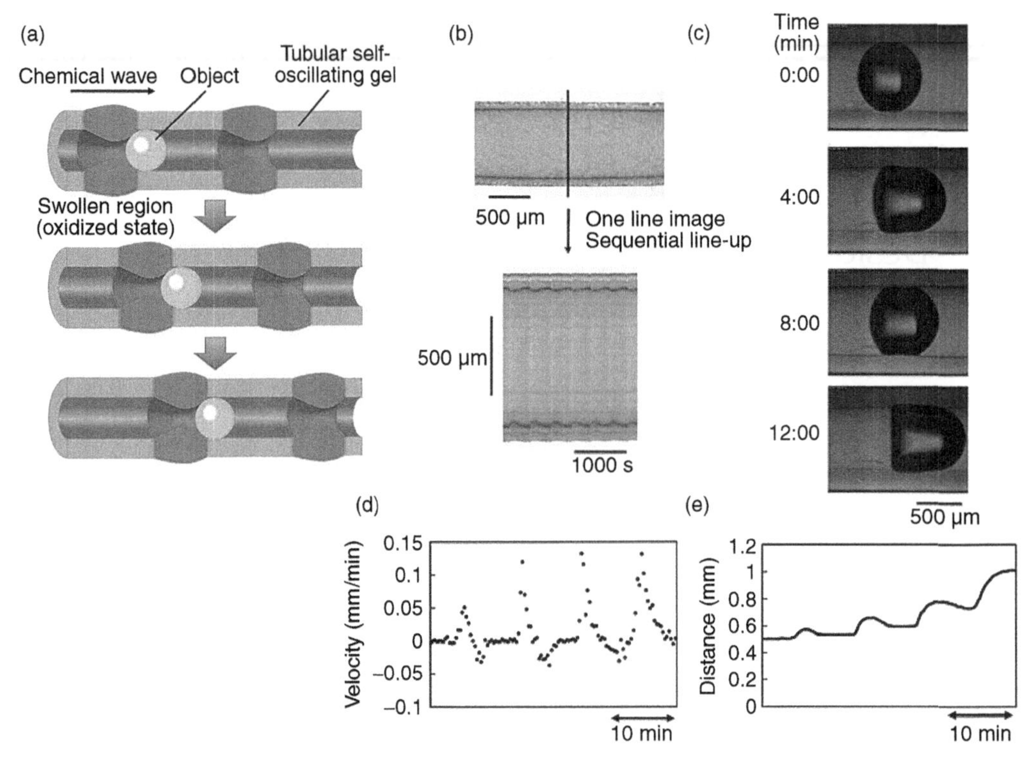

FIGURE 5.1.4 (a) Schematic illustration of autonomous transport by peristaltic pumping of a tubular self-oscillating gel. (b) Time course images of the peristaltic motion of the tubular self-oscillating gel having IPN structure. (c) Behavior of the autonomous transport of a CO_2 bubble in the gel tube by peristaltic pumping. (d) Change in the position of the bubble. (e) The velocity of the bubble.

investigated. First, a tubular self-oscillating gel (poly(NIPAAm-*co*-Ru(bpy)$_3$) gel) adhered to the inner surface of a glass capillary was prepared, and the periodic inner diameter changes during the BZ reaction were analyzed. Second, by removing the gel from the glass capillary, a tubular gel that can swell and deswell freely without a mechanical restraint was prepared. In this case, to improve the mechanical strength of the gel as well as the swelling kinetics, 2-acrylamide-2′-methylpropane sulfonic acid (AMPS) as another component was added into the polymer network. The tubular poly(NIPAAm-*co*-APMS-*co*-Ru(bpy)$_3$) with a microaggregated structure was obtained due to the effect of poor solvent in the polymerization process. The gel exhibited peristaltic motion with a deformation of the outer side in a catalyst-free BZ reaction solution. Third, a tubular self-oscillating gel with an interpenetrating network (IPN) structure composed of self-oscillating and nonoscillating polymers was prepared to cause peristaltic motion only at the inner surface of the gel tube. The tubular IPN gel exhibited the peristaltic motion and a significant change in outer diameter was not observed. As above, these tubular self-oscillating gels exhibited various types of peristaltic motion.

In addition, it was demonstrated that an object could be autonomously transported in the gel tube by the peristaltic pumping motion, which was similar to that of an intestine. Figure 5.1.4c shows the behavior of a CO_2 bubble in the tubular poly(NIPAAm-*co*-Ru(bpy)$_3$) gel. When the bubble became large enough to contact the inner surface of the gel tube, it started to move intermittently by repeated deformation and restoration in the direction of the chemical wave propagation. When the chemical wave reached the contact point, the bubble was squashed and deformed by swelling of the gel layer at that point. Then, the bubble was mechanically pushed forward by the peristaltic pumping mechanism. After the wave passed through, the gel layer deswelled, and the squashed bubble returned to its initial round shape. Due to the decrease in pushing force and negative pressure, the bubble moved backward slightly. After that, the movement of the bubble stopped for a while. Thus, the movement was intermittent. By repeating this process, the bubble was transported in the gel tube autonomously. It is obvious that a net movement of the bubble occurs by repeating backward and forward movements. Potential applications in artificial intestines, artificial digestive tracts, etc., can be envisioned.

Furthermore, we demonstrated that we can cause autonomous pulsatile flow in a tubular gel by utilizing the peristaltic motion of the tubular self-oscillating gel like an intestine (Fig. 5.1.5) [51]. The autonomous flow was proved by using latex beads as tracer particles and analyzing the motion. Pulsatile flow was observed to synchronize with the peristaltic motion of the tubular gel. It was demonstrated that the velocity of the fluid increased locally around the swollen region with the propagation of the chemical wave. The flow velocity of the tracer particles exhibited the maximum value during the swelling process. Further, the dimensionless Reynolds number (Re) and Womersley number (α) were theoretically estimated, which indicated that the flow state in the tubular gel was completely laminar flow. Thus, a new possibility of the self-oscillating gel as an autonomous chemomechanical gel pump has been demonstrated.

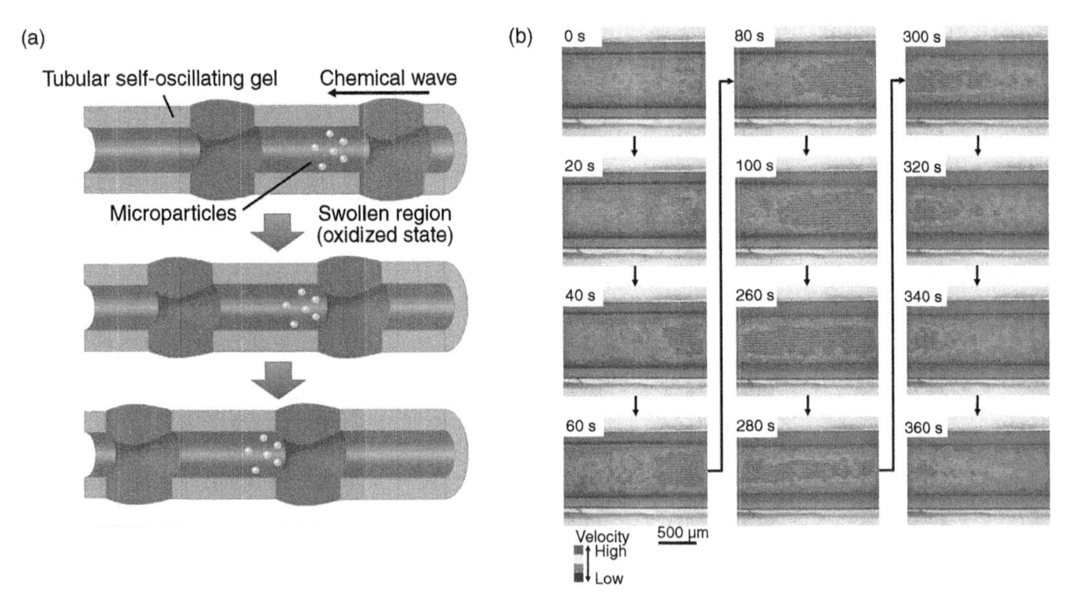

FIGURE 5.1.5 (a) Schematic illustration of autonomous pulsatile flow by peristaltic motion of a tubular self-oscillating gel. (b) Distribution of the velocity vector in the tubular self-oscillating gel during the autonomous peristaltic motion.

5.1.4.3 Self-Oscillating Polymer Brushes

Recently, surface modification techniques for polymer chains have progressed a great deal with the development of a new polymer synthesis method. In particular, surface-initiated atom transfer radical polymerization (SI-ATRP) is one of the most effective modification methods for preparing a well-defined dense polymer brush structure, or polymer brush, on solid substrates. Thus, a self-oscillating polymer brush prepared by SI-ATRP can be expected to create a novel self-oscillating surface with autonomous function, which will lead to potential applications in transporting systems for nanomaterials of flow control in microfluidics.

We prepared self-oscillating polymer brush on glass substrates and the inner surface of a glass capillary (Fig. 5.1.6) [52]. The figure shows an image observed by using a fluorescence microscope, which shows that the self-oscillating polymer brush was successfully grafted onto the inner surface of a glass capillary. The catalyst-free BZ reaction solution was fed into the glass capillary, and the BZ reaction was observed by fluorescence microscope. Spatiotemporal image analyses were performed in different locations of the glass capillary, and the oscillating profiles of fluorescence intensity were compared. Oscillation of the fluorescence intensity occurred at each position with a phase difference. This finding suggests that the chemical wave propagated in the self-oscillating polymer brush layer on the inner surface of a glass capillary. Further, in order to improve self-oscillating behaviors, the correlation between the nanostructure of the polymer brush and the self-oscillating profiles has been investigated. It has been indicated that a suitable nanostructure design

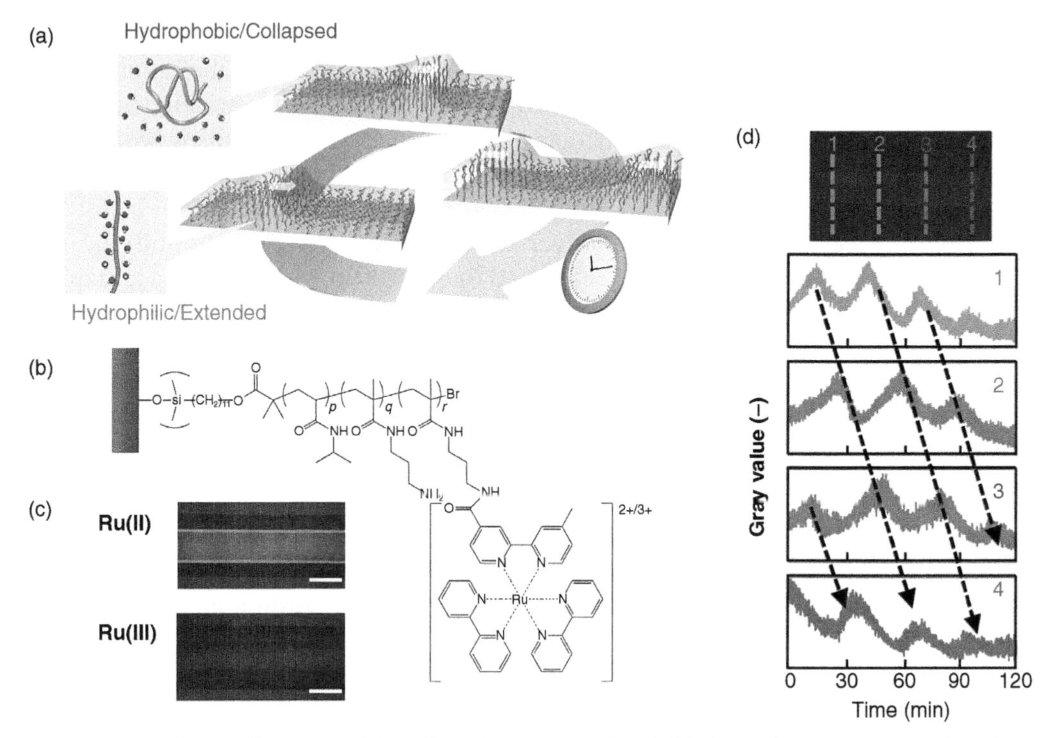

FIGURE 5.1.6 (a) Schematic illustration of the self-oscillating polymer brush. (b) Chemical structure of the self-oscillating polymer brush. (c) Images of glass capillary modified with the self-oscillating polymer observed by fluorescence microscope. (d) Oscillating profile of fluorescence intensity at each position for the self-oscillating polymer brush on the inner surface of the glass capillary.

of the polymer brush existed for the autonomous function [53]. A self-oscillating surface to generate spontaneous periodic changes was demonstrated using synthetic polymers as a novel functional surface, which has potential applications in systems such as nanotransport systems.

5.1.5 Self-Oscillating Functional Fluids

5.1.5.1 Transmittance and Viscosity Oscillation of Polymer Solutions and Microgel Dispersions

In the case of the uncross-linked self-oscillating linear polymer, that is, poly(NIPAAm-*co*-Ru(bpy)$_3$), the polymer chain undergoes periodic soluble–insoluble changes spontaneously, and the transmittance of the polymer solution oscillates autonomously synchronized with the redox changes of the copolymerized Ru(bpy)$_3$ [54]. Furthermore, we prepared submicron-sized poly(NIPAAm-*co*-Ru(bpy)$_3$) gel particles by surfactant-free aqueous precipitation polymerization and analyzed the oscillating behavior of the microgel dispersions in the BZ reaction [55]. The microgel dispersions also exhibited transmittance oscillation because of swelling–deswelling changes of the microgels. When the temperature increased to near the volume-phase transition temperature of the microgels in the reduced state, the microgels showed dispersing–flocculating oscillation as well as swelling–deswelling oscillation. In the cases of both the polymer solution and the microgel dispersion, viscosity oscillation was observed with optical transmittance [56–58]. Especially in the case of the microgel dispersion, it was found that viscosity oscillation exhibits two waveforms; a simple pulsatile waveform and a complex waveform with two peaks per period caused by dispersing–flocculating oscillation. It is expected that these polymer solutions and microgel dispersions can be applied as novel functional fluids.

5.1.5.2 Autonomous Viscosity Oscillation by Reversible Complex Formation of Terpyridine-Terminated Branched-PEG in the BZ Reaction

Autonomous viscosity oscillations of a polymer solution were also realized based on the different mechanisms [59,60]. We reported autonomous viscosity oscillations of the polymer solutions coupled with metal–ligand association/dissociation between Ru and terpyridine (tpy), driven by the BZ reaction. It was well known that mono-tpy coordination is stable when the Ru is oxidized ($Ru(tpy)^{3+}$), whereas bis-tpy coordination is stable when the Ru center is reduced ($Ru(tpy)_2^{2+}$) (Fig. 5.1.7a). For the polymer design, the tpy ligand for Ru catalyst was attached to the terminals of poly(ethylene glycol) (PEG) with different numbers of branches (linear-, tetra, and octa-PEG) (Fig.5.1.7b). In the oxidized state, these

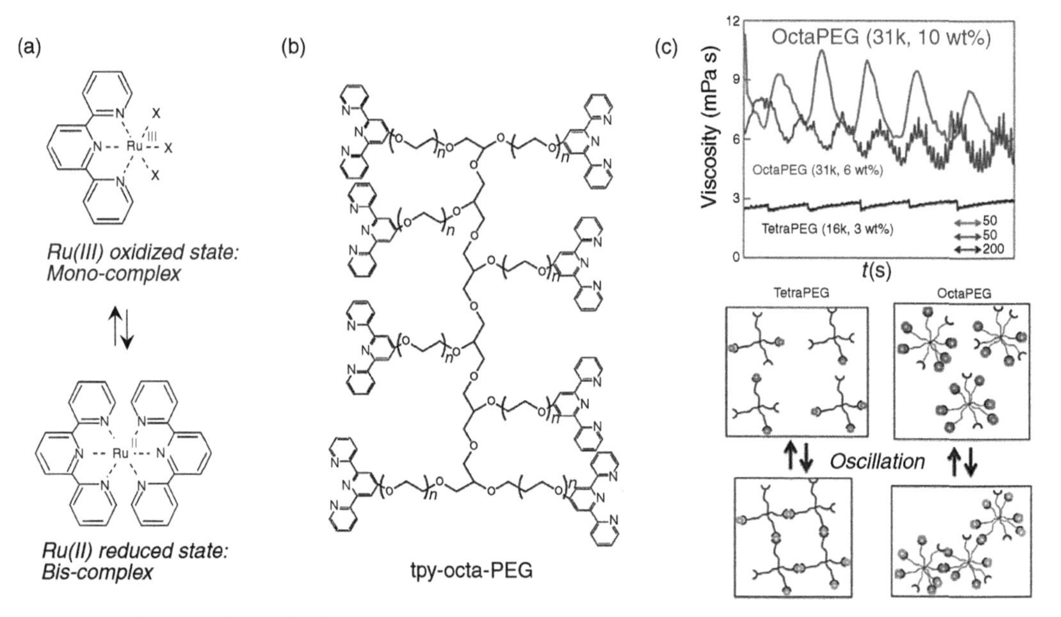

FIGURE 5.1.7 (a) Reversible complex formation of Ru-terpyridine during the BZ reaction. (b) Chemical structure of the terpyridine terminated octa-PEG. (c) Oscillating profile of viscosity of the aqueous solution containing $Ru(tpy)_2$-tetra or $Ru(tpy)_2$-octa PEG, HNO_3, $NaBrO_3$, and MA at 25°C

polymers exhibited as solutions. In contrast, when the Ru center was reduced, gels were obtained for the tetra- and octa-PEG because of the formation of a three-dimensional polymer network through Ru-tpy coordination. By increasing the number of PEG branches, the number of cross-linking points necessary for gelation was successfully decreased. This was qualitatively explained by the tree-like structure theory stating a rate of reaction of cross-linking points for a branched polymer at the gelation point. Furthermore, the gelation kinetics of the octa-PEG was approximately for times faster than those of the tetra-PEG system.

The polymer solution exhibited self-oscillation of absorbance and viscosity when the BZ substrates were added to the solutions of Ru-tpy-modified tetra-/octa-PEG (Fig. 5.1.7c). This indicated that the Ru-tpy attached to the polymer ends could serve as a mental catalyst for the BZ reaction. The viscosity oscillation profiles of the tetra- and octa-PEG were compared under the optimized conditions for each system. As expected, the octa-PEG was much more effective than the tetra-PEG in providing a large oscillation amplitude as well as a higher baseline viscosity. For the octa-PEG, the baseline viscosity and the amplitude were approximately twice as high and 10 times larger, respectively, than for the tetra-PEG system. This is likely because the number of cross-linking points necessary for gelation was decreased by increasing the branch number of PEG, as predicted from the tree-like structure theory. As a result, the maximum value of cross-linking points in oscillation is closer to that necessary for gelation. Thus, viscosity oscillation occurred in the region of higher viscosity with a large amplitude.

5.1.6 Self-Oscillating Block Copolymers

5.1.6.1 Self-Oscillating Micelles

Recently, we designed a novel block copolymer that could undergo spontaneous unimer–micelle oscillation under constant conditions [61]. The target block copolymer (PEO-*b*-P(NIPAAm-*r*-Ru(bpy)$_3$)) was successfully prepared by reversible addition fragmentation chain transfer (RAFT) random copolymerization of NIPAAm and a vinyl monomer with a Ru(bpy)$_3$ side chain from poly(ethylene oxide) (PEO)-based macrochain transfer agent (Fig. 5.1.8a). The aggregation behavior of PEO-*b*-P(NIPAAm-*r*-Ru(bpy)$_3$) diblock copolymer was first investigated in both reduced and oxidized state of Ru(bpy)$_3$. The average hydrodynamic radius (R_h) increased sharply above a certain temperature, indicating that self-assembly from unimer to micelle occurs at a specific temperature. Importantly, an approximately 2.5°C difference in aggregation temperature was observed between the oxidized state and the reduced state (Fig. 5.1.8b). This is because the hydrophilicity of the second block increased because of the increase in charge.

Using this difference in transition temperatures, a dynamic unimer–micelle transition under the conditions of the BZ reaction was demonstrated. By adding the BZ substrates (HNO_3, $NaBrO_3$, and MA) into the block copolymer solution, the oscillating behavior of the block copolymer under the constant conditions was analyzed. The scattering intensity and

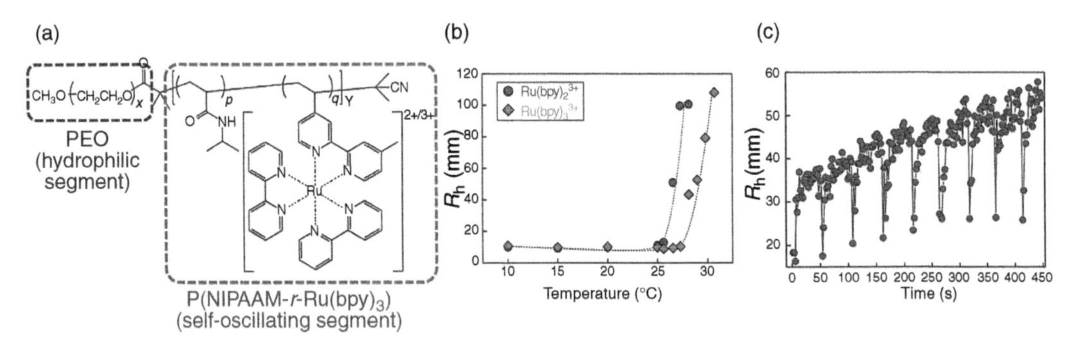

FIGURE 5.1.8 (a) Chemical structure of PEO-*b*-P(NIPAAM-*r*-Ru(bpy)$_3$). (b) Hydrodynamic radius (R_h) of the diblock copolymer in the reduced and the oxidized states of Ru(bpy)$_3$ side chain as a function of temperature. (c) Oscillating profile of the of R_h the diblock copolymer determined by time-resolved DLS measurements.

R_h were measured as a function of time with the aid of time-resolved dynamic light scattering (DLS). Figure 5.1.8c shows the oscillating profiles of the scattering intensity for the 0.5 wt% block copolymer solution at a temperature (26°C). The baseline of the scattering intensity increased with time, indicating that the size of the micelles essentially increased during the oscillation process. The figure shows the oscillating profiles of the average R_h calculated from the fitting of the autocorrelation function, which was collected every 2 s. These results clearly show that the size of the scattering particles rhythmically oscillates in synchrony with the BZ reaction. This is the first report of a synthetic block copolymer that exhibits "temporal structure," undergoing self-oscillation between unimer and micelle, as an example of a dissipative structure.

5.1.6.2 Self-Oscillating Vesicles: Spontaneous Structural Changes of Synthetic Diblock Copolymers

Furthermore, we have demonstrated autonomous cyclic changes in the formation–fragmentation of vesicles by the block copolymer [62]. In this case, the block ratio of hydrophilic segments was set to be lower than the previous study [61] to obtain vesicles as an equilibrium structure. The image of the vesicle recorded by florescence microscope clearly shows an intense ring around the self-assembled structure, indicating the presence of a bilayer vesicle membrane where Ru(bpy)$_3$ is selectively located. From DLS measurements, periodic changes of the scattering intensity with larger amplitude were obtained, suggesting that oscillation occurs between the two states; large aggregates with a high light scattering ability and small particles with a low scattering ability (Fig. 5.1.9a). It was revealed that R_h values also periodically oscillated with an amplitude of over 100 nm. This result suggests that structural changes occur between vesicles and their fragmented states (i.e., unimers).

In situ real-time observation of the self-oscillating behaviors of vesicles was carried out by using blight-field optical microscopy with a time-lapse mode. The images provide confirmation that a rhythmical self-oscillation between association and dissociation of

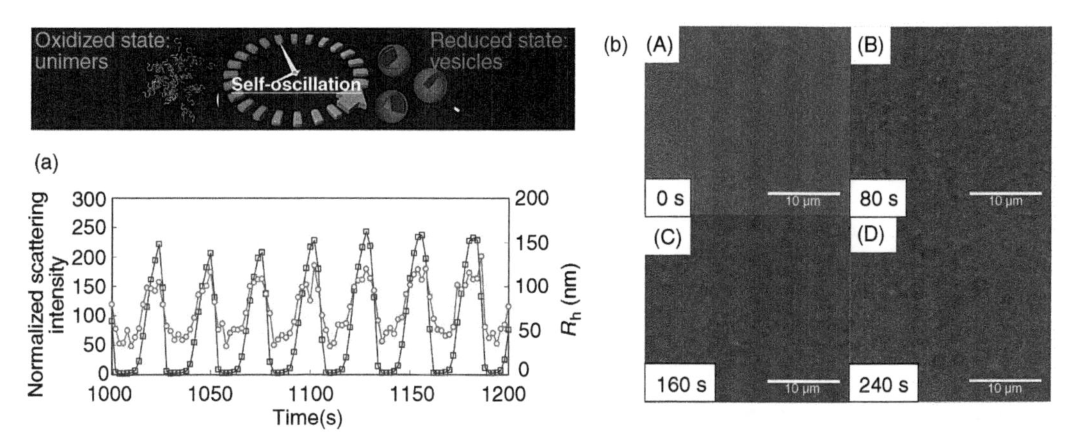

FIGURE 5.1.9 Self-oscillating vesicles. (a) Time evolution of normalized scattering intensity [dark gray (blue in the web version) plots] and R_h [light gray (red in the web version) plots] of the diblock copolymer aqueous solution during the BZ reaction. (b) Snapshots of transition from fragmented states (unimers) to vesicles.

vesicles occurs that is coupled with the BZ reaction (Fig. 5.1.9b). In an association process, each vesicle exhibited Brownian motion and gradually increased its size. On the other hand, vesicles quickly disappeared within a few seconds in the fragmentation process. During the process of vesicle growth accompanying the reduction of $Ru(bpy)_3^{3+}$, the autonomous fusion of two vesicles to form a large vesicle was also observed, similar to a biological process occurring at the cell membrane. Thus, for the first time, autonomous cycling between the formation and fragmentation of artificial vesicles has been realized.

5.1.6.3 Self-Beating Artificial Cells: Design of Cross-Linked Polymersomes Showing Self-Oscillating Motion

As a more advanced biomimetic materials system, we designed cross-linked polymersomes that show autonomous shape and volume oscillations, like a biological cell membrane [63]. The target polymersomes were prepared by thermosensitive micellization of a diblock copolymer followed by cross-linking the vesicular core. The thermosensitive diblock copolymer PEO-*b*-P(NIPAAm-*r*-NAPMAm) was prepared by RAFT random copolymerization from PEO macroinitiators. $Ru(bpy)_3$ groups and vinylidene groups were then introduced into the P(NIPAAm-*r*-NAPMAm) segment through the coupling reaction between the primary amine groups of NAPMAm and the *N*-hydroxysuccinimidyl (NHS) esters of $Ru(bpy)_3$ or methacrylate (NHS-MA). Thus, a well-defined cross-linkable diblock copolymer PEO-P(NIPAAm-*r*-NAPMAm-*r*-NAPMAmRu$(bpy)_3$-*r*-NAPMAmMA) was obtained as the precursor for the cross-linked polymersomes (Fig. 5.1.10a). To prepare the cross-linked polymersomes, the diblock copolymer was dissolved in an aqueous solution and the temperature was kept above the aggregation temperature. Using UV-light irradiation, the vesicular core was cross-linked.

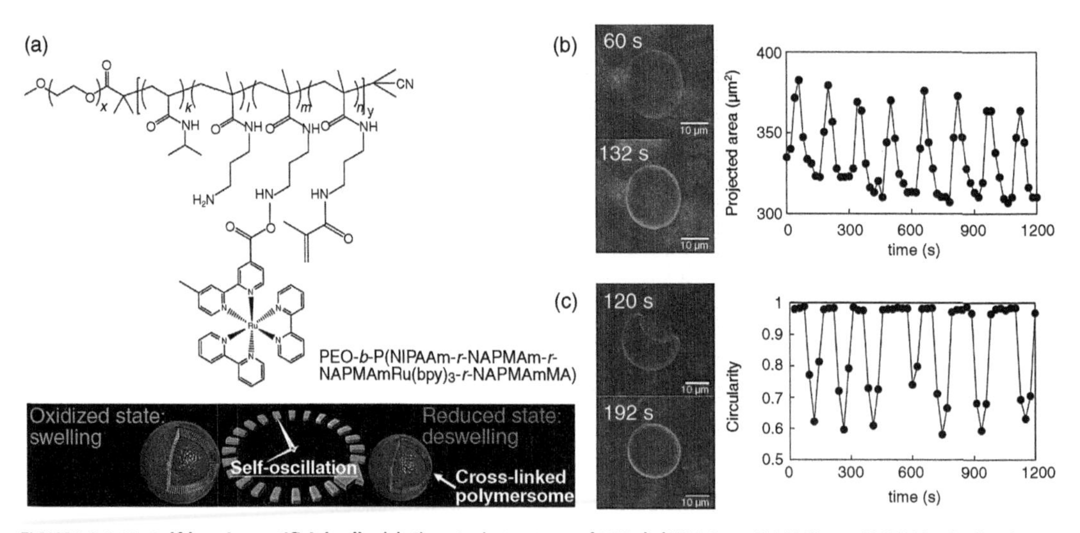

FIGURE 5.1.10 Self-beating artificial cells. (a) Chemical structure of PEO-*b*-(NIPAAm-*r*-NAPMAm-*r*-NAPMAmRu(bpy)$_3$-*r*-NAPMAmMA). (b) Autonomous volume oscillations of a cross-linked polymersome during the BZ reaction (right). Snapshots of the oscillating behaviors detected using a dark-field optical microscope (left). Changes in the projected area of the polymersome with time. (c) Autonomous buckling/unbuckling oscillations during the BZ reaction (right). Snapshots of the oscillating shape behaviors by optical microscope (left). Oscillating profile of the circularity.

Figure 5.1.10b shows snapshots of the microscope images and changes in projected area of the cross-linked polymersome during the BZ reaction. As expected, rhythmic volume oscillation similar to that of a biological cell membrane was observed at 25°C. It is also noted that the volume change ratio of the cross-linked polymersomes was larger than that of conventional self-oscillating gels. This is likely because of the characteristics of the polymersomes; the small sizes and hollow structures of the polymersomes provided a large space where the vesicle membrane can afford to move freely. Interestingly, during the BZ reaction, some polymersomes showed periodic shape changes, that is, self-oscillations between buckled and unbuckled states (Fig. 5.1.10c). The degree of deformation can be expressed as circularity. This phenomenon could be related to hydration-induced buckling instability, when the tangential stress is induced by membrane hydration. If the stress exceeds the threshold of instability, the membrane would buckle inward to relax the stress. On the contrary, in the reduced state, the membrane is dehydrated. Since the membrane dehydration induces tangential stress in the opposite direction, the polymersomes recover from the buckled state to the unbuckled state. As a result, drastic shape oscillation occurred. This is the first realization of synthetic cross-linked polymersomes that exhibit a self-beating motion.

5.1.7 Conclusions and Future Trends

As mentioned above, novel "self-oscillating" polymer gels that exhibit oscillation like heart muscle under constant external conditions have been developed. Since the first report in 1996, those polymer gels have been systematically studied as well as their applications to smart materials. Herein, our recent progress on the self-oscillating materials was summarized. In future, these polymer gels will attract much more attention as a subject not only for fundamental study but also for application study in the research field of polymer science, materials science, physical chemistry, theoretical simulation, and biophysics. The future applications for biomaterials would be also envisioned.

References

[1] T. Tanaka, Phys. Rev. Lett. 40 (1978) 820.

[2] R. Yoshida, Curr. Org. Chem. 9 (2005) 1617.

[3] A. Lendlein, V.P. Shastri, Adv. Mater. 22 (2010) 3344.

[4] M.W. Urban (Ed.), Handbook of Stimuli-Responsive Materials, Wiley-VCH, Weinheim, 2011.

[5] D. Bhattacharyya, T. Schafer (Eds.), Responsive Membranes and Materials, John Wiley & Sons, Ltd, West Sussex, UK, 2013.

[6] R.M. Ottenbrite, K. Park, T. Okano, N.A. Peppas (Eds.), Biomedical Applications of Hydrogels Handbook, Springer, New York, 2010.

[7] T. Okano, Adv. Mater. 21 (2009) 3404.

[8] T. Miyata, Supramolecular Design for Biological Applications, in: N. Yui (Ed.), CRC Press, Boca Raton, 2002, pp. 191–225.

[9] A.S. Hoffman, Adv. Drug. Deliv. Rev. 65 (2013) 10.

[10] R. Yoshida, K. Uchida, Y. Kaneko, K. Sakai, A. Kikuchi, Y. Sakurai, T. Okano, Nature 374 (1995) 240.

[11] Y. Kaneko, K. Sakai, A. Kikuchi, R. Yoshida, Y. Sakurai, T. Okano, Macromolecules 28 (1995) 7717.

[12] A. Harada, Y. Takashima, Chem. Rec. 13 (2013) 420.

[13] J.P. Gong, Y. Katsuyama, T. Kurokawa, Y. Osada, Adv. Mater. 15 (2003) 1155.

[14] Y. Okumura, K. Ito, Adv. Mater. 13 (2001) 485.

[15] K. Haraguchi, T. Takeshima, Adv. Mater. 14 (2002) 1120.

[16] T. Sakai, Y. Akagi, T. Matsunaga, M. Kurakazu, U. Chung, M. Shibayama, Macromol. Rapid. Commun. 31 (2010) 1954.

[17] G.P. Misra, R.A. Siegel, J. Control. Release 81 (2002) 1.

[18] G. Rabai, K. Kustin, I.R. Epstein, J. Am. Chem. Soc. 111 (1989) 3870.

[19] R. Yoshida, H. Ichijo, T. Hakuta, T. Yamaguchi, Macromol. Rapid. Commun. 16 (1995) 305.

[20] R. Yoshida, T. Yamaguchi, H. Ichijo, Mater. Sci. Eng. C 4 (1996) 107.

[21] R. Yoshida, T. Takahashi, H. Ichijo, T. Yamaguchi, J. Am. Chem. Soc. 118 (1996) 5134.

[22] R. Yoshida, Adv. Mater. 22 (2010) 3463.

[23] R. Yoshida, T. Ueki, NPG Asia Mater. 6 (2014) e107.

[24] R.J. Field, M. Burger (Eds.), Oscillators and Traveling Waves in Chemical Systems, John Wiley & Sons, New York, 1995.

[25] I.R. Epstein, J.A. Pojman, An Introduction to Nonlinear Chemical Dynamics: Oscillators, Waves, Patterns, and Chaos, Oxford University Press, New York, (1998).

[26] R.J. Field, E. Körös, R.M. Noyes, J. Am. Chem. Soc. 94 (1972) 8649.

[27] T. Amemiya, T. Ohmori, T. Yamaguchi, J. Phys. Chem. A 104 (2000) 7336.

[28] R. Yoshida, T. Tanaka, S. Onodera, T. Yamaguchi, E. Kokufuta, J. Phys. Chem. A 104 (2000) 7549.

[29] S. Maeda, Y. Hara, R. Yoshida, S. Hashimoto, Angew. Chem. Int. Ed. 47 (2008) 6690.

[30] Y. Takeoka, M. Watanabe, R. Yoshida, J. Am. Chem. Soc. 125 (2003) 13320.

[31] S. Sasaki, S. Koga, R. Yoshida, T. Yamagichi, Langmuir 19 (2003) 5595.

[32] D. Suzuki, T. Kobayashi, R. Yoshida, T. Hirai, Soft Matter 8 (2012) 11447.

[33] R. Mitsunaga, K. Okeyoshi, R. Yoshida, Chem. Commun. 49 (2013) 4935.

[34] M. Hidaka, R. Yoshida, J. Control. Release 150 (2011) 171.

[35] T. Masuda, A. Terasaki, A.M. Akimoto, K. Nagase, T. Okano, R. Yoshida, RSC Adv. 5 (2015) 5781.

[36] T. Ueki, M. Watanabe, R. Yoshida, Angew. Chem. Int. Ed. 51 (2012) 11991.

[37] T. Ueki, K. Matsukawa, T. Masuda, R. Yoshida, Polymer Preprints, Japan, 63 (2014) 6710.

[38] O. Tabata, H. Kojima, T. Kasatani, Y. Isono, R. Yoshida, Proceedings of the International Conference on MEMS 2003, 2003, pp. 12–15.

[39] O. Tabata, H. Hirasawa, S. Aoki, R. Yoshida, E. Kokufuta, Sens. Actuat. A 95 (2002) 234.

[40] S. Maeda, H. Hara, T. Sakai, R. Yoshida, S. Hashimoto, Adv. Mater. 19 (2007) 3480.

[41] S. Nakata, M. Yoshii, S. Suzuki, R. Yoshida, Langmuir 30 (2014) 517.

[42] V.V. Yashin, A.C. Balazs, Science 314 (2006) 798.

[43] V.V. Yashin, S. Suzuki, R. Yoshida, A.C. Balazs, J. Mater. Chem. 22 (2012) 13625.

[44] O. Kuksenok, A.C. Balazs, Adv. Funct. Mater. 23 (2013) 4601.

[45] V.V. Yashin, O. Kuksenok, A.C. Balazs, Prog. Polym. Sci. 35 (2010) 155.

[46] Y. Murase, S. Maeda, S. Hashimoto, R. Yoshida, Langmuir 25 (2008) 8427.

[47] Y. Murase, M. Hidaka, R. Yoshida, Sens. Actuat. B 149 (2010) 272.

[48] Y. Murase, R. Takeshima, R. Yoshida, Macromol. Biosci. 11 (2011) 1713.

[49] R. Yoshida, Y. Murase, Colloids Surf. B 99 (2012) 60.

[50] Y. Shiraki, R. Yoshida, Angew. Chem. Int. Ed. 51 (2012) 6112.

[51] Y. Shiraki, A.M. Akimoto, T. Miyata, R. Yoshida, Chem. Mater. 26 (2014) 5441.

[52] T. Masuda, M. Hidaka, Y. Murase, A.M. Akmoto, K. Nagase, T. Okano, R. Yoshida, Angew. Chem. Int. Ed. 52 (2013) 7468.

[53] T. Masuda, A. M. Akimoto, K. Nagase, T. Okano, R. Yoshida, Chem. Mater. in press (doi: 10.1021/acs/chemmater.5b03228).

[54] R. Yoshida, T. Sakai, S. Ito, T. Yamaguchi, J. Am. Chem. Soc. 124 (2002) 8095.

[55] D. Suzuki, T. Sakai, R. Yoshida, Amgew. Chem. Int. Ed. 47 (2008) 917.

[56] Y. Hara, R. Yoshida, J. Chem. Phys. 128 (2008) 224904.

[57] D. Suzuki, H. Taniguchi, R. Yoshida, J. Am. Chem. Soc. 131 (2009) 12058.

[58] H. Taniguchi, D. Suzuki, R. Yoshida, J. Phys. Chem. B 114 (2010) 2405.

[59] T. Ueno, K. Bundo, Y. Akagi, T. Sakai, R. Yoshida, Soft Matter 6 (2010) 6072.

[60] T. Ueki, Y. Takasaki, K. Bundo, T. Ueno, Y. Akagi, T. Sakai, R. Yoshida, Soft Matter 10 (2014) 1349.

[61] T. Ueki, M. Shibayama, R. Yoshida, Chem. Commun. 49 (2013) 6947.

[62] R. Tamate, T. Ueki, M. Shibayama, R. Yoshida, Angew. Chem. Int. Ed. 53 (2014) 11248.

[63] R. Tamate, T. Ueki, R. Yoshida, Adv. Mater. 27 (2015) 837.

5.2

Soft Shape-Memory Materials

Koichiro Uto, Cole A. DeForest, Deok-Ho Kim

DEPARTMENT OF BIOENGINEERING, UNIVERSITY OF WASHINGTON, SEATTLE, WA, USA

CHAPTER OUTLINE

5.2.1 Introduction

Mother Nature displays numerous examples of materials that can autonomously change their shape in response to external stimuli. This is seen in both the conifer pinecone and the wheat awn, where microscopic fibril orientation change accompanied by macroscopic close–open shape transition is induced by depending on hydration level (Fig. 5.2.1a and b) [1]. Despite their biological nature, this shape-changing effect is possible via noncell-mediated processes; the microarchitecture of these biological systems ultimately governs their ability to change dynamically their macroscopic shape. In nonbiological systems, researchers have created a variety of materials that have the ability to "memorize" a temporary given shape, and then "recover" to an original permanent shape when triggered by external stimuli. This "shape-memory effect" (SME) is characteristic of all shape-memory materials. SME is an extremely broad phenomenon, and a wide range of materials including polymers [2,3,4], metal alloys [5], ceramics [6,7], supramolecular systems [8,9], and their composites [10], as well as crystalline porous coordination polymers [11] have each been shown to exhibit SME. Since molecular conformational changes within these artificial systems result in macroscopic structural actuations, these shape-memory materials are not so dissimilar from living systems that change shape in response to external stimuli including the pinecone (Fig. 5.2.1c and d).

The most noteworthy and extensively researched shape-memory materials are "shape-memory alloys" (SMAs). Ölander first discovered and reported in 1932 a novel metallic transformation of gold-cadmium (AuCd) alloy, whose pseudoelasticity triggered unusual macroscopic deformation [12]. The discovery of the SME in equiatomic nickel-titanium (NiTi) alloy, which is well known as nitinol, represented a paradigm shift in the SMA field,

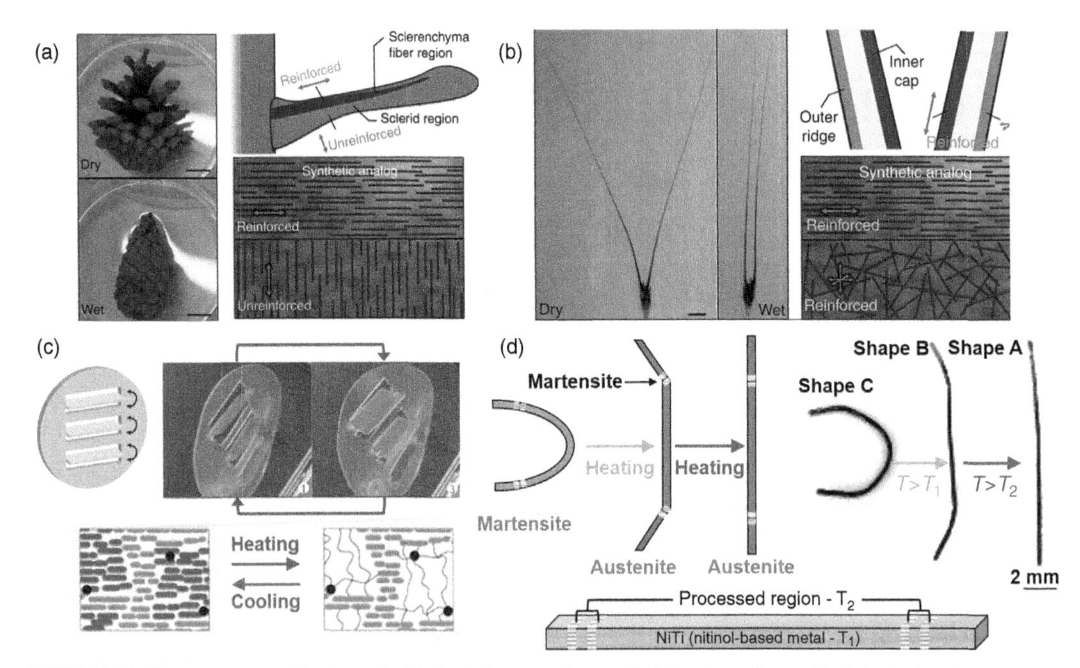

FIGURE 5.2.1 Shape-memory effect seen in Mother Nature and an artificial system. (a and b) Biological systems: (a) conifer pinecone and (b) wheat awn that smartly use fiber orientation to induce shape change [1]. (c and d) Artificial systems: (c) reversible shape-memory plastic [4] and (d) shape-memory alloys that can also actuate by changing molecular structure in response to stimulus [5].

representing a major body of both academic and industrial research. "Shape-memory polymers" (SMPs) were described just a few years later, marked by their first mention in a US patent applied by Vernon and Vernon in 1941 [13,14]. They discovered an "elastic memory" property in thermoplastic synthetic resins made of methacrylic acid ester developed for dental restoration. In this thermally induced SME, they demonstrated that polymeric materials could change shape upon pressure application and then recover their original shape upon heating. Over half a century later, "shape-memory hydrogels" (SMH) [15,16] and "biodegradable polymers" [17,18] have further represented a paradigm shift in soft shape-memory materials (Fig. 5.2.2). Since then, the area of soft shape-memory materials based on polymer and supramolecular systems has attracted tremendous attention, marked by an exponential increase in relevant scientific publications. The reasons for this impressive development are many and accompanied with some important findings including reversible SMH [19], light-induced SME [20], surface SME [21], triple-/multi-SME [22,23], temperature memory [10] as well as two-way (reversible) SME [24,25] as shown in Fig. 5.2.2. In conjunction with the rapid evolution of material science and increasingly sophisticated fabrication techniques, unique and highly functionalized soft shape-memory materials that match capabilities of SMAs and ceramics have gradually emerged. Therefore, it is no doubt that soft shape-memory materials will continue to become increasingly valuable and prominent for a broad scope of applications.

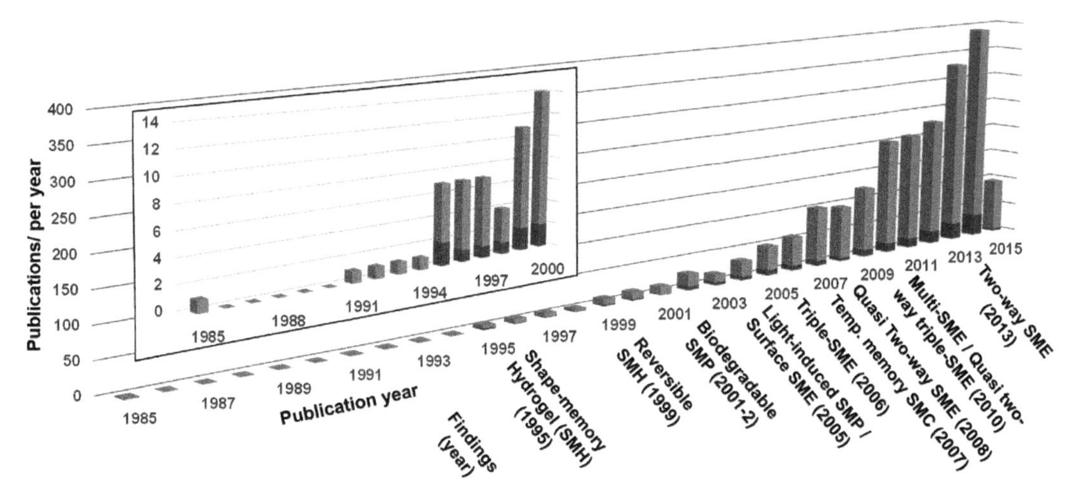

FIGURE 5.2.2 Evolution of published papers in the field of soft shape-memory systems. It shows the results for publication of a topic search for "shape-memory" polymer(s) (light gray [orange in the web version]) and gel(s) (dark gray [blue in the web version]) but not alloy(s) in ISI web of knowledge performed on May 4, 2015. It also shows some key findings addressing shape-memory polymer systems.

In this chapter, we focus on recent efforts to design and fabricate soft shape-memory materials, including both polymeric and supramolecular systems. We first classify these materials based on their micro- and nanostructure (Section 5.2.2). We then highlight how soft shape-memory materials have been applied to biomedical applications as implantables (Section 5.2.3.1), drug delivery devices (Section 5.2.3.2), and tissue engineering scaffolds (Section 5.2.3.3). In addition, we briefly discuss future trends for utilizing soft shape-memory materials for biomedical applications (Section 5.2.4).

5.2.2 Classification of Shape-Memory Materials

5.2.2.1 Polymer Network Architecture

Polymer network structures offer several parameters to tailor properties such as the chain length (molecular weight), branching (molecular shape), or composition (molecular connecting and positioning) in multicopolymer systems. In other words, the properties and functionalities are determined by material nanoarchitectonics. Generally, SMPs have been categorized by the difference in chemical structures and morphologies of the forming network, for examples chemically (or physically) cross-linked semicrystalline (or glassy) polymers. This classification is strongly related to the molecular design of SMPs, and is very useful in describing SMP systems based on thermal phase changes, known as thermally induced SME. The transition temperature (melting temperature [T_m] and glass transition temperature [T_g]) in SMPs can be tuned by precious designing of network structure (Fig. 5.2.3a). In this regard, the T_m of chemically cross-linked poly(ε-caprolactone) (PCL) can be adjusted to physiological temperature range by tailoring the nanoarchitectonics

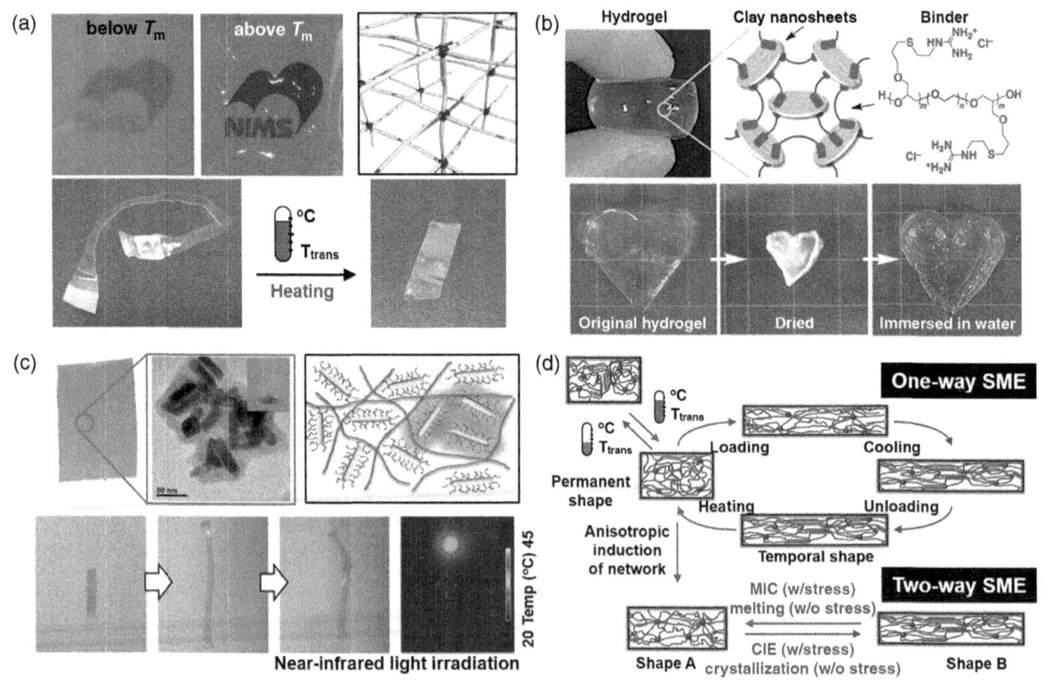

FIGURE 5.2.3 Classification of soft shape-memory materials from the viewpoint of nanoarchitectonics. (a–c) Structures and (d) molecular mechanism. (a) Chemically cross-linked polymer network, (b) supramolecular network with clay nanosheets [29], and (c) inorganic/polymer composite network system, and their shape-memory profiles [30]. (d) The nanoscale molecular mechanism for one-way and two-way SME of a cross-linked semicrystalline polymer system.

of PCL [26,27]. In addition, molecular network structures influence not only the thermal properties but also the mechanical properties and biodegradability. Therefore, there is no doubt that the concept of material nanoarchitectonics in SMP systems is crucial to the design of soft shape-memory materials especially for biomedical applications. The relationship between chemical structure and their functions in SMPs has been well addressed and widely reviewed by the Bowman group [28].

5.2.2.2 Supramolecular Network Architecture

The SME is based on the combination of structural and morphological property, and the majority of soft shape-memory materials contain permanent chemical and physical cross-linking points in their network structure as described previously. On the other hand, the supramolecular system has shown potential in a range of applications in the biomedical field due to its versatile and dynamic nature resulting from noncovalent interactions. In this regard, an alternative methodology for creating soft shape memory by reversible noncovalent interactions as cross-linking points has attracted much attention. Anthamatten and coworkers first reported that reversible noncovalent interactions can be used efficiently to fix mechanically deformed states at low temperature [31]. In this system, they utilized multiple hydrogen bonding between ureidopyrimidinone moieties to make a temporal shape, and the supramolecular material clearly showed the thermally induced SME due to the dynamic nature of hydrogen bonding. In addition, nanoscale inclusion complex formation between cyclodextrin and poly(ethylene glycol) has been employed as a molecular switch to actuate SME in the supramolecular system [32]. Despite these successes, distinct applications utilizing supramolecular interactions have not yet been fully realized, due in part to poor network mechanical properties. Recently, Aida et al. successfully fabricated moldable supramolecular hydrogels consisting of a polymeric binder carrying guanidinium ion pendants and clay nanosheets [29]. The hydrogel demonstrated excellent material properties, having formed through a multivalent salt bridge involving hydrogen bonding and electrostatic interactions. Interestingly, a supramolecular gel network can remember its shape even after drying and rewetting (Fig. 5.2.3b). High water content, mechanically tough, and shape-memory supramolecular gels with well-organized nanoarchitectonics offer different potentials over polymer network systems. Although the supramolecular shape-memory material has a relatively short history, its structural versatility and diversity should be applicable for designing a new class of biomaterials.

5.2.2.3 Composite System

As discussed above, most SMPs utilize reversible thermal phase transition induced by heating above T_m and T_g or cooling below the crystallization temperature (T_c) and T_g. However, such direct heating or cooling is often incompatible with biomedical applications *in vivo*; our bodies can only accommodate a narrow physiological range of temperatures. Instead, the transition temperature of these materials must be engineered to match that of body temperature. Another rational strategy to overcome this issue is to utilize endogenous heating that generates heat from inside material by indirect heating. In view of this, the hybridization with SMPs and other materials such as inorganic materials including (nano)particles and (nano)wires is called shape-memory composites (SMCs) and is often used to endow a special triggering switch and multifunctionality to SMPs. Through appropriately designed material, various stimuli including magnetic, optical, and electrical energies can be applied as a source to convert into thermal energy to induce phase transition. For example, remote activation of bulk and surface SMEs via near-infrared (NIR) light irradiation by using gold nanorods (AuNRs)-embedded PCL composites has been demonstrated (Fig. 5.2.3c) [30,33]. To achieve an efficient photothermal effect in response to NIR light, a high and homogeneous dispersion of AuNRs in the cross-linked PCL matrix is necessary. In fact, PCL modification with AuNRs was efficient to enhance nanoscale dispersibility and miscibility in the PCL matrix. This composite is just one example of many SMCs, and there are many excellent review articles covering SMP composites [34,35]. From those reviews, the relationship between nanostructures of composites and their functionality is highly relevant, suggesting the importance of material nanoarchitectonics in SMCs.

5.2.2.4 Molecular Mechanism

Though various molecular or nanoscale switches can be designed into shape-memory materials to trigger phase transition, we will focus our discussion of the molecular mechanism of SME to thermally induced changes. The most common class of shape-memory material to date is a thermally induced one-way dual type. The terms "thermally induced," "one-way," and "dual" imply a stimulation method to induce SME, irreversible shape change, and the total number of programmable shapes. Therefore, one-way dual SME refers to materials that are able to shift their shape from a temporary shape to a permanent shape in an irreversible fashion. On the other hand, more sophisticated two-way and/or triple (or multi-) SMEs have also been developed recently [4,22–25]. Strictly speaking, the programming process to make a temporary shape is crucial to achieve a two-way reversible system. In a cross-linked glassy or semicrystalline SMP, how the skeleton of crystallized geometry is built and the conformation orientation of the switching domain in the polymer network is created are key factors to determine whether the system is "one-way" or "two-way" (Fig. 5.2.3c). In similar way, how many different switching domains are introduced into the polymer network or how broad transition is produced by material design are key elements to create "triple" or "multi-" SME systems. For more information, the reader is referred to a recent review by Xie and coworkers that describes the design criteria and principle regarding the new behavior of SMPs [36]. From the viewpoint of the molecular mechanism of SMPs, it is also noticed that the materials nanoarchitectonics plays an important role in deciding whether the system is a "one-way" or "two-way" or "dual," "triple," or "multi-" SME.

5.2.2.5 Material Textures and Forms

So far, we have discussed the properties of soft shape-memory materials as a function of their nanoarchitectonics. At the same time, material microarchitectonics, also known as material forms, should be tailored to specific applications as SME in material was generally treated with bulk phenomenon. As such, designing an SMP object at the submicron to microscale is challenging. In particular, the synthesis of well-regulated nanoscale structures built up as meso- or macroscopic materials remains challenging. Recent rapid evolution in SMPs has been developed in efforts to meet various requirements in diverse potential applications. As a result, not only traditional film, tube, and sponge (foam) forms, but also microparticles, surface as well as micro/nanofiber that exhibit SMEs at mesoscopic to microscopic scales, have attracted much attention (Fig. 5.2.4).

Although these forms have different object scales from nano- (nm) to centimeter (cm) and various dimensions from one-dimensional (1D) fiber to three-dimensional (3D) sponge, it is possible to fabricate these material forms with excellent shape-memory properties [37,38]. Despite unique material textures and forms with multiscale, the underlying molecular principle of SMEs is largely equivalent to that of bulk systems, suggesting similar design criteria and principles. Structural flexibility and diversity originated from material microarchitectonics may certainly promote soft shape memory for many new applications.

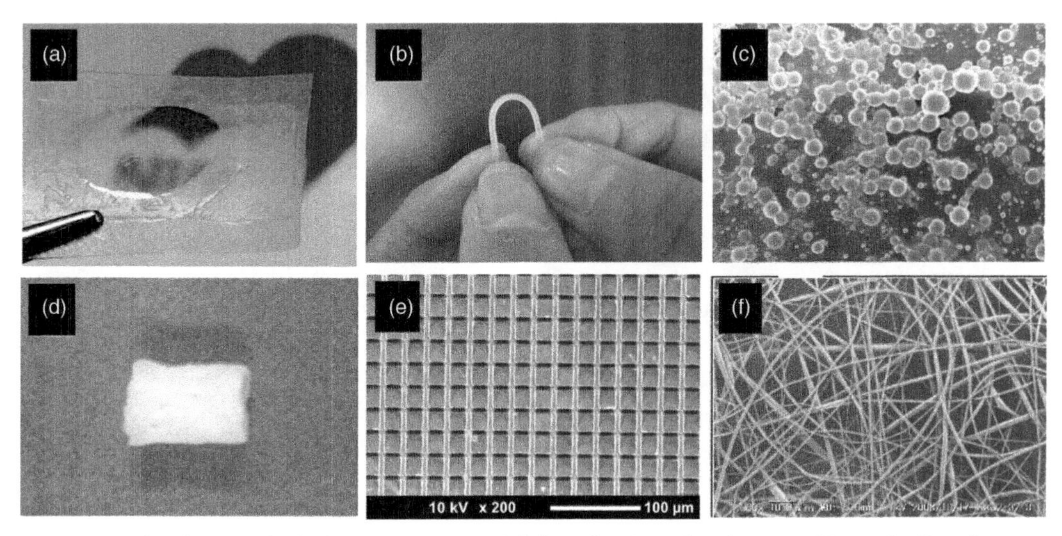

FIGURE 5.2.4 Classification of soft shape-memory materials from the viewpoint of macroarchitectonics (forms). Variants in shape-memory forms such as (a) film, (b) tube, (c) particle, (d) sponge (foam), (e) surface, and (f) fiber types. SMP platforms have various material dimensions from 1D (fiber) and 2D (surface) to 3D (sponge).

5.2.3 Biomedical Applications of Shape-Memory Materials

Representing a novel smart material, soft shape-memory materials are uniquely suited for applications in medicine and biotechnology. In 2002, Lendlein and Langer first demonstrated the concept of biodegradable thermally responsive SMP sutures [17]. In combination with publishing the excellent review article on "designing materials for biology and medicine" by Langer and Tirrell [39], many researchers are utilizing SMPs to introduce biocompatible and biodegradable implant materials through minimally invasive surgical procedures. In this section, we overview recent studies on soft shape-memory materials for biomedicine.

5.2.3.1 Implantable Devices

SMPs have most notably been promoted because of their potential in minimally invasive surgery, where a compacted device could be passed through a smaller incision and deployed to its full shape once inside the body [40]. For biomedical devices, the heating of polymer to activate SMEs has been proposed by body, temperature, optical/laser heating, and remote inductive heating [41]. As each of these thermal activation methods is possible within the body, control over SMP geometry is possible with implantable devices.

Cerebral aneurysms treated by traditional endovascular methods using noble metal (platinum)-based coils have a tendency to be unstable, due to chronic inflammation, compaction of coils, or growth of the aneurysm. In addition, with physical limitation, mechanical mismatch between hard metal and the thinned, weakened wall, aneurysms exhibit a potential for rupture. Maitland et al. addressed this issue and developed a new filling

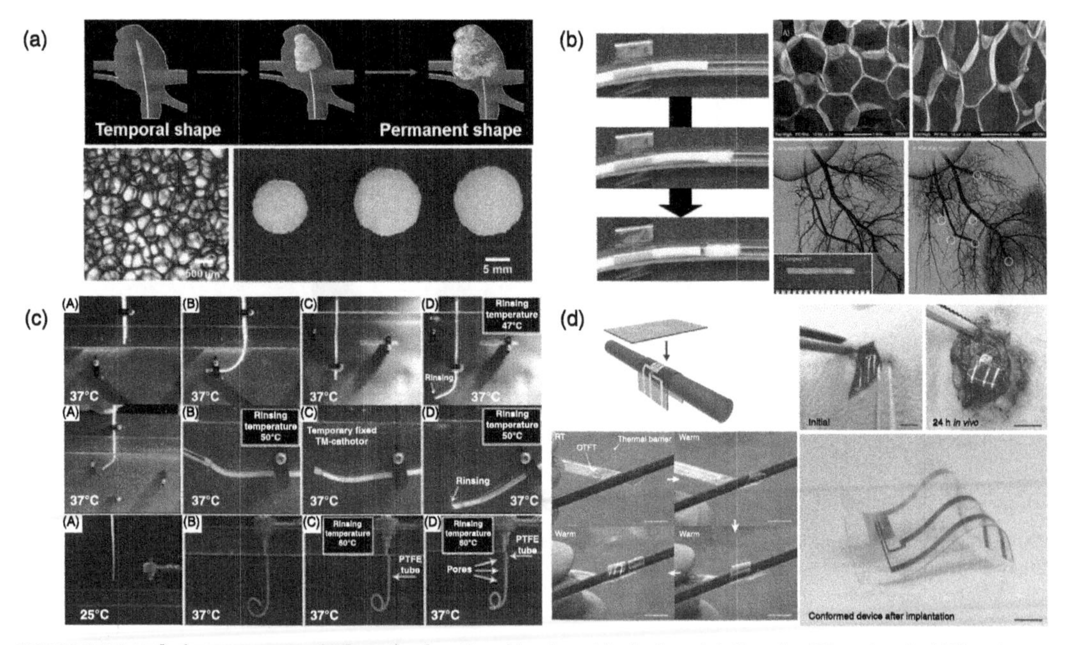

FIGURE 5.2.5 Soft shape-memory platform for functional implantable devices. (a) Closed-cell low density [42] and (b) opened-cell SMP foam devices for aneurysm filling [43]. Both SMP foam devices can deliver to the aneurysm via a catheter as a crimped temporary shape. These foams enable expansion within the aneurysm, as it recovers to its permanent shape via stimuli, and finally treated aneurysm with fully expanded foam. The reticulated foam device (b) is also capable of achieving rapid vascular occlusion in an *in vivo* porcine model. (c) Intelligent catheters based on temperature-memory effect in SMPs. Although these catheters are composed of the same material, they can operate in different ways such as (top) individually programmable, (middle) *in situ* programmable, and (bottom) intelligent drainage catheter [44]. (d) SMP-based implantable electronics. By combining SMPs and organic thin-film transistors (OTFTs), a unique form of adaptive electronics is developed, which changes their mechanical properties from rigid and planar to soft and compliant, in order to enable soft and conformal wrapping around 3D objects, including biological tissue [45].

method for the treatment of intracranial aneurysms using polyurethane-based SMP foams (Fig. 5.2.5a) [42]. The SMP foam with a crimped temporary shape is capable of expanding to fill the aneurysm sac. In particular, their developed low-density SMP foams displayed only a small expansion force, suggesting a decreased risk of aneurysm rupture upon treatment. However, the SMP foam was predominantly a closed cell structure with limited potential for full healing, which involves blood clotting and cell migration throughout the foam's inner volume space. The development of a more open-cell microstructure might further improve the healing response. To overcome this issue, they successfully fabricated low-density SMP foams with reticulated pore structure (Fig. 5.2.5b) [43]. Nondestructive reticulation of SMP foams was achieved by using a gravity-driven floating NiTi alloy pin array coupled with vibratory agitation of the foam and additional chemical etching. It was clearly demonstrated that reticulation of SMP foams resulted in a reduced elastic modulus and increased permeability while retaining their shape-memory property. They also showed the capability of a rapid vascular occlusion device in an *in vivo* experiment using a porcine model. Although further study is needed to definitively prove the advantage of reticulate structures in their system, well-regulated microarchitectonics should improve the efficacy of aneurysm healing response.

In the previously described approaches, catheters can be utilized to deliver developed SMP foams to diseased areas. Catheters are essential medical devices that can be inserted into the body cavity, duct, or vessel to treat diseases and perform a surgical procedure. Lendlein and coworkers developed a new type of intelligent catheter based on a multiblock copolymer [44]. Importantly, they cleverly adopted the temperature memory effect (TME), which is the capability of a polymer to remember the temperature where they were deformed recently, into the system [4,10]. To achieve this actuation, they used the multiblock copolymer consisting of PCL and poly(ω-pentadecalactone) selected as switching and hard segment forming components, respectively. They finally demonstrated three concepts including individually programmable, *in situ* programmable, and intelligent drainage TM-catheters to show the working principle of TME for application potential in minimally invasive medical devices (Fig. 5.2.5c). Therefore, this concept should prove powerful as TME in soft shape-memory materials enables the realization of various response temperatures with the same polymer material by simple regulation of thermomechanical processing, without requiring synthesis of the new material.

Soft electronic devices are capable of addressing health care problems that require chronic device implantation. In view of this, intimate conformability is essential for obtaining stable interfaces on complex surfaces such as tissues and organs. SMPs may have the potential to contribute in this field. Someya et al. developed a unique form of adaptive electronics that softly conforms or deploys into a 3D shape in response to a stimulus by exploiting the functional features of soft shape-memory materials [45]. They first fabricated SMP substrates composed of 1,3,5-triallyl-1,3,5-triazine-2,4,6(1H,3H,5H)-trione, tricyclodecane dimethanol diacrylate, and *tris*[2-(3-mercaptopropionyloxy) ethyl] isocyanurate, integrated with organic thin film transistors (OTFTs) (Fig. 5.2.5d). The resulting hybrids can change their mechanical properties from rigid and planar, to soft and compliant via SMEs, in order to enable soft and conformal wrapping around 3D objects such as biological tissue. These acutely physiologically stable and active OTFTs have the potential to address challenging biomedical problems by enabling new means of creating intimate interfaces between body tissue and high performance, robust bioelectronics.

5.2.3.2 Drug-Releasing Devices

Polymeric materials have been developed into multiplatform technologies to offer biomedical materials with multifunctionality [39]. For example, in addition to a unique structural role, SMP medical devices offer biodegradability and enable controlled therapeutic drug release. Since Wache et al. first reported the development of an SMP stent as a new vehicle for drug delivery in 2003 [46], there has been much effort to design drug-eluent stents (DESs). A drug-loaded, degradable SMP stent has been demonstrated by Lendlein's group. They successfully demonstrated a first example of the potential application of such SMPs as ureteral stents [47], and the potential of drug-loaded SMPs as injectable or implantable self-anchoring implant rods, which could enable spatial fixation for a local drug release [48].

The development of releasing systems involving multiple therapeutics, macromolecular drugs, remote control, and/or spatiotemporal control over payload delivery has been addressed as a recent trend in the field of SMPs (Fig. 5.2.6). Wang et al. reported an SMP-DES developed by chemically cross-linked copolymer networks of poly(ethylene glycol) and PCL. By optimizing the molecular composition and weight of copolymers, they successfully adjusted their transition temperature to match that of body temperature. They loaded two different drugs (mitomycin C and curcumin) into their SMP network to potentially prevent in-stent restenosis of the vessel; both short- and long-term therapeutic effect was achieved by controlled dual drug release (Fig. 5.2.6a) [49]. Additionally, Zhou and

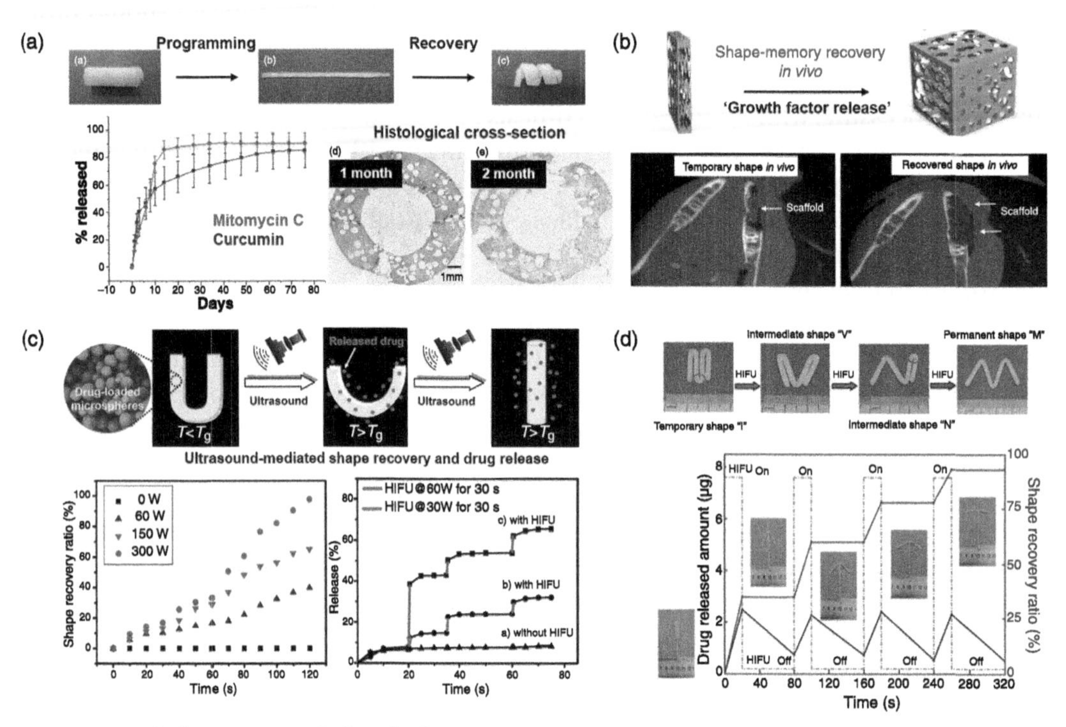

FIGURE 5.2.6 Soft shape-memory platform for functional drug delivery devices. (a) Biodegradable SMP-DES. SMP-DES shows shape recovery in response to temperature change and dual drug (mitomycin C/curcumin) release property [49]. (b) Shape-memory porous nanocomposite scaffold. This device enables the loading of growth factor BMP-2 during calcium cross-linking of sodium alginate. *In vivo* shape-memory recovery process of the BMP-2-loaded porous nanocomposite scaffold is clearly demonstrated by using cone beam computed topography [50]. (c) Biodegradable cylindrical shape-memory rod made of SMP microspheres. Shape recovery and payload protein release effects can be modulated by applying the ultrasound [51]. (d) HIFU-enabled spatial and temporal control of shape recovery and release of loaded drugs. Spatially and temporally controllable shape recovery and copper sulfate release in response to HIFU application is demonstrated [52].

coworkers reported a delivery of a macromolecular object using a smart porous nanocomposite scaffold to repair a mandibular bone defect (Fig. 5.2.6b) [50]. The fabricated scaffold consists of chemically cross-linked PCL and hydroxyapatite nanoparticles that is an SMC system, and succeeded in preparing highly interconnected pores of scaffold using a sugar-leaching method. Furthermore, to load macromolecular objects into the system, they adopted a coating layer of calcium alginate and bone morphogenetic protein-2 (BMP-2) on the porous SMP framework. The developed SMP scaffold displayed good shape-memory recovery in both *in vitro* and *in vivo* environments, and they found that it promoted new bone generation in the rabbit mandibular bone defect model.

Zhang and coworkers recently reported biodegradable shape-memory cylindrical rods offering a unique structure [51]. In this research, chitosan functionalized poly(lactic acid-*co*-glycolic acid) microspheres containing lysozyme as a model payload were first prepared by the emulsion method, and a macroscopic cylindrical-shaped rod was then fabricated by directly sintering the drug-loaded macrospheres (Fig. 5.2.6c). By employing high-intensity focused ultrasound (HIFU), the temporal and simultaneous regulation of SMEs and payload release of the 3D cylindrical rod were remotely operated. Moreover, these two processes are controllable and could be manipulated by varying acoustic power and insonation pulse duration. Additionally, Xia and Zhao proposed a new concept and modality enabling the simultaneous control of SMEs and release of loaded drug by utilizing a unique feature of HIFU [52]. To achieve this, they selected poly(methyl methacrylate-*co*-butyl acrylate) copolymer as a matrix component because of the biocompatibility and easy tunability of its transition temperature. They clearly showed that the HIFU-triggered shape recovery process can be spatially and temporarily controlled, allowing the SME to manifest in selected regions on demand, endowing SMPs with the capability of adopting multiple intermediate shapes and synchronizing the release of loaded drugs in a switchable manner (Fig. 5.2.6d). From these studies, it is clear that drug-releasing ability is applicable for not only medical device applications but also tissue engineering and regenerative medicine, suggesting the importance of combinations with other functionalities.

5.2.3.3 Tissue Engineering

The advent of biodegradable SMPs spurred the investigation of their use as a vehicle for tissue engineering. Tissue can be grown on collapsible SMP scaffolds *in vitro* and then delivered into the body using minimally invasive techniques to initiate repair or reconstruction of tissue organs. In addition to the biocompatibility and biodegradability of scaffold, the shape memory will surely open the door to new applications in tissue engineering.

Success in bone tissue engineering, especially in the treatment of critical-sized craniomaxillofacial bone defects, requires conformal matching between the scaffold and the tissue defects. Toward this, Grunlan et al. developed an SMP scaffold exhibiting an open porous structure and a "self-fit" ability [53]. They produced a porous cross-linked PCL network by the solvent casting/particulate leaching method using a fused salt template. To enhance the bioactivity, a polydopamine coating was conducted onto the wall of porous cross-linked PCL frameworks. The scaffold became malleable and showed "self-fit" ability after pressing into an irregular model defect (Fig. 5.2.7a). In addition, they successfully demonstrated that polydopamine-coated scaffolds exhibited superior bioactivity, osteoblast adhesion, proliferation, osteogenic gene expression, and extracellular matrix deposition after hydroxyapatite mineralization. In this system, polydopamine coating is an additional value to the SMP scaffold but clearly showed enhancement bioactivity without loss of original SMP property.

Cell responsiveness to its surrounding mechanical cues has been the subject of active research. In spite of a considerable amount of ongoing research, current efforts are centered on rather static patterns. Due to the dynamic nature of the regeneration processes, static substrates seem to be deficient in mimicking changing physiological conditions, such as development, wound healing, and disease. Surface SMEs can provide a dynamic change of micro- and nanotopographical property to adhered cells [27,56,57], and may have the potential to be powerful tools for regulating cell functions and fate. In this

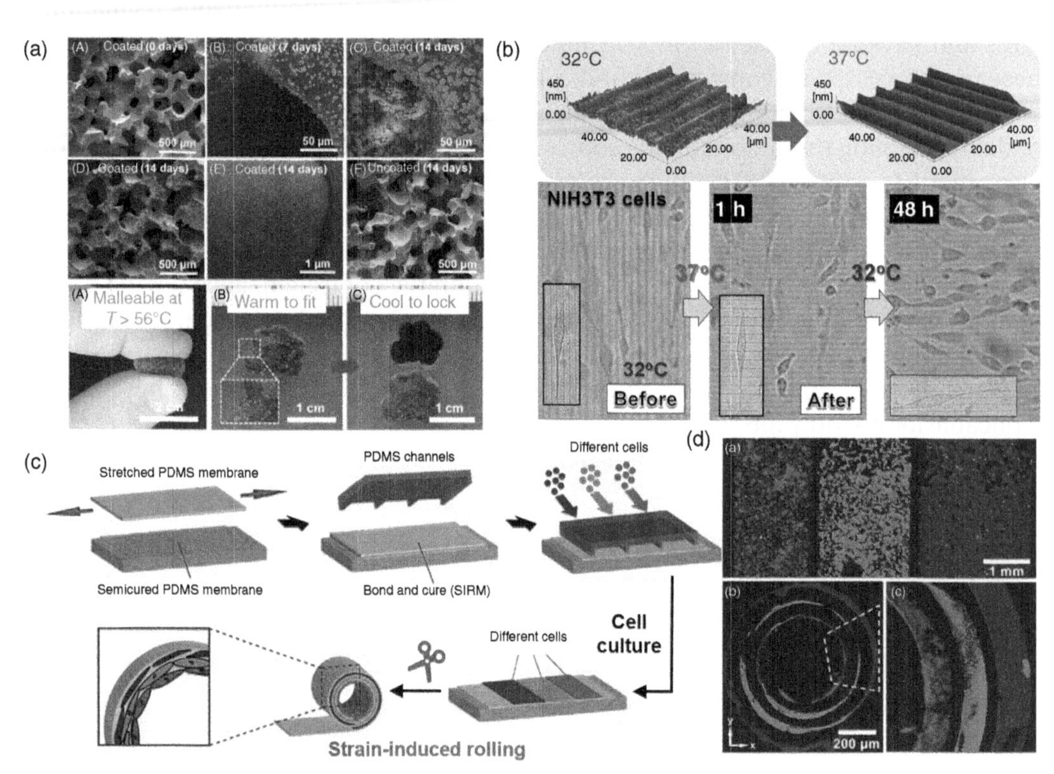

FIGURE 5.2.7 Soft shape-memory platform for functional tissue engineering scaffolds. (a) Bioactive self-fitting SMP scaffold for bone tissue engineering. SMP scaffold can be used as a template for apatite mineralization, and exhibits an open porous structure and the capacity to conformally "self-fit" into irregular defects [53]. (b) Surface shape-memory platform for mechanobiological control of cell functions and fate. Shape-memory surface transition can dynamically regulate cellular morphology, orientation, and movement [54]. (c) Stress-induced rolling bilayer membrane for 3D vascular tissue engineering. This platform enables one-pot fabrication of tubular structures with multipole cell types forming different layers of the tube walls [55].

approach, the adjusting transition temperature to physiological temperature range is a most important technical issue. Uto et al. successfully designed cross-linked PCL tailored nanoarchitectonics, providing dynamic mechanical cues in response to 5°C temperature difference (32°C and 37°C) [26,27]. They also demonstrated that orientation modes as well as rotational movement of cells could be dynamically regulated in a desired manner using surface SMEs (Fig. 5.2.7b) [54].

Soft shape-memory material is also applicable as a scaffold to 3D vascular tissue engineering. Zhang et al. proposed a versatile, one-pot strategy for depositing different types of cells in 3D to mimic tubular structure in vascular tissue [55]. Their strategy to fabricate tubular structures with layered walls made of multiple types of cells is called the stress-induced rolling membrane (SIRM) technique. The SIRM device is fabricated by bonding two elastic membranes together (Fig. 5.2.7c). After mechanical scratching of substrate, flat-to-tube shape transition was induced by rolling, generated from the device's internal stress. They found that the 3D vascular mimic structures composed of both randomly or highly oriented endothelial cells, smooth muscle cells, and fibroblasts was fabricated in a one-pot process by using SIRM technique. This technique may not consist of SMEs, but this unique idea should be incorporated into designing soft shape-memory materials. Furthermore, this strategy will enrich the toolbox for 3D micro-/nanofabrication by initially patterning in 2D and transforming into 3D.

5.2.4 Conclusions and Perspectives

Although our understanding of design principles and mechanisms in soft shape-memory material, including polymer and supramolecular systems, has been rapidly and dramatically improved, there are only a few examples of materials exhibiting SMEs commercially available. In conjunction with rapid technological evolution of this field and interdisciplinary study, unique and highly functionalized soft shape-memory material and actuation principles have started to appear. The recent developed concept, which is a thermally driven reversible and bidirectional shape-memory effect (rbSME) platform, is useful in the creation of future biomedical devices [25], although the actuation temperature range, accuracy, and operation mode must continue to be improved. In addition, deformable, programmable micro-optics has been developed by combining surface SMEs and micro-optics [58]. Since it has been clearly demonstrated that these rewritable and switchable optics worked as SMP holograms, they may prove applicable to the biomedical field as new thermal actuated smart devices. Origami-inspired nanotechnology and manufacturing is another hot topic in materials science. By combining with SMPs and origami-inspired technology, a new concept sequential self-folding robot was developed [59,60]. Composite sheets composed of laminating several layers including SMPs work as building blocks to achieve highly sophisticated robotic movements. These results may indicate the importance of not only materials design but also system design into how assembled architectonics are operated. Here, we picked up and discussed on a number of featured and unique examples, but many other materials and principles have been extensively reported. However, there is no doubt that the unique characteristics and functions of shape-memory materials are a direct result of material nanoarchitectonics, and that soft polymer and supramolecular systems satisfy a different set of applications than those of hard shape-memory systems such as alloys and ceramics. Moreover, SMPs are one of the most fascinating polymer classes, and will accelerate the development more rapidly and discursively. In this situation, to establish more practical and valuable systems using soft shape-memory materials, we should always ask how can nanoarchitectonics express functions and the principle be used technically.

References

[1] R.M. Erb, J.S. Sander, R. Grisch, A.R. Studart, Nat. Commun. 4 (2013) 1712.

[2] A. Lendlein, S. Kelch, Angew. Chem. Int. Ed. 41 (12) (2002) 2034–2057.

[3] C. Liu, H. Qin, P.T. Mather, J. Mater. Chem. 17 (16) (2007) 1543–1558.

[4] M. Behl, K. Kratz, U. Noechel, T. Sauter, A. Lendlein, Proc. Natl. Acad. Sci. 110 (31) (2013) 12555–12559.

[5] M.I. Khan, A. Pequegnat, Y.N. Zhou, Adv. Eng. Mater. 15 (5) (2013) 386–393.

[6] M.V. Swain, Nature 322 (6076) (1986) 234–236.

[7] A. Lai, Z. Du, C.L. Gan, C.A. Schuh, Science 341 (6153) (2013) 1505–1508.

[8] X. Yan, F. Wang, B. Zheng, F. Huang, Chem. Soc. Rev. 41 (18) (2012) 6042–6065.

[9] R. Dong, Y. Pang, Y. Su, X. Zhu, Biomater. Sci. 3 (17) (2015) 937–954.

[10] P. Miaudet, A. Derré, M. Maugey, C. Zakri, P.M. Piccione, R. Inoubli, et al., Science 318 (5854) (2007) 1294–1296.

[11] Y. Sakata, S. Furukawa, M. Kondo, K. Hirai, N. Horike, Y. Takashima, et al., Science 339 (6116) (2013) 193–196.

[12] A. Ölander, J. Am. Chem. Soc. 54 (10) (1932) 3819–3833.

[13] Vernon LB, Vernon HM, Inventors Patent US2,234,993, 1941.

[14] Vernon LB, Vernon HM, Inventors Patent US2,234,994, 1941.

[15] Y. Osada, A. Matsuda, Nature 376 (6537) (1995) 219.

[16] Z. Hu, X. Zhang, Y. Li, Science 269 (5223) (1995) 525–527.

[17] A. Lendlein, R. Langer, Science 296 (5573) (2002) 1673–1676.

[18] A. Lendlein, A.M. Schmidt, R. Langer, Proc. Natl. Acad. Sci. 98 (3) (2001) 842–847.

[19] T. Miyata, N. Asami, T. Uragami, Nature 399 (6738) (1999) 766–769.

[20] A. Lendlein, H. Jiang, O. Junger, R. Langer, Nature 434 (7035) (2005) 879–882.

[21] B.A. Nelson, W.P. King, K. Gall, Appl. Phys. Lett. 86 (10) (2005) 103108.

[22] I. Bellin, S. Kelch, R. Langer, A. Lendlein, Proc. Natl. Acad. Sci. 103 (48) (2006) 18043–18047.

[23] T. Xie, Nature 464 (7286) (2010) 267–270.

[24] T. Chung, A. Romo-Uribe, P.T. Mather, Macromolecules 41 (1) (2008) 184–192.

[25] M. Behl, K. Kratz, J. Zotzmann, U. Nöchel, A. Lendlein, Adv. Mater. 25 (32) (2013) 4466–4469.

[26] K. Uto, K. Yamamoto, S. Hirase, T. Aoyagi, J. Control. Release 110 (2) (2006) 408–413.

[27] M. Ebara, K. Uto, N. Idota, J.M. Hoffman, T. Aoyagi, Adv. Mater. 24 (2) (2012) 273–278.

[28] G.J. Berg, M.K. McBride, C. Wang, C.N. Bowman, Polymer 55 (23) (2014) 5849–5872.

[29] S. Tamesue, M. Ohtani, K. Yamada, Y. Ishida, J.M. Spruell, N.A. Lynd, et al., J. Am. Chem. Soc. 135 (41) (2013) 15650–15655.

[30] Q. Shou, K. Uto, M. Iwanaga, M. Ebara, T. Aoyagi, Polym. J. 46 (8) (2014) 492–498.

[31] J. Li, J.A. Viveros, M.H. Wrue, M. Anthamatten, Adv. Mater. 19 (19) (2007) 2851–2855.

[32] S. Zhang, Z. Yu, T. Govender, H. Luo, B. Li, Polymer 49 (15) (2008) 3205–3210.

[33] Q. Shou, K. Uto, W.-C. Lin, T. Aoyagi, M. Ebara, Macromol. Chem. Phys. 215 (24) (2014) 2473–2481.

[34] J. Leng, X. Lan, Y. Liu, S. Du, Prog. Mater. Sci. 56 (7) (2011) 1077–1135.

[35] M. Behl, M.Y. Razzaq, A. Lendlein, Adv. Mater. 22 (31) (2010) 3388–3410.

[36] Q. Zhao, H.J. Qi, T. Xie, Prog Polym Sci. 49–50 (2015) 79–120.

[37] F. Friess, U. Nöchel, A. Lendlein, C. Wischke, Adv. Healthc. Mater. 3 (12) (2014) 1986–1990.

[38] D.I. Cha, H.Y. Kim, K.H. Lee, Y.C. Jung, J.W. Cho, B.C. Chun, J. Appl. Polym. Sci. 96 (2) (2005) 460–465.

[39] R. Langer, D.A. Tirrell, Nature 428 (6982) (2004) 487–492.

[40] I.V.W. Small, P. Singhal, T.S. Wilson, D.J. Maitland, J. Mater. Chem. 20 (17) (2010) 3356–3366.

[41] M. Ebara, Y. Kotsuchibashi, K. Uto, T. Aoyagi, Y.-J. Kim, R. Narain, et al. Shape-memory materials. Smart biomaterials, NIMS Monographs, Springer, Japan, 2014, pp. 285–373 Chapter 7.

[42] J.N. Rodriguez, F.J. Clubb, T.S. Wilson, M.W. Miller, T.W. Fossum, J. Hartman, et al., J. Biomed. Mater. Res. 102 (5) (2014) 1231–1242.

[43] J.N. Rodriguez, M.W. Miller, A. Boyle, J. Horn, C.-K. Yang, T.S. Wilson, et al., J. Mech. Behav. Biomed. Mater. 40 (0) (2014) 102–114.

[44] K. Kratz, U. Voigt, A. Lendlein, Adv. Funct. Mater. 22 (14) (2012) 3057–3065.

[45] J. Reeder, M. Kaltenbrunner, T. Ware, D. Arreaga-Salas, A. Avendano-Bolivar, T. Yokota, et al., Adv. Mater. 26 (29) (2014) 4967–4973.

[46] H.M. Wache, D.J. Tartakowska, A. Hentrich, M.H. Wagner, J. Mater. Sci. Mater. Med. 14 (2) (2003) 109–112.

[47] A.T. Neffe, B.D. Hanh, S. Steuer, A. Lendlein, Adv. Mater. 21 (32–33) (2009) 3394–3398.

[48] C. Wischke, A.T. Neffe, S. Steuer, A. Lendlein, J. Control. Release 138 (3) (2009) 243–250.

[49] C.-S. Yang, H.-C. Wu, J.-S. Sun, H.-M. Hsiao, T.-W. Wang, ACS Appl. Mater. Interfaces 5 (21) (2013) 10985–10994.

[50] X. Liu, K. Zhao, T. Gong, J. Song, C. Bao, E. Luo, et al., Biomacromolecules 15 (3) (2014) 1019–1030.

[51] M. Bao, Q. Zhou, W. Dong, X. Lou, Y. Zhang, Biomacromolecules 14 (6) (2013) 1971–1979.

[52] G. Li, G. Fei, H. Xia, J. Han, Y. Zhao, J. Mater. Chem. 22 (16) (2012) 7692–7696.

[53] D. Zhang, O.J. George, K.M. Petersen, A.C. Jimenez-Vergara, M.S. Hahn, M.A. Grunlan, Acta Biomater. 10 (11) (2014) 4597–4605.

[54] M. Ebara, K. Uto, N. Idota, J.M. Hoffman, T. Aoyagi, Int. J. Nanomed. 9 (Suppl. 1) (2014) 117–126.

[55] B. Yuan, Y. Jin, Y. Sun, D. Wang, J. Sun, Z. Wang, et al., Adv. Mater. 24 (7) (2012) 890–896.

[56] K.A. Davis, K.A. Burke, P.T. Mather, J.H. Henderson, Biomaterials 32 (9) (2011) 2285–2293.

[57] D.M. Le, K. Kulangara, A.F. Adler, K.W. Leong, V.S. Ashby, Adv. Mater. 23 (29) (2011) 3278–3283.

[58] H. Xu, C. Yu, S. Wang, V. Malyarchuk, T. Xie, J.A. Rogers, Adv. Funct. Mater. 23 (26) (2013) 3299–3306.

[59] S. Felton, M. Tolley, E. Demaine, D. Rus, R. Wood, Science 345 (6197) (2014) 644–646.

[60] M.T. Tolley, S.M. Felton, S. Miyashita, D. Aukes, D. Rus, R.J. Wood, Smart Mater. Struct. 23 (9) (2014) 094006.

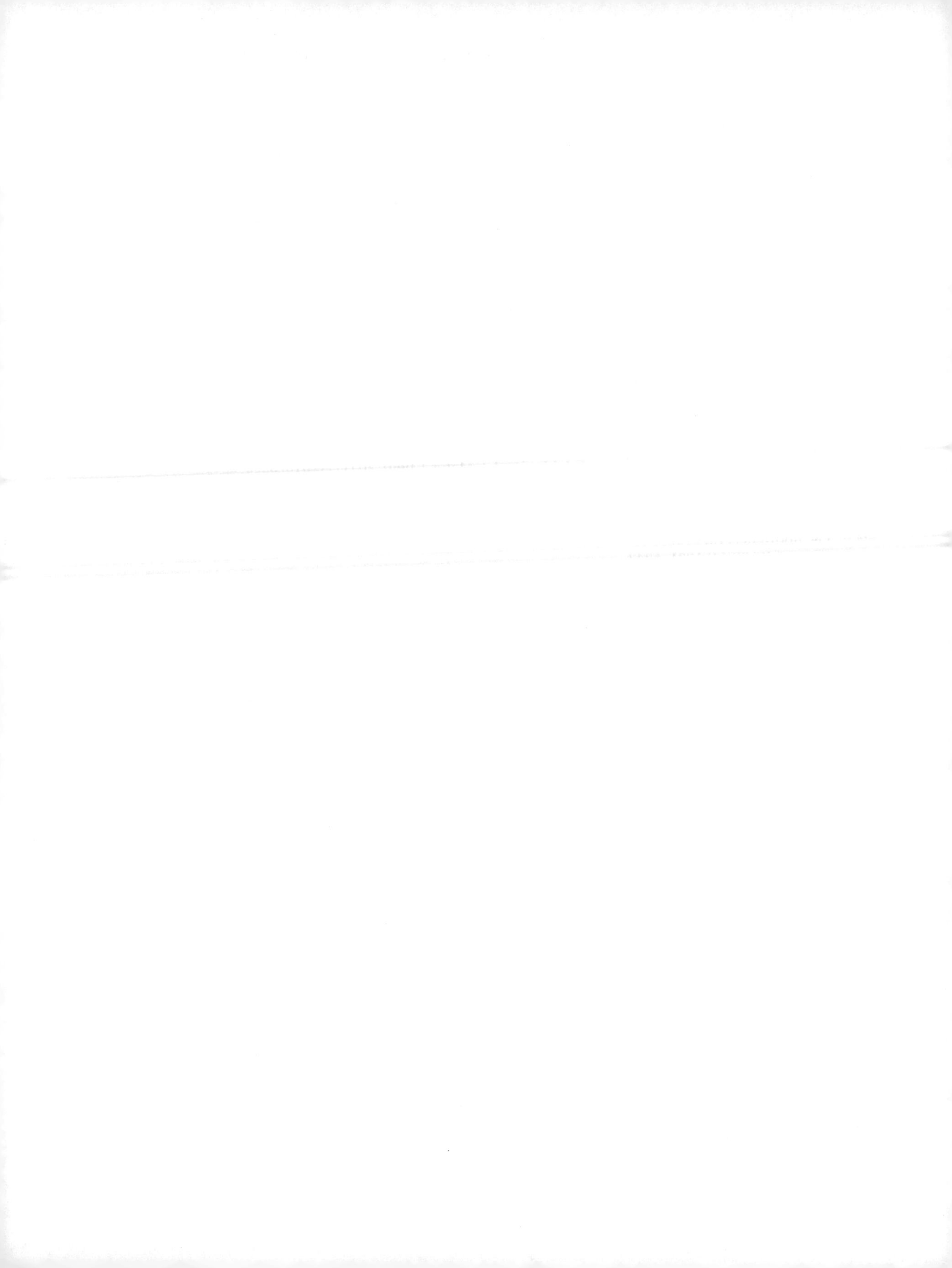

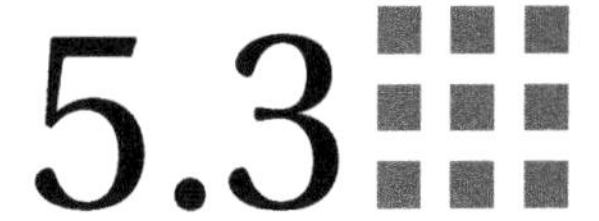

Cell Surface Engineering via Methacryloyl-Derivatized Carbohydrates

Yasuhiko Iwasaki

DEPARTMENT OF CHEMISTRY AND MATERIALS ENGINEERING, FACULTY OF CHEMISTRY, MATERIALS AND BIOENGINEERING, KANSAI UNIVERSITY, OSAKA, JAPAN

CHAPTER OUTLINE

5.3.1 Introduction

Cell-mediated therapies have been considered attractive approaches for medical treatment because cells have the advantages of biocompatibility, flexible morphologies, bioactivity, and tissue homing [1,2]. Cells are the smallest units of living bodies and are involved in various disease processes, including infection, inflammation, and metastasis; therefore, they can offer multiple advantages for targeting diseases. Furthermore, using autologous cells can reduce the immune response, such as immune clearance and foreign body reactions that are observed when synthetic materials are introduced into a living body. Although cells have highly therapeutic functions themselves, conjugation of drugs, fluorochromes, contrast agents, and nanoparticles onto/into cells can make cell-mediated therapies more effective. Cell surface engineering is a new strategy for cell immobilization and has been studied considering the structure of the cell membrane. The well-known fluid-mosaic model for the structure of a cell was proposed by Singer and Nicolson [3]. According to this model, amphiphilic phospholipids are arranged in a bilayer structure and proteins are located in or on it. The distribution of these components is asymmetric, that is, negatively charged phospholipids such as phosphatidylserine are predominantly found on the inner, cytoplasmic side of the membrane, whereas neutral, zwitterionic phosphorylcholine lipids such as phosphatidylcholines are more commonly located in the outer leaflet [4]. The outermost surface of the cell membrane is densely covered with carbohydrates, and these carbohydrates contribute to most of the communications between living cells and their environments [5]. Given the presence of such a diverse range of components in the cell membrane, several approaches for cell surface immobilization can be proposed.

Metabolic delivery of unnatural functional groups into carbohydrates is one of the most robust cell surface engineering methods. In this chapter, surface modification of living cells through a glycosylation pathway and the biointerfacial aspects of the immobilized molecules are described. In addition, a new strategy for the preparation of biofunctional polymeric materials using unnatural carbohydrates generated on mammalian cells is introduced.

5.3.2 Surface Modification of Mammalian Cells

Surface modification of living cells has been the subject of study for a variety of biological applications such as imaging, transfection, and control of cell surface interactions [6–8]. Several processes have been proposed to achieve modification; they can be mainly divided into direct and metabolic immobilization methods. For direct cell surface immobilization, lipophilic anchors [9–11], chemical immobilization [12,13], ligand–receptor interactions [14], and fusion [15,16] have been performed, as shown in Fig. 5.3.1.

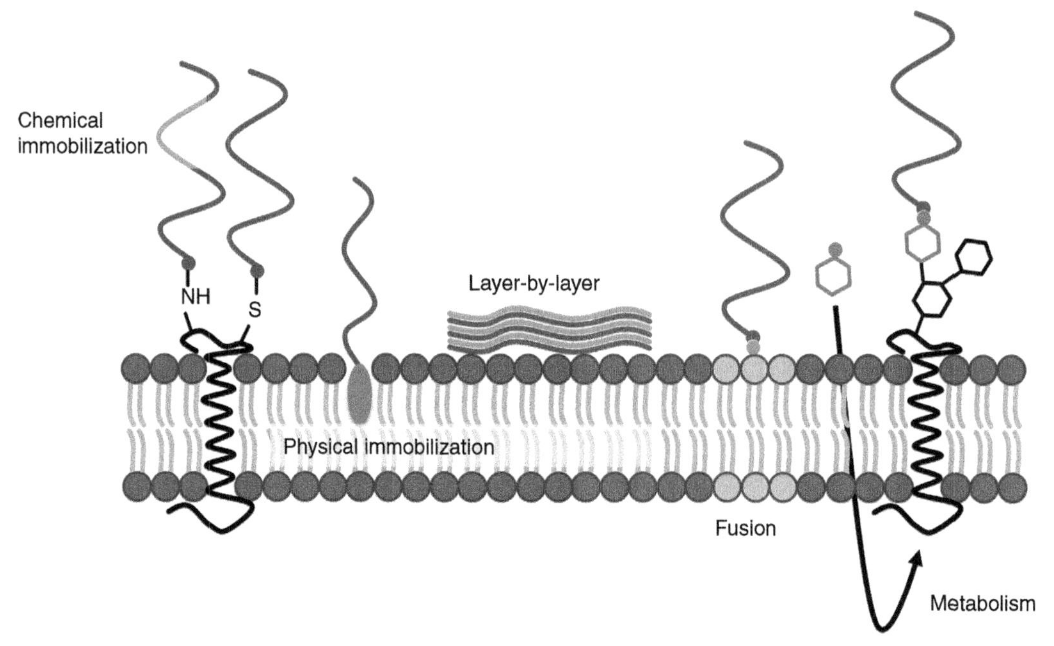

FIGURE 5.3.1 Schematic of processes for cell surface immobilization.

5.3.3 Metabolic Surface Engineering of Living Cells

Metabolic labeling is one of the most robust methods for the surface engineering of living mammalian cells [17–19]. Sialic acid is the terminal residue of the oligosaccharides that cover the mammalian cell surface. The biosynthesis of sialic acid, beginning with uridine diphosphate (UDP)-*N*-acetyl glucosamine (UDP-GlcNAc), occurs via five consecutive reactions [20]. In the first reaction, UDP-GlcNAc 2-epimerase catalyzes the formation of *N*-acetyl mannosamine (ManNAc) from UDP-GlcNAc. Reutter et al. demonstrated the feasibility of metabolic sialic acid engineering with *N*-propanoyl-D-mannosamine (ManNProp), a one-carbon extension to the *N*-acyl position of *N*-acetyl-D-mannosamine (ManNAc) [21,22]. Recently, various types of ManNAc derivatives bearing nonreactive alkyl *N*-acyl groups, fluorinated substituents, and bioorthogonal functional groups have been synthesized and applied to cell surface immobilization and imaging glycosylation [23]. Since the initial demonstration of cell surface engineering with *N*-levulinoylmannosamine (ManLev) [24], this technique has been applied to the development of targeted imaging reagents [25,26] and methods for gene transfer [8]. The tagging technique has led to great progress in cell biology and biomedical science [17,19,27]. It has also been reported that cell surface modification with monosaccharides can be achieved in a living animal [28,29]. The metabolic delivery of nonnatural functional groups into sialic acid was verified by using flow cytometry [24], Western blot analysis [28], and liquid chromatography–mass spectrometry [30].

5.3.4 Metabolic Delivery of Methacryloyl Groups into Carbohydrates

In order to expand metabolic glycoengineering to the biomacromolecular field, *N*-methacryloyl mannosamine (ManM), a mannosamine derivative bearing a methacryloyl group, has been synthesized [31]. The methacryloyl group is one of the most useful groups for polymer synthesis. In addition to undergoing polymerization, the C=C bond of the methacryloyl group can participate in various organic reactions. ManM was synthesized using a process similar to that employed for the synthesis of ManLev [32], but with methacrylic acid rather than levulinic acid. The chemical structure and hydrogen-1 nuclear magnetic resonance spectrum of ManM, which was obtained as a mixture of anomers, are shown in Fig. 5.3.2. Three days of cultivation is typically required to deliver unnatural functional groups into carbohydrates via glycosylation [32]. Thus, the proliferation of human promyelocytic leukemia (HL-60) cells was investigated to determine the cultivation period in the presence and absence of ManM. Figure 5.3.3 shows the proliferation of HL-60 cells cultured in RPMI-1640 medium with 10% fetal bovine serum with and without 5 mM ManM. An increase in the concentration of the HL-60 cells was observed after 48 h of cultivation. It has been reported that the doubling time for HL-60 cells is approximately 30–40 h and varies with passage level [33]. The proliferation behavior of the HL-60 cells cultured in

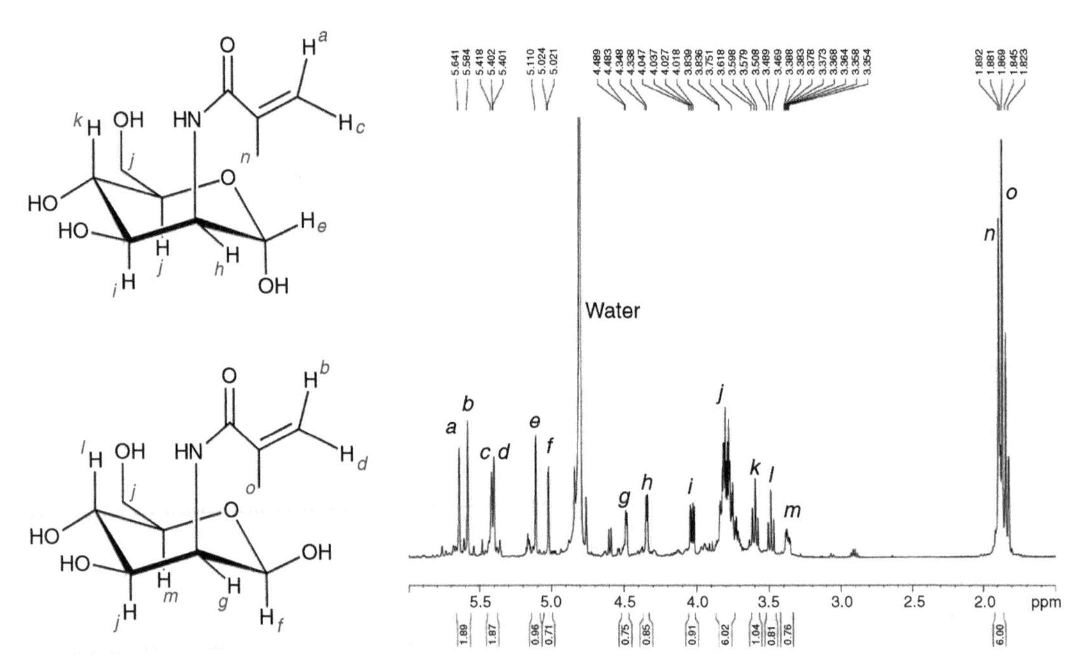

FIGURE 5.3.2 Chemical structure and ¹H-NMR spectrum of ManM.

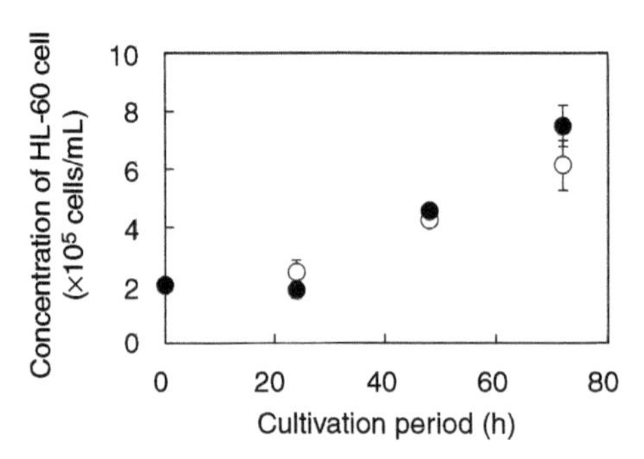

FIGURE 5.3.3 Proliferation of HL-60 cells cultured in RPMI-1640 medium with 10% fetal bovine serum alone (●) and containing 5 mM ManM (○).

RPMI-1640 medium with 10% fetal bovine serum corresponded to that previously reported in the literature. Furthermore, the proliferation of HL-60 cells cultured in the presence of 5 mM ManM was not significantly different from that in RPMI-1640 medium with 10% fetal bovine serum for each cultivation period [34].

Confirmation of delivery of the methacryloyl groups to the cell surface was performed using the thiol-ene reaction. After 3 days of HL-60 cell cultivation in the presence of 5 mM ManM, the cells were rinsed three times with the cell culture medium. RPMI-1640 medium containing 2.5 wt% thiol-terminated 4-arm poly(ethylene glycol) ($PEG_4$10K-SH) and photoinitiator was then added to the cells, and the tissue culture dish was exposed to UV light for 15 min at 37°C. Figure 5.3.4a shows the differential interference contrast (DIC) and laser scanning confocal (LSC) micrographs for ManM-treated and -untreated HL-60 cells after immobilization with $PEG_4$10K-SH. The cells were also treated with Alexa Fluor® 488 C5-maleimide and DRAQ-5TM after PEGylation in order to stain the $PEG_4$10K-SH immobilized on the cell surfaces and nuclei, respectively. It can be seen that the fluorescence micrographs were significantly different for the cells treated with ManM. In addition, the outline of the ManM-treated cells can be clearly seen on the LSC micrograph. Furthermore, each cell in the LSC micrograph matched the corresponding cells in the DIC micrograph. However, when the cells were not treated with ManM, none of the cells were bordered with green fluorescence. These results indicated that the methacryloyl groups were delivered to the surfaces of the HL-60 cells via ManM treatment and the functional groups participated in the thiol-ene reaction. Importantly, no adverse effect of the thiol-ene reaction with $PEG_4$10K-SH was observed. It can also be seen in Fig. 5.3.4b that there was good agreement between the LSC and flow cytometric data.

Next, in order to demonstrate the efficacy of this cell surface engineering approach, cell microarrays were prepared using a micropatterned poly(2-methacryloyloxyethyl phosphorylcholine [MPC]) (PMPC) polymer brush surface as the substrate. PMPC brushes were prepared on a silicon (Si) wafer via surface-initiated atom transfer radical polymerization, as previously described elsewhere [35]. Selective decomposition of the initiators immobilized on the Si wafer using UV light irradiation resulted in micropatterning of the

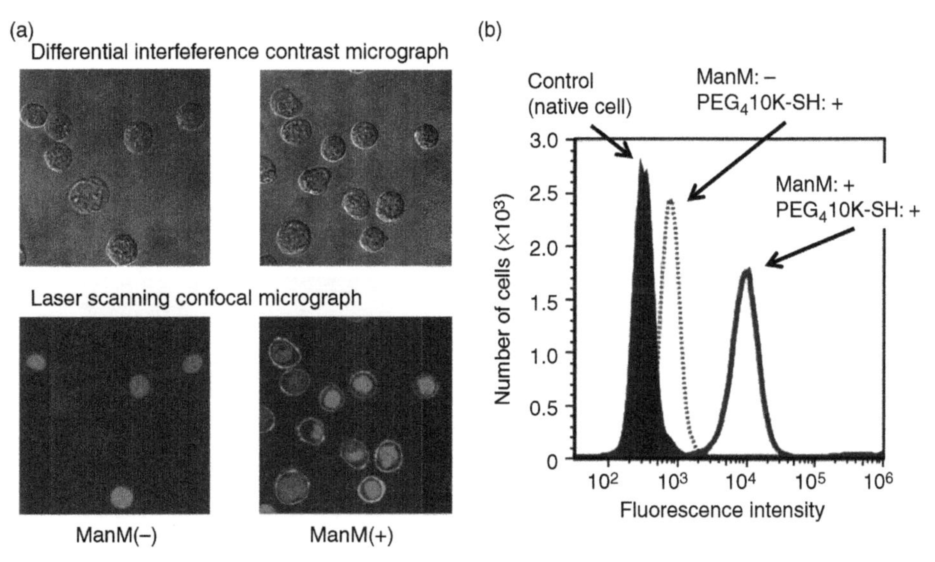

FIGURE 5.3.4 (a) Microscopic images of ManM-treated and -nontreated HL-60 cells after contact with 4-arm $PEG_4$10K-SH and Alexa Fluor 488 C5-maleimide. (b) Flow cytometric data for HL-60 cells after surface immobilization.

wafer surface via the formation of regions of PMPC brushes with different, well-controlled sizes.

To introduce binding sites on the cell surfaces that would bind to avidin adsorbed on the micropatterned substrate, the thiol-ene reaction was performed using $PEG_4$10K-SH and 2-biotinamidoethyl methacrylate, as shown in Fig. 5.3.5a. After the reaction, the suspension of modified cells was placed in contact with the avidin-patterned surface for 30 min at 37°C in RPMI-1640 containing 10% fetal bovine serum. Subsequently, the surface was rinsed with the culture medium and placed in contact with calcein AM. As shown in Fig. 5.3.5b, the surface modified HL-60 cells selectively attached to the region on the Si wafer that was covered with avidin. In addition, the adherent cells were stained with calcein AM, indicating that their viability was preserved, even after the attachment. Furthermore, when HL-60 cells without ManM treatment were placed in contact with the same substrate, the number of adherent cells was significantly reduced. It was also found that the thiol-ene reaction does not occur with ManM-treated cells that have been exposed to 0.1 U/mL sialidase.

This process may be advantageous for the functionalization of cell surfaces because the synthetic polymers are immobilized at the topmost surfaces of the cells. In addition, the methacryloyl group is the most desirable group for polymer synthesis and should be effective for the preparation of cell-based polymer materials.

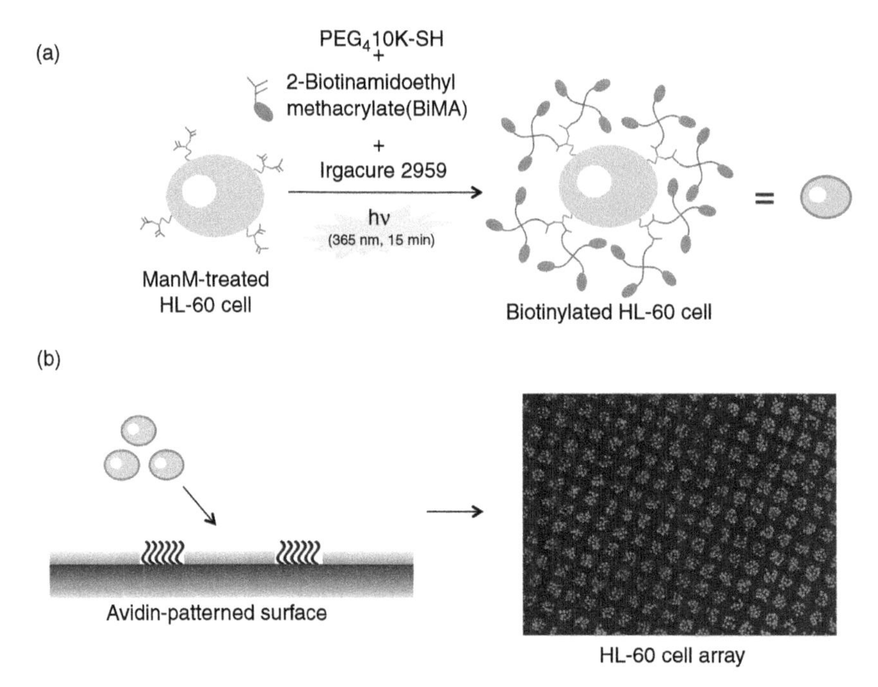

FIGURE 5.3.5 (a) Biotinylation of HL-60 cells and cell microarray preparation. (b) Cell microarray formed on an avidin-patterned surface. The cells were stained with calcein AM. Scale bar represents 100 μm.

5.3.5 Surface Modification of Mammalian Cells With Thermoresponsive Polymers [36]

Although chemical ligations on mammalian cell surfaces have been performed using unnatural functional groups delivered to carbohydrates [37], the number of studies of mammalian cell surface modifications with synthetic polymers remains limited [31]. In order to control biointerfacial aspects with environmental stimuli, thermoresponsive polymers were immobilized on mammalian cell surfaces.

Certain *N*-substituted acrylamide polymers exhibit phase separation characteristics with associated changes in their properties upon heating above a certain lower critical solution temperature (LCST) [38–40]. Polymers based on *N*-isopropyl acrylamide (NIPAM) are the best-known examples. The homopolymer has an LCST of 32°C in aqueous solution [41]. NIPAM can also be polymerized with a wide variety of comonomers, and with the appropriate choice of comonomer, the LCST can be controlled to near physiological temperatures [42,43]. Poly(*N*-isopropylacrylamide) (PNIPAM) polymers have therefore recently been investigated for use in drug delivery [44,45], biomolecule separation [46], and tissue engineering [47] applications.

In order to obtain thiol-terminated PNIPAM (PNIPAM-SH), NIPAM was polymerized via reversible addition-fragmentation chain transfer polymerization followed by treatment with ethanolamine.

Figure 5.3.6a is a schematic representation of the surface modification of HL-60 cells with PNIPAM. HL-60 cells were first exposed to ManM (5 mM) for 3 days in order to deliver methacryloyl groups to the carbohydrates of the cells. RPMI-1640 medium containing 2.5

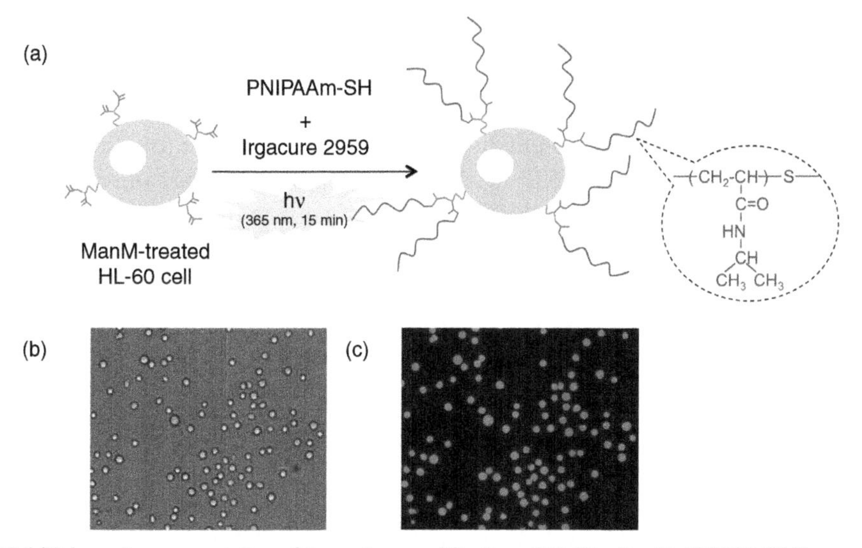

FIGURE 5.3.6 (a) Schematic representation of the surface modification of HL-60 cells with PNIPAM. (b) Phase-contrast and (c) fluorescence micrographs of HL-60 cells immobilized with PNIPAM. For (c), the cells were stained with calcein-AM. The micrographs were taken below the LCST of PNIPAM.

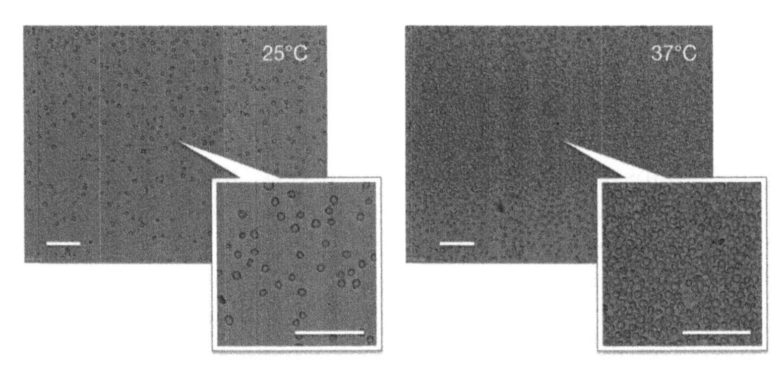

FIGURE 5.3.7 Temperature-assisted aggregation of PNIPAM-immobilized HL-60 cells. Bars represent 100 μm.

wt% thiol-terminated PNIPAM and 0.05 wt% Irgacure 2959 was then added to the cells, and then the tissue culture dish was exposed to UV light (365 nm) for 15 min at 4°C. This protocol was adapted from a previous report that described the surface modification of HL-60 with thiol-terminated 4-arm PEG [34].

The phase-contrast image of the HL-60 cells, as shown in Fig. 5.3.6b, revealed that the round cell shape was preserved after immobilization of PNIPAM. Furthermore, every cell was stained with calcein-AM (Fig. 5.3.6c), indicating that cell viability was preserved, even after the immobilization of the PNIPAM.

The thermoresponsive nature of the PNIPAM-immobilized cells was determined via phase-contrast microscopic observation. Figure 5.3.7 shows phase-contrast micrographs of PNIPAM-immobilized HL-60 cells at 25 and 37°C. At 25°C, the cells were homogeneously scattered, as would be expected for typical nonadhesive HL-60 cells. In contrast, cellular aggregation occurred at 37°C, which is above the LCST of PNIPAM. Okano and coworkers recently reported that the intracellular uptake and cytotoxicity of solubilized PNIPAM-based polymers are extremely low [48,49]. PNIPAM-SH was immobilized at 4°C, at which temperature it was completely soluble in the cell culture media. Notably, under these experimental conditions, PNIPAM-SH cannot spontaneously penetrate inside the cells. Thus, the aggregation of the HL-60 cells at 37°C is due to dehydration of the PNIPAM-immobilized surfaces of the cells. In addition, when native HL-60 cells (without ManM treatment) were also treated with PNIPAM-SH in the presence of a photoinitiator and UV irradiation, they did not aggregate at 37°C. Therefore, the methacryloyl groups delivered to the cell surface functioned as tags for the immobilization of PNIPAM.

5.3.6 Preparation of Glycol Protein-Conjugated Hydrogels [50]

The complex structure of cell membranes can be considered the most sophisticated structure generated in nature. All of the components are dynamically arranged in the plasma membrane and regulate highly specific biointerfacial interactions. Cell surface engineering with synthetic molecules thus provides robust materials with bioactivities governed by cell surface molecules.

To characterize the polymerization ability of methacryloyl-functionalized glycoproteins, redox-initiated free radical polymerization with MPC was performed. MPC is a highly hygroscopic monomer and useful for creating biocompatible materials because the phosphorylcholine unit avoids nonspecific interaction with plasma proteins and cells [51]. The increase in size of the glycoproteins after reaction with MPC was determined by Western blot analysis. ManM-treated and -untreated HL-60 cells were disrupted via ultrasonication, and any insoluble substances were precipitated by centrifugation. The separate precipitates were then dissolved in RIPA lysis buffer, mixed with a given amount of MPC, and subjected to radical polymerization via redox initiation. Figure 5.3.8 shows Western blot analysis data for the P-selectin glycoprotein ligand-1 (PSGL-1) of ManM-treated and -untreated HL-60 cells after polymerization. PSGL-1 is a disulfide-bonded homodimeric mucin-like glycoprotein expressed on leukocytes that interacts with both P- and E-selectin [52]. It consists of two identical 120-kDa glycoprotein chains and has numerous sialylated, fucosylated O-linked oligosaccharide branches, many of which terminate in the sLex determinant [53]. The even number lanes of Fig. 5.3.8 are the blot results for lysates from the native HL-60 cells (without ManM treatment). Bands of monomeric and dimeric PSGL-1 of similar size were observed, regardless of the MPC concentration. In contrast, the increase in size of the PSGL-1 ManM-treated cells due to conjugation was qualitatively recognized after polymerization (odd number lanes). The original bands from the monomeric and dimeric PSGL-1 faded as the concentration of MPC increased, and the electrophoretic mobility of PSGL-1 was completely reduced due to the large hydrodynamic size when the concentration of MPC was greater than 500 mM. In addition

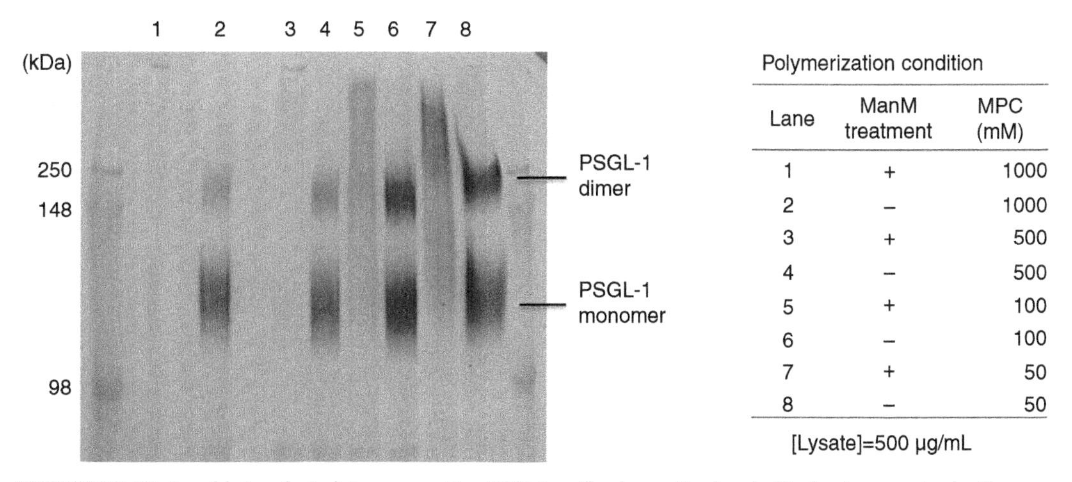

Polymerization condition

Lane	ManM treatment	MPC (mM)
1	+	1000
2	–	1000
3	+	500
4	–	500
5	+	100
6	–	100
7	+	50
8	–	50

[Lysate]=500 μg/mL

FIGURE 5.3.8 Western blot analysis data representing PSGL-1 antibody reactive bands. The lysate was mixed with various concentrations of 2-MPC, and polymerization was performed using a redox initiator. Odd-numbered lanes: ManM-treated HL-60 cells; even-numbered lanes; untreated HL-60 cells. *Reprinted from Ref. [50], with permission from American Chemical Society, Copyright 2013.*

to these results based on MPC polymerization, similar results were observed using the thiol-ene reaction. Conjugation of PSGL-1 to HL-60 cells with thiol-terminated PEG [31] and PNIPAM [36] was also verified by Western blot analysis. Thus, alternative functions, such as selective adhesion and thermoresponsive association, were provided to these HL-60 cells. Both free-radical polymerization and the thiol-ene reaction are therefore robust processes for the preparation of cell-based polymeric materials and the chemical modification of glycoproteins.

Next, the addition of *N,N′*-methylenebisacrylamide to the polymerization solution resulted in the formation of hydrogels containing the glycoproteins. In the preparation of the hydrogels, the final MPC and protein concentrations were adjusted to 2.5 M and 1000 μg/mL, respectively. The concentration of MPC was optimized by referring to the literature [54]. Figure 5.3.9a and b present photographs of MPC hydrogels after staining with Coomassie Brilliant Blue (CBB) and periodic acid–Schiff (PAS) reagents, respectively. The CBB and PAS staining methods are commonly used to stain proteins and carbohydrates, respectively. Before staining, the hydrogels were rinsed with RIPA lysis buffer and phosphate buffered saline in order to remove any unbound glycoproteins. The hydrogels prepared without cell lysate (Fig. 5.3.9a and d) and with untreated HL-60 cell lysate (Fig. 5.3.9b and e) were not stained with either CBB or PAS. In contrast, the dyes remained in the hydrogels prepared using the ManM-treated HL-60 cell lysate (Fig. 5.3.9c and f). These results indicated that the glycoproteins were covalently immobilized in the hydrogels prepared with the lysate from the ManM-treated HL-60 cells. Furthermore, no aggregation or precipitation of the glycoproteins was observed in the hydrogels, possibly due to their covalent conjugation to very hydrophilic polymer chains.

Finally, IL-1α stimulated and nonstimulated human umbilical vein endothelial cells (HUVECs) were placed in contact with the hydrogels to investigate selectin-mediated cell

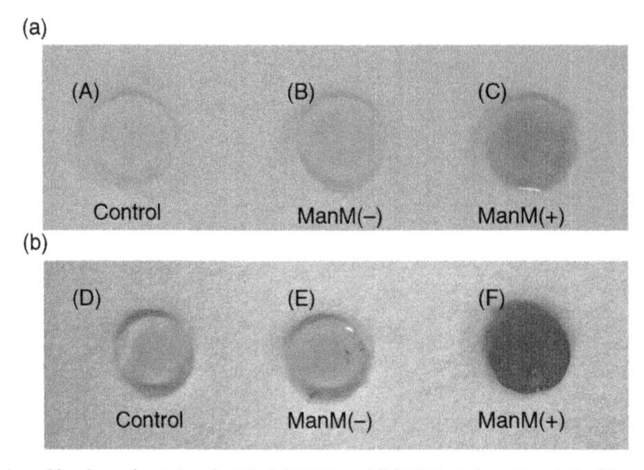

FIGURE 5.3.9 Photographs of hydrogels stained with (a) CBB and (b) PAS stains. *Reprinted from Ref. [50], with permission . Copyright 2013 American Chemical Society.*

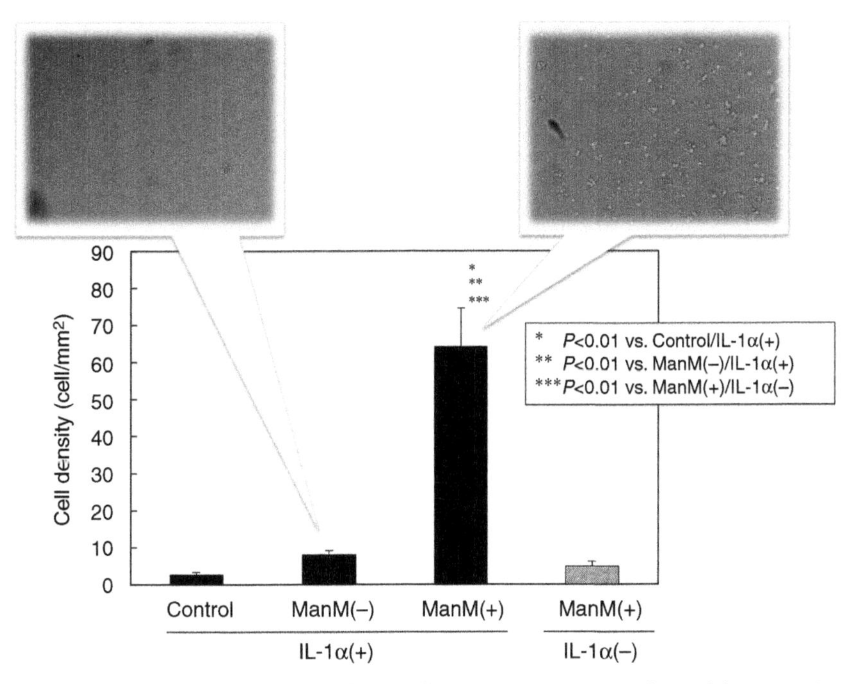

FIGURE 5.3.10 Density of adherent HUVEC cells on hydrogels. $^{*}P < 0.01$ versus control/IL-1α (+); $^{**}P < 0.01$ versus ManM(–)/IL-1α(+); $^{***}P < 0.01$ versus ManM(+)/IL-1α(–). *Reprinted from Ref. [50], with permission from Copyright 2013 American Chemical Society.*

adhesion. The density of the adherent cells on the hydrogels is summarized in Fig. 5.3.10. On the MPC hydrogels (no lysate) and hydrogels prepared with the lysate from the untreated HL-60 cells (without ManM treatment), very few IL-1α stimulated HUVECs were observed. In contrast, a large number of IL-1α-stimulated HUVECs adhered to the hydrogels prepared with the lysate from the ManM-treated HL-60 cells. In addition, the nonstimulated HUVECs did not adhere to the hydrogels prepared with the lysate from the ManM-treated HL-60 cells. The results of this cell adhesion study confirmed that glycoproteins of mammalian cells were transferred to synthetic hydrogels with preservation of their ability to bind to the selectin expressed on the surfaces of the HUVECs.

Preparation of hydrogel-bearing natural glycoproteins from leukemia cells was also successful, and the selectin-mediated adhesion of cytokine-stimulated endothelial cells on the hydrogel was observed [50]. In living systems, selectin-mediated cell adhesion is considered an essential step leading to inflammation, reperfusion injury, rheumatoid arthritis, metastasis, infection, and so forth [55,56]. Novel synthetic materials that regulate these bioresponses can be obtained through cell surface modification as described here. Metabolic oligosaccharide engineering with ManM is a robust process for the creation of biointeractive synthetic materials because conventional radical polymerization is the most practical polymerization method for the polymerization of glycoprotein monomers. Moreover, metabolic oligosaccharide engineering can be applied to a wide variety of cells, which is important because the relative dimensions, concentrations, and chemistries of all membrane components can vary depending on cell type and disease [57]. Polymeric materials obtained via metabolic oligosaccharide engineering can, in fact, be designed to uniquely interact with specific substrates.

5.3.7 Conclusions and Future Perspectives

In this chapter, the delivery of methacryloyl groups to carbohydrates on living mammalian cell surfaces was described. Because the delivery of methacryloyl groups into the carbohydrates of cell surfaces is tolerated in various types of cells, a great variety of biological applications for this technology are possible, such as the control of cell surface characteristics and cell-mediated drug delivery. There have been many ManNAc analogs used for the installation of nonnatural functional groups into cell surface glycans, but ManM may have a higher impact due to its utility for the synthesis of new polymeric materials bearing components generated from cell membranes. They will be useful in molecular separation, biosensors, and the development of biomedical materials

References

[1] M.T. Stephan, D.J. Irvine, Nano Today 6 (2011) 309.

[2] Y. Su, Z. Xie, G.B. Kim, C. Dong, J. Yang, ACS Biomater. Sci. Eng. 1 (2015) 201.

[3] S.J. Singer, G.L. Nicolson, Science 175 (1972) 723.

[4] J.A. Virtanen, K.H. Cheng, P. Somerharju, Proc. Natl. Acad. Sci. USA 95 (1998) 4964.

[5] R.A. Dwek, Chem. Rev. 96 (1996) 683.

[6] S. Boonyarattanakalin, S.E. Martin, Q. Sun, B.R. Peterson, J. Am. Chem. Soc. 128 (2006) 11463.

[7] I. Chen, M. Howarth, W. Lin, A.Y. Ting, Nat. Methods 2 (2005) 99.

[8] J.H. Lee, T.J. Baker, L.K. Mahal, J. Zabner, C.R. Bertozzi, D.F. Wiemer, M.J. Welsh, J. Biol. Chem. 274 (1999) 21878.

[9] K. Kato, K. Umezawa, D.P. Funeriu, M. Miyake, J. Miyake, T. Nagamune, Biotechniques 35 (2003) 1014.

[10] D. Rabuka, M.B. Forstner, J.T. Groves, C.R. Bertozzi, J. Am. Chem. Soc. 130 (2008) 5947.

[11] Y. Teramura, Y. Kaneda, H. Iwata, Biomaterials 28 (2007) 4818.

[12] C.L. Stabler, X.L. Sun, W. Cui, J.T. Wilson, C.A. Haller, E.L. Chaikof, Bioconjug. Chem. 18 (2007) 1713.

[13] J.K. Armstrong, H.J. Meiselman, T.C. Fisher, Am. J. Hematol. 56 (1997) 26.

[14] J.L. Panza, W.R. Wagner, H.L. Rilo, R.H. Rao, E.J. Beckman, A.J. Russell, Biomaterials 21 (2000) 1155.

[15] D. Dutta, A. Pulsipher, W. Luo, H. Mak, M.N. Yousaf, Bioconjug. Chem. 22 (2011) 2423.

[16] W. Luo, A. Pulsipher, D. Dutta, B.M. Lamb, M.N. Yousaf, Sci. Rep. 4 (2014) 6313.

[17] O.T. Keppler, R. Horstkorte, M. Pawlita, C. Schmidt, W. Reutter, Glycobiology 11 (2001) 11R.

[18] J.A. Prescher, C.R. Bertozzi, Cell 126 (2006) 851.

[19] J. Du, K.J. Yarema, Adv. Drug. Deliv. Rev. 62 (2010) 671.

[20] S. Hinderlich, R. Stäsche, R. Zeitler, W. Reutter, J. Biol. Chem. 272 (1997) 24313.

[21] H.J. Grünholz, E. Harms, M. Opetz, W. Reutter, M. Cerný, Carbohydr. Res. 96 (1981) 259.

[22] H. Kayser, R. Zeitler, C. Kannicht, D. Grunow, R. Nuck, W. Reutter, J. Biol. Chem. 267 (1992) 16934.

[23] J. Du, M.A. Meledeo, Z. Wang, H.S. Khanna, V.D. Paruchuri, K.J. Yarema, Glycobiology 19 (2009) 1382.

[24] L.K. Mahal, K.J. Yarema, C.R. Bertozzi, Science 276 (1997) 1125.

[25] G.A. Lemieux, K.J. Yarema, C.L. Jacobs, C.R. Bertozzi, J. Am. Chem. Soc. 121 (1999) 4278.

[26] Y. Iwasaki, H. Maie, K. Akiyoshi, Biomacromolecules 8 (2007) 3162.

[27] J.E. Hudak, C.R. Bertozzi, Chem. Biol. 21 (2014) 16.

[28] J.A. Prescher, D.H. Dube, C.R. Bertozzi, Nature 430 (2004) 873.

[29] D. Soriano Del Amo, W. Wang, H. Jiang, C. Besanceney, A.C. Yan, M. Levy, Y. Liu, F.L. Marlow, P. Wu, J. Am. Chem. Soc. 132 (2010) 16893.

[30] S.J. Luchansky, S. Argade, B.K. Hayes, C.R. Bertozzi, Biochemistry 43 (2004) 12358.

[31] Y. Iwasaki, H. Matsuno, Macromol. Biosci. 11 (2011) 1478.

[32] K.J. Yarema, L.K. Mahal, R.E. Bruehl, E.C. Rodriguez, C.R. Bertozzi, J. Biol. Chem. 273 (1998) 31168.

[33] R. Gallagher, S. Collins, J. Trujillo, K. McCredie, M. Ahearn, S. Tsai, R. Metzgar, G. Aulakh, R. Ting, F. Ruscetti, R. Gallo, Blood 54 (1979) 713.

[34] Y. Iwasaki, T. Ota, Chem. Commun. 47 (2011) 10329.

[35] R. Iwata, P. Suk-In, V.P. Hoven, A. Takahara, K. Akiyoshi, Y. Iwasaki, Biomacromolecules 5 (2004) 2308.

[36] Y. Iwasaki, M. Sakiyama, S. Fujii, S. Yusa, Chem. Commun. 49 (2013) 7824.

[37] J.A. Prescher, C.R. Bertozzi, Nat. Chem. Biol. 1 (2005) 13.

[38] N. Monji, C.A. Cole, A.S. Hoffman, J. Biomater. Sci. Polym. Ed. 5 (1994) 407.

[39] A. Yamazaki, F.M. Winnik, R.M. Cornelius, J.L. Brash, Biochim. Biophys. Acta 1421 (1999) 103.

[40] I. Idziak, D. Avoce, D. Lessard, D. Gravel, X.X. Zhu, Macromolecules 32 (1999) 1260.

[41] M. Heskins, J.E. Guillent, J. Macromol. Sci. Chem. A2 (1968) 1441.

[42] Y.G. Takei, T. Aoki, K. Sanui, N. Ogata, T. Okano, Y. Sakurai, Bioconjug. Chem. 4 (1993) 341.

[43] H. Feil, Y.H. Bae, J. Feijen, S.W. Kim, Macromolecules 26 (1993) 2496.

[44] A. Kikuchi, T. Okano, Adv. Drug. Deliv. Rev. 54 (2002) 53.

[45] P. Techawanitchai, M. Ebara, N. Idota, T. Aoyagi, Colloids Surf. B 99 (2012) 53.

[46] J. Kobayashi, A. Kikuchi, K. Sakai, T. Okano, Anal. Chem. 75 (2003) 3244.

[47] A. Kikuchi, T. Okano, J. Control. Release 101 (2005) 69.

[48] E. Ayano, M. Karaki, T. Ishihara, H. Kanazawa, T. Okano, Colloids Surf. B 99 (2012) 67.

[49] J. Akimoto, M. Nakayama, K. Sakai, T. Okano, Biomacromolecules 10 (2009) 1331.

[50] Y. Iwasaki, A. Matsunaga, S. Fujii, Bioconjug. Chem. 25 (2014) 1626.

[51] Y. Iwasaki, K. Ishihara, Sci. Technol. Adv. Mater. 13 (2012) 064101.

[52] P.A. Aeed, J.-G. Geng, D. Asa, L. Raycroft, L. Ma, Å.P. Elhammer, Glycoconjug. J. 15 (1998) 973.

[53] K.R. Snapp, H. Ding, K. Atkins, R. Warnke, F.W. Luscinskas, G.S. Kansas, Blood 91 (1998) 154.

[54] Y. Kiritoshi, K. Ishihara, J. Biomater. Sci. Polym. Ed. 13 (2002) 213.

[55] E.E. Simanek, G.J. McGarvey, J.A. Jablonowski, C.-H. Wong, Chem. Rev. 98 (1998) 833.

[56] S.R. Barthel, J.D. Gavino, L. Descheny, C.J. Dimitroff, Expert Opin. Ther. Targets 11 (2007) 1473.

[57] M.D. Mager, V. LaPointe, M.M. Stevens, Nat. Chem. 3 (2011) 582.

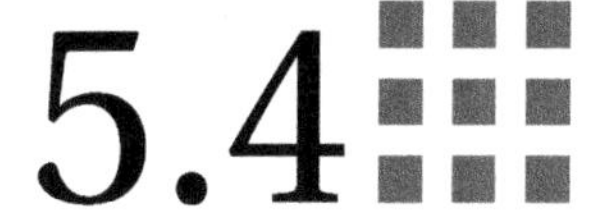

Fibrous Materials

Rio Kurimoto, Eri Niiyama, Mitsuhiro Ebara

INTERNATIONAL CENTER FOR MATERIALS NANOARCHITECTONICS (MANA), NATIONAL INSTITUTE FOR MATERIALS SCIENCE (NIMS), TSUKUBA, JAPAN

CHAPTER OUTLINE

5.4.1 Introduction

Almost all of the tissues and organs in the human body, such as the bone, skin, tendon, and cartilage, are synthesized and hierarchically organized into fibrous structures with nano-/microsized fibers [1]. Therefore, fibrous materials have a major role to play in the rapidly expanding fields of biomedicine including biomaterials, tissue engineering, and regenerative medicine. In particular, a well-defined nanofibrous structure is very similar to the extracellular matrix (ECM) [2]. Polymeric fibers have been investigated extensively over the last decade and have a high potential for commercialization. A large number of various polymeric materials were used to create nanofibrous sheets in various forms such as textiles, nonwovens, and composite materials. Nanofibers exhibit special properties mainly due to their extremely high surface-to-weight ratio compared to conventional nonwovens. Low-density, large surface area to mass, high pore volume, and tight pore size make the nanofiber nonwoven appropriate for a wide range of filtration applications.

Polymeric nanofibers can be processed by a number of techniques such as self-assembly, drawing, template synthesis, phase separation, and electrospinning (Fig. 5.4.1). Self-assembly by a bottom-up method for the preparation of nanofibers from polymers, peptides, and macromolecules is a versatile and powerful technique to construct well-defined nanostructures. This is accomplished by spontaneous and automatic organization of molecules into desired structures through various types of intermolecular interaction [3]. Drawing, a direct writing technique, is an optimized method for the fabrication of single fibers using a viscous polymer solution with volatile organic solvents. A continuous long linear fiber can be obtained by the drawing method, and the fiber diameter relies

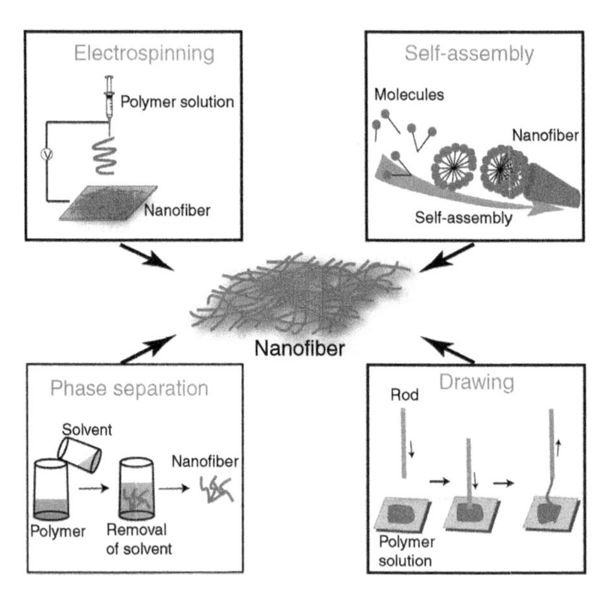

FIGURE 5.4.1 Fabrication method of nanofibers, electrospinning, self-assembly, phase separation, and drawing.

on the size of the needle (micropipette), polymer solution flow rate, and temperature, which affect the viscosity of the polymer and the evaporation rate of the solvent. Phase separation is a method that has long been used to fabricate porous polymer fibrous membranes or sponges by inducing the separation of a polymer solution into two different phases, namely, the polymer-poor phase (low polymer concentration) and polymer-rich phase (high polymer concentration). This enables the preparation of a three-dimensional nanofibrous structure with interconnected pores. On the other hand, electrospinning has gained popularity over the last decade, and an electrical force is used to induce the formation of nonwoven polymer fibers from a polymer solution with the fiber diameters on the nanometer to micrometer scale or greater [4,5]. In electrospinning, the "Taylor cone" of a polymer solution droplet forms at the end of a capillary tip when electrical forces are applied [5]. When the electric field reaches a critical level at which the repulsive electric force overcomes the surface tension force, a charged jet of the solution is ejected from the tip of the "Taylor cone." As the jet diameter decreases when the jet flies to the collector, the radial forces from charged ions exceed the cohesive forces of the jet solution, causing it to split into many fibers. Furthermore, these divided fibers repel each other, leading to chaotic trajectories and bending instability. At the same time, the solvent evaporates and the polymer solidifies on the collector. Thus, continuous fibers are laid to form a nonwoven sheet.

Generally, one of the most important characteristics of fibers is morphology. The morphologies of fibers or nanofibers are easily observed using operating microscope, a fluorescence microscope, scanning electron microscope (SEM), transmission electron microscope (TEM), and atomic force microscope (AFM) (Fig. 5.4.2). Among them, SEM is most commonly used to confirm the morphologies or observe fracture surfaces

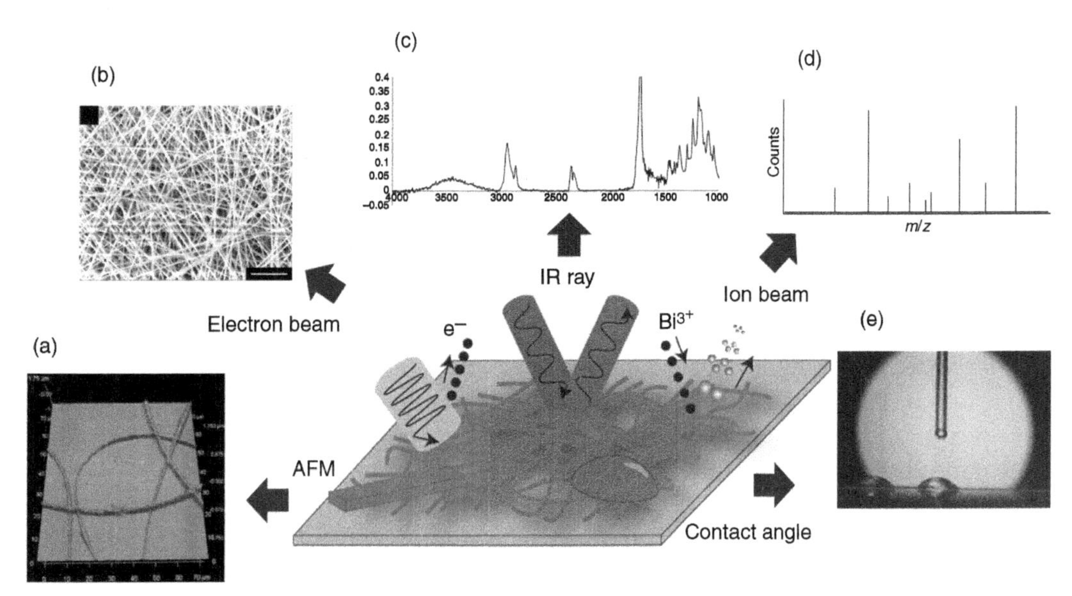

FIGURE 5.4.2 Characterization methods of polymeric fibrous materials. (a) AFM, (b) SEM, (c) IR, (d) TOF-SIMS, and (e) contact angle measurement.

(cross-section). There are two observation modes, namely, the secondary electron (SE) image mode and backscattered electron (BSE) mode [6]. Usually, the SE image mode offers the highest resolution and the most convenient operation procedures. From SE images of fibers, their diameter, diameter distribution, and pore size can be calculated. The BSE mode enables the observation of additives in the fibers even when they are completely embedded in the fibers because electrons reflected from the sample by elastic scattering are more easily detected in the BSE mode than electrons emitted from deeper regions of the sample in the SE mode [7]. Likewise, TEM is very useful and commonly used for the confirmation of embedded additives at a very high magnification compared with SEM in the BSE mode. Wang et al. observed fibers and magnetic field-responsive fibers using SEM (SE and BSE modes), a fluorescence microscope, and TEM [7]. Another interesting characteristic of nanofibers is their many pores of subnanometer to micrometer sizes or their high porosity. Although SEM and TEM are useful for the investigation of pores and their size, we were able to obtain only surface values. The typical methods for evaluation of the size, density, and distribution of whole pores are mercury intrusion porosimetry, liquid extrusion porosimetry, and capillary flow porosimetry.

5.4.2 Physical Signal-Responsive Fibers

In this section, physical stimuli-responsive fibers will be introduced, which are composed of polymers responsive to temperature, light/UV, or electric/magnetic field, which enable "on/off" switching and reversible property changes of nanofibers.

5.4.2.1 Temperature-Responsive Fibers

The most widely used temperature-responsive polymers are poly(*N*-isopropylacrylamide) (PNIPAAm) and its derivations. A PNIPAAm solution, which undergoes a sharp and reversible phase transition from monophasic below a specific temperature to biphasic above it, generally exhibits the so-called lower critical solution temperature (LCST). The PNIPAAm has an LCST of 32°C in aqueous solution. Rockwood et al. and Okuzaki et al. reported the preparation of PNIPAAm nanofibers by electrospinning under optimized conditions using different solvents [8,9]. However, because of the solubility of the NIPAAm homopolymer in an aqueous solution prepared below the LCST, the resulting nanofibers rapidly dissolve in water, whereas the nanofibers prepared above the LCST disperse and aggregate in water because of the lack of interpolymer and interfiber cross-links that keep the nanofibers in the swollen state. From this regard, temperature-responsive polymer-grafted chitosan (CTS) nanofibers were reported [10]. First, a CTS-graft-PNIPAAm copolymer was also synthesized by using 1-ethyl-3-(3-dimethylaminopropyl)carbodiimide and *N*-hydroxy succinimide as grafting agents to graft carboxyl-terminated PNIPAAm chains onto the CTS biomacromolecules. And then, CTS-*g*-PNIPAAm with or without bovine serum albumin was fabricated into nanofibers through electrospinning using poly(ethylene oxide) (PEO) as a fiber-forming facilitating additive. The CTS-*g*-PNIPAAm/PEO nanofibers showed a pH- and temperature-dependent swelling behavior. The drug release study showed that the nanofibers provided controlled release of the entrapped protein.

The authors successfully prepared chemically cross-linked temperature-responsive electrospun nanofibers by thermal curing [11]. As a member of the NIPAAm family, *N*-hydroxymethylacrylamide (HMAAm) was copolymerized with NIPAAm by free-radical copolymerization because temperature-responsive HMAAm can be cross-linked by self-condensation at high temperatures (above 110°C). As a result of cross-linking, very stable nanofibers in aqueous solution were obtained and manipulated as a bulk material. By extension of the above-mentioned examples, the authors successfully prepared temperature-responsive electrospun nanofibers by photocuring [12]. The temperature-responsive nanofiber mats were prepared using the copolymers NIPAAm and 2-carboxyisopropylacrylamide conjugated to 4-aminobenzophenone, a photoinitiator. The crosslinked temperature-responsive nanofibers were obtained by UV irradiation for 30 min (Fig. 5.4.3). Chemically cross-linked nanofibers were also reported by

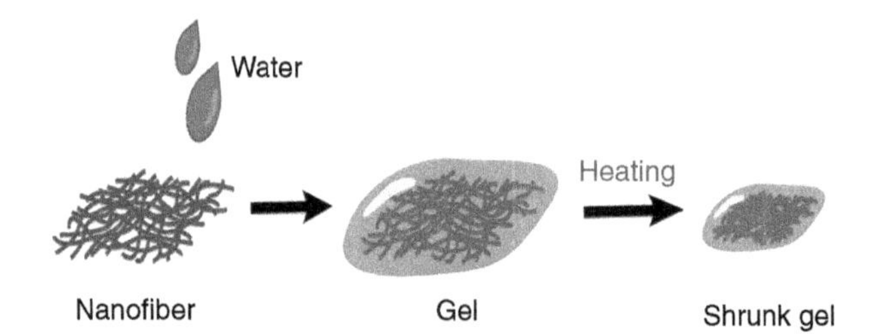

FIGURE 5.4.3 Schematic illustration of nanofibers that can change their phase by each environment.

Maeda et al. [13]. First, poly(NIPAAm-*co*-AAc) was synthesized. The obtained polymer was mixed with β-cyclodextrin. This polymer solution was electrospun into nanofibers and dried at 140°C for 24 h for thermal curing. This fiber mat rapidly shrinks in response to temperature changes over the LCST. The response of this mat is over 100 times faster than that of the typical PNIPAAm hydrogels.

5.4.2.2 Photoresponsive Fibers

Since the light stimulus can be imposed instantly and delivered in specific amounts with high accuracy, light-sensitive fibers may possess special advantages over others. The representative photoresponsive phenomenon is photochromism, which is the reversible transformation of a chemical species between two isomeric forms by absorption of visible light or UV light. In addition to color changes, these transformations are accompanied by changes in the physical and chemical properties of the species involved, such as alterations in the dipole moment, refractive index, and geometrical structure. Importantly, these dynamic transformations can generate coincident changes in the optical, chemical, electrical, and bulk properties of systems that incorporate them. Photochromic molecules, therefore, play a pivotal role in photoresponsive systems, which are capable of capturing optical signals and then converting them, through their isomerization, to useful properties. Benedetto et al. studied photochromism using spiropyran (SP)-embedded electrospun nanofibers [14]. The photochromism reaction of SP proceeds with electrocyclic ring opening followed by a molecular rotation; consequently, SP (off-state) changes to its open form, merocyanine (on-state). Sur et al., on the other hand, prepared peptide amphiphile nanofiber matrices by incorporation of a photolabile artificial amino acid to control bioactivity (Fig. 5.4.4) [15]. The peptide amphiphiles self-assembled into cylindrical nanofibers. Cell adhesion is dynamically controlled by rapid photolytic removal of the RGDS peptide from the nanofiber. This dynamic temporal control of cell–material interactions can become an important component in the design of new artificial matrices based on nanostructures for regenerative medicine research. Lim et al. reported on the light-responsive microfibers containing photothermal magnetite nanoparticles prepared using microcapillary devices [16]. Since the magnetite nanoparticles incorporated into temperature-responsive microfibers generated heat upon the absorption of visible light, volume changes in the microfibers triggered by both visible light irradiation and temperature were demonstrated.

5.4.2.3 Electric Field-Responsive Fibers

An electrical field in the form of an external stimulus offers numerous advantages (e.g., availability of equipment). This form of an external stimulus also allows for precise control over the magnitude of the current, the duration of electrical pulses, and the interval between pulses. Poly(vinyl alcohol) (PVA) is one of the well-known electroactive polymers with good thermal stability, chemical resistance, water permeability, and biocompatibility. Xia et al. demonstrated electric-field induced actuation of PVA microfibers (Fig. 5.4.5) [17].

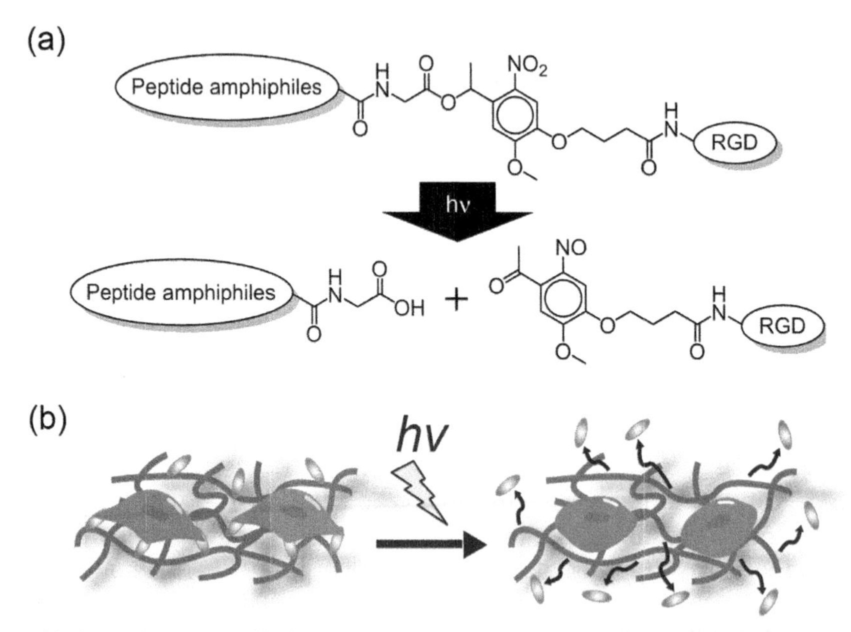

FIGURE 5.4.4 (a) Chemical structures of a photo-cleavable linker. (b) Schematic diagram of the photodynamic control of bioactivity for investigating the dynamic nature of native ECM as scaffolds.

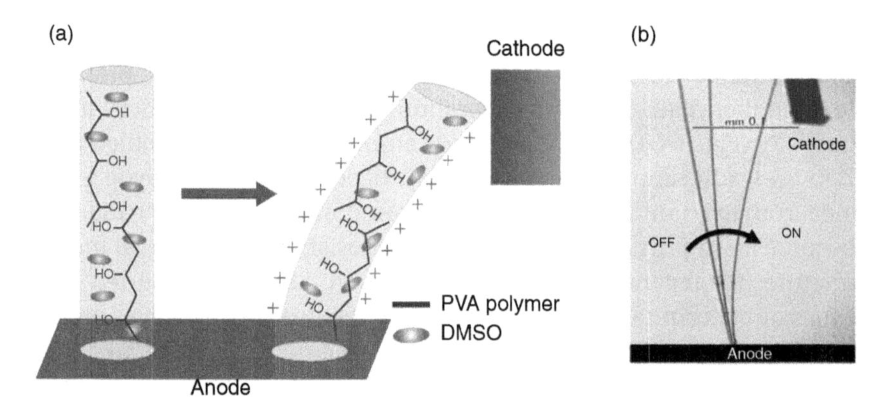

FIGURE 5.4.5 (a) Schematic representation of electric field-responsive movement of PVA fiber swollen with DMSO. (b) Actuations of PVA fibers induced by applying a 1-kV dc electric field. Bending process for a single fiber clamped at the anode.

During spinning of the fibers, dimethyl sulfoxide (DMSO) was used as the solvent, and this greatly influenced the fiber properties because the remaining DMSO made it easier for the PVA fibers to become positively charged and then bend toward the cathode. The actuation behavior depended mainly on the mechanical and dielectric properties, which are related to the chemical structures of the fibers. It is clear that hydroxyl and carbon–oxygen double bonds are important factors influencing the electroactive characteristics of PVA fibers. Shi et al. prepared hybrid hydrogels composed of bacterial cellulose nanofibers and sodium alginate as a dual stimuli-responsive release system [17]. The pH and electric field stimuli-responsive swelling properties and drug release behaviors of the hybrid hydrogels were investigated. When electric field charged from 0 V to 0.5 V, the hydrogels showed an increasing swelling ratio from 8 times to 14 times their dry weight. In addition, the drug release from the hydrogels could be enhanced with an applied electric stimulus. Zhou et al. demonstrated directional electromechanical properties of poly(3,4-ethylenedioxythiophene)/poly(4-styrene sulfonate) composite films containing aligned poly(vinyl pyrrolidone)/poly(methyl methacrylate) nanofiber assemblies [18]. The composite film incorporating the aligned nanofiber assemblies exhibited anisotropic electromechanical properties due to the anisotropic electromechanical properties within the composite film.

5.4.2.4 Magnetic Field-Responsive Fibers

When designing a magnetic-responsive fiber, several factors need to be considered, including the magnetic properties, field strength, or field geometry. Gao et al. demonstrated the decoration of magnetite nanoparticles onto the surface of the cross-linked nanofibers. The nanofibers with magnetite showed a magnetic responsiveness to the applied magnet [19]. Wu et al. developed magnetite–carbon nanofiber hybrids in order to align carbon nanofibers in epoxy using a relatively weak magnetic field [20]. A weak magnetic field ($\sim$50 mT) can align these nanofiber hybrids to form a chain-like structure in epoxy resin. Upon curing, the epoxy nanocomposites showed greatly improved electrical conductivity in the alignment direction and significantly higher fracture toughness when the composites are aligned normal to the crack surface, compared to those containing randomly oriented ones. The authors, on the other hand, reported on alternating magnetic field (AMF)-responsive nanofibers. The nanofibers are composed of a chemically cross-linkable temperature-responsive polymer with an anticancer drug and magnetic nanoparticles, which serve as a trigger of drug release and a source of heat, respectively (Fig. 5.4.6) [21]. By chemical cross-linking, the nanofiber mesh shows switchable changes in the swelling ratio in response to alternating "on/off" switches of AMF because the self-generated heat from the incorporated magnetic nanoparticles induces the deswelling of polymer networks in the nanofibers. Correspondingly, the "on/off" release of drug from the nanofibers is observed in response to AMF. The nanofiber mesh induced the apoptosis of cancer cells due to a synergistic effect of chemotherapy and hyperthermia.

5.4.3 Chemical Signal-Responsive Fibers

5.4.3.1 pH-Responsive Fibers

While physical stimuli are advantageous because they allow local and remote control, they result in a discontinuous response when the stimulus is turned "off." In other words, only the illuminated region is active, and continuous illumination is necessary. In the human body, however, the appearance of numerous bioactive molecules is tightly controlled to maintain a normal metabolic balance via the feedback system called homeostasis.

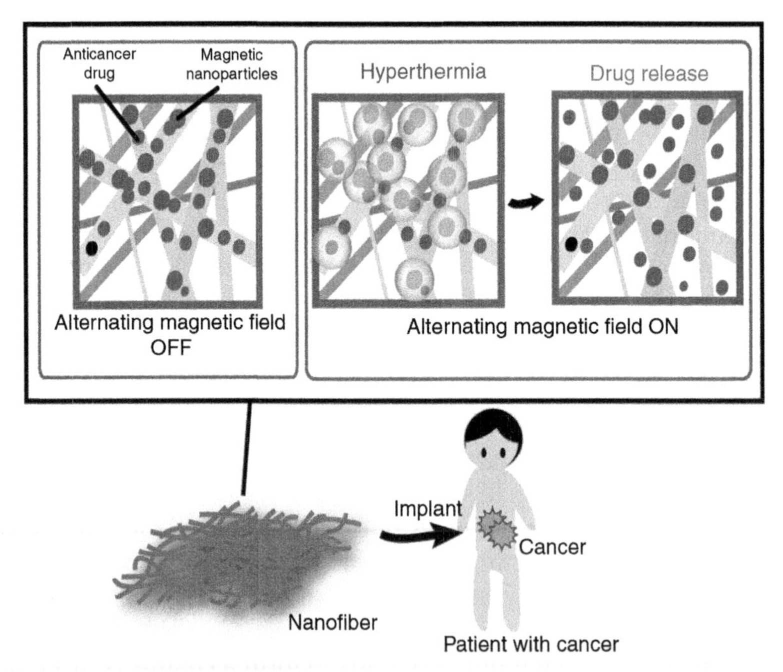

FIGURE 5.4.6 Schematic illustration of nanofibers that can apply chemotherapy and hyperthermia by the heating of incorporating magnetic nanoparticles and releasing of drug.

For example, the human body exhibits variations in pH along the gastrointestinal tract, tumoral areas, inflamed or infected tissues, and the endosomal lumen. Therefore, pH-responsive polymers that show dynamic responses to environmental pH have attracted much attention. The pH-responsive polymers are polyelectrolytes that bear in their structure weak acidic or basic groups that either accept or release protons in response to changes in environmental pH. The pH-responsive polymers can be generated by conjugation of acidic or basic groups to the polymer backbone of polyelectrolytes that undergo ionization similarly to acidic or basic groups of monoacids or monobases.

Gestos et al. prepared pH-responsive electrospun nanofibers using poly(acrylic acid) (PAA), which has the merits of biocompatibility and cross-linkability without the need for additional cross-linkers [22]. The carboxylic groups not only play a role in pH responsiveness but also function as cross-linkers under UV irradiation. Therefore, the UV treatment time strongly affects the extent of swelling induced by pH switching. The 5-min UV-treated PAA nanofibers swelled at both pH 3 and pH 8, and their swelling ratios decreased with increasing UV treatment time to 25 min. The 25-min UV-treated fiber attained swelling ratios of 0.91 at pH 3 and 2.0 at pH 8. Wang et al. prepared pH-responsive fibers using a polybase material: a monodisperse triblock copolymer consisting of poly(methyl methacrylate)-block-poly(2-(diethylamino)ethyl methacrylate)-block-poly(methyl methacrylate) (PMMA-*b*-PDEA-*b*-PMMA) [23]. The fibers expanded at pH 7.3 and contracted at pH 3.5 because the triblock copolymer exhibited contrasting pH-responsive behaviors:

the polybase charge is neutral above pH 5 (collapsed) and positive below pH 5 (expanded). The fibers showed greater responsiveness than the control film because the surface area of the fibers significantly increased. This increased the rate of diffusion of the solvated hydrogen ions throughout the polymer matrix; thus, the responsiveness consequently increased. Jin and Hsieh carried out a similar study of electrospun nanofibers prepared from PAA and PVA mixture solution [24]. According to cross-link temperature and pH, the equilibrium swelling in planar dimensions, that is, thickness and mass, was clearly demonstrated. With increasing cross-linking network density, the equilibrium swelling in planar dimensions, that is, thickness and mass, decreased at the same pH. Furthermore, the equilibrium swelling of nanofibers increased with increasing pH.

5.4.3.2 Biomolecules-Responsive Fibers

Since the stimulus-responsive fibers are becoming increasingly important in biomedical and biomaterial applications, recently, there has been increasing interest in fibers with functionality that induces responses upon exposure to biological small molecules or biomacromolecules. In particular, polymers that respond to glucose have received considerable attention because of their potential application in sensing proteins. Heo et al. successfully evaluated *in vivo* glucose-sensitive fibers (Fig. 5.4.7) [25,26]. They designed and synthesized a unique fluorescent monomer based on diboronic acid that enables reversible responsiveness to glucose without any reagents or enzymes. This glucose-responsive

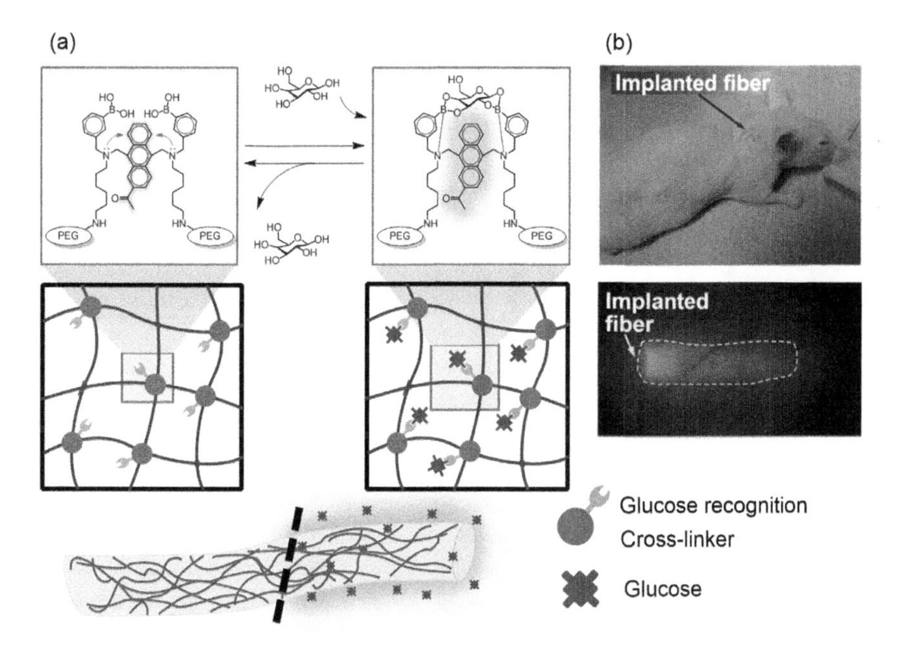

FIGURE 5.4.7 (a) Fluorescence intensity changes depending on the abundance of glucose. (b, c) Schematic diagram of glucose responsibility in hydrogel fibers. (d) The fluorescence of a fiber-shaped sensor implanted under the skin can be detected through the skin.

fluorescent monomer (GF monomer) was modified from a glucose-responsive fluorescent dye (GF dye). The principle underlying the glucose responsiveness of the GF dye is briefly explained as follows: the GF dye comprises a diboronic acid moiety and an anthracene moiety that act as the specific glucose-recognition site and the fluorogenic site, respectively. Sawada et al. developed calcium ion (Ca^{2+})-responsive hydrogels composed of designed β-sheet peptides [27,28]. As the novel designed peptide, E1Y9, has a Glu residue to interact with Ca^{2+}, the peptide in the sol-state self-assembled into hydrogels in the presence of Ca^{2+}. The hydrogels showed a high cell-adhesive ability that was similar in magnitude to fibronectine. Thus, the novel peptide-based nanofiber hydrogels can facilitate development studies for three-dimensional cell culturing for tissue engineering.

On the other hand, the authors have innovated a nanofiber mesh for the removal of toxins from the blood, which they are hopeful may be incorporated into wearable blood purification systems for kidney failure patients (Fig. 5.4.8) [29]. We made their nanofiber mesh using two components: a blood-compatible primary matrix polymer made from polyethylene-*co*-vinyl alchohol, and several different forms of zeolites. Zeolites have

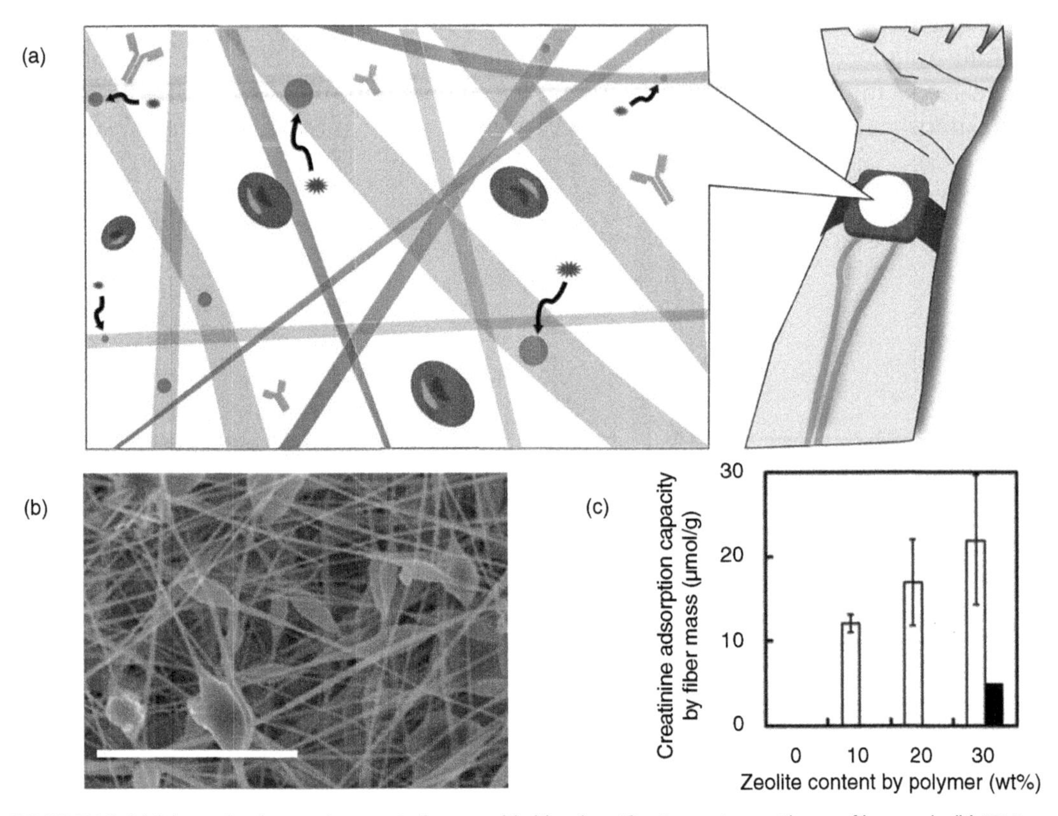

FIGURE 5.4.8 (a) Schematic of a novel concept of a wearable blood purification system with nanofiber mesh. (b) SEM image of a nanofiber mesh containing zeolite. (c) Creatinine adsorption increased depending on the zeolite content in the nanofiber meshes.

microporous structures capable of adsorbing toxins such as creatinine from blood. Different zeolites have different pore sizes meaning they can be used to selectively adsorb specific solutes. Our result demonstrated that a 16-g mesh is enough to remove all the creatinine produced in one day by the human body. Although the new design is still in its early stages and not yet ready for production, nanofiber-based biomaterials will soon be a feasible, compact, and cheap alternative to dialysis for kidney failure patients across the world.

5.4.4 Conclusions and Future Trends

As described in this chapter, fibrous materials are becoming increasingly important today. Especially, smart nanofiber-based technologies are becoming the premier tool for a wide range of applications in the areas of medicine and biotechnology. This chapter mainly addressed the developments of smart nanofibers. Although the concepts of these smart nanofibers are sound, the practical applications require significant improvements in the fiber properties. The synthesis of new polymers and cross-linkers with more biocompatibility and better biodegradability would be essential for successful applications. It is also expected that principles from the expanding research area of supramolecular chemistry will be applied to design novel types of nanofibers with tailored properties, which can preferably be prepared in an aqueous environment. Also, protein engineering might contribute to the development of nanofiber systems with very precise control over their microstructure, and thus their properties. Concurrent developments in the design of new responsive polymers along with structure–property evaluations are vital for practical applications of smart hydrogels.

References

[1] W. Zheng, W. Zhang, X. Jiang, Adv. Eng. Mater. 12 (2010) B451.

[2] G.A. Di Lullo, S.M. Sweeney, J. Korkko, L. Ala-Kokko, J.D. San Antonio, J. Biol. Chem. 277 (2002) 4223.

[3] T. Kato, Science 295 (2002) 2414.

[4] N. Bhardwaj, S.C. Kundu, Biotechnol. Adv. 28 (2010) 325.

[5] R.L. Dahlin, F.K. Kasper, A.G. Mikos, Tissue Eng. Part B – Rev. 17 (2011) 349.

[6] G.D. Danilatos, J. Microsc. – Oxford 162 (1991) 391.

[7] H. Wang, Y. Li, L. Sun, Y. Li, W. Wang, S. Wang, S. Xu, Q. Yang, J. Coll. Interface Sci. 350 (2010) 396.

[8] D.N. Rockwood, D.B. Chase, R.E. Akins Jr., J.F. Rabolt, Polymer 49 (2008) 4025.

[9] H. Okuzaki, K. Kobayashi, H. Yan, Synthetic Metals 159 (2009) 2273.

[10] H. Yuan, B. Li, K. Liang, X. Lou, Y. Zhang, Biomed. Mater. 9 (2014) 055001.

[11] Y.-J. Kim, M. Ebara, T. Aoyagi, Sci. Technol. Adv. Mater. 13 (2012) 064203.

[12] Y.-J. Kim, M. Ebara, T. Aoyagi, Angew. Chem. – Int. Ed. 51 (2012) 10537.

[13] S. Maeda, T. Kato, H. Kogure, N. Hosoya, Appl. Phys. Lett. 106 (2015) 171909.

[14] F. Di Benedetto, E. Mele, A. Camposeo, A. Athanassiou, R. Cingolani, D. Pisignano, Adv. Mater. 20 (2008) 314.

[15] S. Sur, J.B. Matson, M.J. Webber, C.J. Newcomb, S.I. Stupp, ACS Nano 6 (2012) 10776.

[16] D. Lim, E. Lee, H. Kim, S. Park, S. Baek, J. Yoon, Soft Matter 11 (2015) 1606.

[17] X. Shi, Y. Zheng, G. Wang, Q. Lin, J. Fan, RSC Adv. 4 (2014) 47056.

[18] J. Zhou, T. Fukawa, M. Kimura, Polym. J. 43 (2011) 849.

[19] Q. Gao, J. Takizawa, M. Kimura, Polym. 54 (2013) 120.

[20] S. Wu, R. Ladani, J. Zhang, A. Kinloch, Z. Zhao, J. Ma, X. Zhang, A. Mouritz, K. Ghorbani, C. Wang, Polymer 68 (2015) 25.

[21] Y.-J. Kim, M. Ebara, T. Aoyagi, Adv. Funct. Mater. 23 (2013) 5753.

[22] A. Gestos, P.G. Whitten, G.M. Spinks, G.G. Wallace, Soft Matter 6 (2010) 1045.

[23] L. Wang, P.D. Topham, O.O. Mykhaylyk, J.R. Howse, W. Bras, R.A.L. Jones, A.J. Ryan, Adv. Mater. 19 (2007) 3544.

[24] X. Jin, Y.L. Hsieh, Polymer 46 (2005) 5149.

[25] H. Shibata, Y.J. Heo, T. Okitsu, Y. Matsunaga, T. Kawanishi, S. Takeuchi, Proc. Natl. Acad. Sci. USA 107 (2010) 17894.

[26] Y.J. Heo, H. Shibata, T. Okitsu, T. Kawanishi, S. Takeuchi, Proc. Natl. Acad. Sci. USA 108 (2011) 13399.

[27] K. Fukunaga, H. Tsutsumi, H. Mihara, Biopolymers 100 (2013) 731.

[28] T. Sawada, M. Tsuchiya, T. Takahashi, H. Tsutsumi, H. Mihara, Polym. J. 44 (2012) 651.

[29] K. Namekawa, M.T. Schreiber, T. Aoyagi, M. Ebara, Biomater. Sci. 2 (2014) 674.

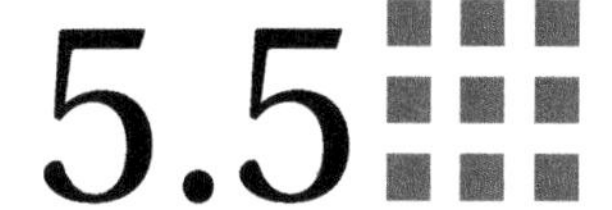

5.5 On/Off Switchable Interfaces

Naokazu Idota

KAGAMI MEMORIAL RESEARCH INSTITUTE FOR MATERIALS SCIENCE AND TECHNOLOGY, WASEDA UNIVERSITY, SHINJUKU, TOKYO, JAPAN

CHAPTER OUTLINE

5.5.1 Introduction

Surface properties are one of the most essential factors in all biomaterials, since biomolecules and cells have to be in contact with the outermost surfaces of substrates. The biological response to substrates always occurs at the interfaces between biomolecules and surfaces [1]. Modification of biomaterials with polymers is thus an attractive technique to adjust the surface properties for biocompatibilities while maintaining the original features of the substrates. For example, synthetic polymer involving poly(ethylene glycol) (PEG) [2], poly(2-hydroxyethyl methacrylate)-*b*-polystyrene [3], and poly(2-methyacryloyloxyethyl phosphorylcoline) [4] have been extensively studied to graft on substrate for use as antithrombogenic materials. These polymer chains exhibit the expanded volume of the random coil through strong interaction with water molecules, which prevent the adsorption of biomolecules [5]. Many researchers have routinely made numerous efforts to develop biocompatible modified surfaces with hydrophilic and/or amphipathic polymers. These surface modifications are a class of static surface properties, which provide continuous biocompatible performance.

On the other hand, cells and proteins exhibit space- and time-dependent dynamic changes in their conformations and functionalities in the human body. Since the 1990s, dynamic switchable surfaces have been comprehensively studied in order to control the biomolecular dynamics by modification with smart polymers [6], which show changes in their conformations and properties in response to external stimuli. Among them, thermoresponsive poly(*N*-isopropylacrylamide) (PNIPAAm) is one of the most successful models to control the interaction between biomolecules and the grafted substrates by temperature alterations [7]. PNIPAAm is well known to show conformational coil-to-globule transition in water around its lower critical solution temperature (LCST), as it is useful to be close to human body temperature. Since the LCST of PNIPAAm is controllable by environmental changes around the polymer chains, multiple smart polymers have been investigated and various stimuli such as pH, light, electric field, or addition of chemicals are used as a trigger to induce the phase transition at a certain temperature by PNIPAAm's LCST shift [8]. In contrast, numerous types of responsive polymers have also been developed to switch their conformation by tuning the stimuli applied. Surface grafting of these smart polymers have been used to control the biomolecular interaction for development of on-demand applications under biologically relevant conditions [9]. The appearance of smart surfaces greatly expands the strategy for design of biomedical materials compared with the previous approach of molecular adsorption in a conventional static concept.

This chapter focuses on the on/off switchable smart polymer-grafted surfaces for biomaterial applications. The phenomena of protein adsorption and cell adhesion were reviewed to understand the interaction with material surfaces, and polymer-grafting techniques were examined for the design of switchable polymer-grafted surfaces. Based on the available knowledge, switchable stimuli-responsive surfaces were categorized into the type of stimuli used as a trigger, and their recent biomedical application, such as cell culture substrates, separation matrices, or drug delivery materials, was studied.

5.5.2 Design of On/Off Switchable Surfaces for Biomaterials

5.5.2.1 Protein Adsorption and Cell Adhesion

In designing biomaterial surfaces, adsorption of biomolecules on substrate surfaces is an important factor to control their biocompatibility, nonfouling, antibacteria, cell adhesion property, biological cascade, and so on. In particular, adsorption of proteins and peptides depends on the surface properties of the substrates, and rapidly occurs as soon as contact occurs among them. The adsorption processes are induced by various physicochemical properties, such as hydrophobicity, polarity, charge species, and structural features [10]. In the surface properties, due to their high-order structure, hydrophobicity is expected to play a main role in protein adsorption through artful balance of intramolecular hydrophobic interaction. When the proteins are attached on solid substrates, their conformation subsequently changes by hydrophobic interaction between the hydrophobic domains of proteins and the substrate. The conformational change leads to the accumulation of proteins to form a stable multilayer, resulting in irreversible protein adsorption on the surfaces. The protein conformation is also important from the point of view of the bioactivity based on their higher-order structures, thus biomolecular adsorption should be considered in the design of switchable surfaces for biomedical application.

In cell adhesion on solid materials, protein adsorption is an essential factor because cells can attach and modify their biological functions through binding extracellular matrices (ECMs) adsorbed on the surfaces. Furthermore, there are two other important steps in the cell adhesion process onto material surfaces, "passive adhesion" and "active adhesion" [11]. Passive adhesion includes the subsequent protein interactions between cells and substrate surfaces, which are reversible, and no intracellular metabolic signaling. Specifically, the control of passive cell adhesion by design of the material surfaces can provide switchable cell-based applications involving manipulation, patterning, and sorting. In contrast, active adhesion means spontaneous activation of cell receptor-mediated interactions after the passive adhesion, and involves cellular metabolic processes such as their morphological changes and signal transduction that depend on the phenotypes. Since the attached cells hardly detach from the substrates due to static surface properties, cell harvest from the surfaces usually requires the addition of enzymatic proteolysis of ECM proteins and chelation of divalent cations. Thus, on/off switchable surfaces should be designed to reverse from active to passive adhesion for noninvasive cell detachment without enzymes and chelating reagents.

5.5.2.2 Polymer Grafting

Significant attention has been routinely directed toward synthesis of polymers with well-defined composition and architecture for industrial and academic fields. Free-radical polymerization is a general method of polymer synthesis because of the wide range of available monomers, tolerance of functional groups, and procedure simplicity. However, this method has the disadvantage of irreversible chain transfer and termination in the preparation of well-defined polymer chains. Since the last two decades, controlled living radical polymerization (CLRP) has been recognized as an important synthesis tool and has rapidly advanced in the development of the techniques, especially on establishing a dynamic equilibration between a minute amount of growing free radical and a large majority of dormant species [12]. These methods are typically classified by dormant chains and free-radical generation; alkyl halides via a catalyzed reaction as atom transfer radical polymerization (ATRP) [13], alkoxyamines by the spontaneous thermal process as nitroxide mediated polymerization [14], and thioesters through the degenerative exchange process as reversible addition fragmentation chain transfer processes [15]. Both living radical polymerizations have the reversible activation/deactivation process with free-radical propagation and termination of a conventional radical polymerization. In these polymerizations, the contribution of termination can be minimized under appropriate conditions, resulting in well-defined polymers with narrow molecular weight distributions being obtained.

In the preparation of polymer-grafted surfaces, numerous grafting techniques have been proposed to simplify the modification process and precisely control their composition and architecture, and they are roughly categorized as "grafting to" and "grafting from" methods [12]. In the "grafting to" approach, synthesized polymers with connectable functional groups, such as carboxyl, amino, and thiol groups, are tethered to activated substrate surfaces through either physical adsorption or chemical reaction. The grafting via chemical reaction technique provides more stable products than the physical adsorption-driven modification due to irreversible covalent bonding. In the "grafting to" methods, a wide variety of surface chemistry for precise control of the polymer architectures, such as Langmuir–Blodgett deposition [16], layer-by-layer method [17], formation of self-assembled monolayers [18], and click chemistry [19] can be used. On the other hand, "grafting to" methods limit interfacial polymer chain densities because of significant decreases in reaction probabilities with the surface functional groups with increasing brush density.

The "grafting from" technique is a direct polymerization from the substrate surfaces by immobilization with initiating functional groups. In this method, monomers easily penetrate through the growing polymer chains grafted on the surfaces, and polymers can be consequently modified even with high density, which is different from the "grafting to" method. While it was difficult to control the architecture of grafted polymers in "grafting from" methods by free-radical polymerizations due to their effect of termination, advanced CLRP techniques allow simultaneous solution of the problems for conventional "grafting to" and "grafting from" methods. Especially, surface-initiated ATRP provides the preparation of high-density polymer brushes because of effective initiation of ATRP initiators immobilized on substrates [13]. In addition, the high-density polymer brushes have been reported to exhibit unique surface properties compared with conventional polymer-grafted surfaces, such as low friction factor, high elastic modulus, and molecular adsorption [20]. Therefore, the versatile grafting methods can provide the control of graft architectures and subsequent development of switchable biomaterial surfaces.

5.5.3 Type of On/Off Switchable Surfaces

5.5.3.1 Thermoresponsive Surfaces

Thermoresponsive polymers have been extensively studied in the field of biomedical applications using smart polymers. Numerous polymers such as PEG-based polymers, polymers with alcohol groups, and amide-substituted polymers are well known to show thermal-induced phase transition in aqueous solution. Substrate surfaces grafted with these polymers also show aqueous wettability changes by temperature alterations. The hydration of grafted polymer chains is a key factor in molecular adsorption, thus switchable wettability of the thermoresponsive polymer-grafted surfaces is desirable in order to control the interaction with biomolecules. PNIPAAm-grafted surfaces have been widely used in on/off switchable materials due to good reversibility of the phase transition with temperature. The temperature dependence of aqueous wettability changes are significantly influenced by the graft architecture of tethered PNIPAAm chains on the surfaces [21]. In particular, chain mobility and graft density of PNIPAAm on the surfaces mainly contribute to the degree of wettability changes and phase transition temperature. Dense polymer brushes on substrate surfaces can be prepared by the surface-initiated ATRP process, and the surfaces are known to exhibit unique properties compared with those prepared by free-radical polymerization [20]. PNIPAAm brushes prepared by surface-initiated ATRP show different phase transition behavior between their outer and inner regions [22]; the mobility of densely packed inner PNIPAAm chains is significantly restricted due to steric hindrance, and the loose outermost region shows drastic conformational changes by temperature alterations. The surface roughness of substrates also significantly affects the aqueous wettability, and PNIPAAm-grafted substrates with micro- or nanogrooves can allow reversible switching between superhydrophilic and superhydrophobic properties [23].

Change from hydrophobic to hydrophilic property by a decrease in temperature of the grafted surfaces below the LCST is useful in biomedical applications, which induces switchable detachment of adsorbed molecules from the surfaces. Since protein adsorption on solid substrates is mainly caused by collapse of various interactions involving hydrophobic interaction and hydrogen bonding, surface wettability of substrates is an important factor to control the protein adsorption. Surface-grafted PNIPAAm develops into the hydration state at low temperature, and the abundant water molecules play a critical role in repelling proteins. As well as wettability control on the PNIPAAm-grafted surfaces, their graft architectures are sensitive to the protein adsorption by temperature alterations. Dependence of static adsorption of human serum albumin at a certain temperature is notable for the grafted surfaces with PNIPAAm layers thicker than 38.1 nm [24]. In addition, PNIPAAm-grafted surfaces with low graft density (<0.08 chains/nm^2) permit adsorption of bovine serum albumin (BSA), which absorbs on surfaces even if the temperature is lower than the LCST [25], and whose distance between grafted chains is roughly equivalent to BSA size.

Other thermoresponsive polymers, such as oligo(ethylene glycol) (OEG) derivatives [26] and elastin-like polypeptides [27], have also been reported to modify substrates for switchable protein adsorption. In cell adhesion, control of protein adsorption is important because cells can also attach to solid substrates mediated by binding with ECM adsorbed on the surfaces. Okano et al. have been developing an enzyme-free cell harvest system using PNIPAAm-grafted surfaces [28]. In this system, confluent cells, which are cultured on PNIPAAm-grafted surfaces at 37°C, can be harvested as a continuous cell sheet with intact ECM containing adhesive proteins from the surfaces by decreasing the temperature to 25°C. Therefore, the cell sheets can be directly patched to diseased parts without any sutures, and be used as a cell source of tissue reconstruction (details are found in Chapter 3.2). As well as the control of protein adsorption, thermoresponsive OEG derivatives, poloxamers, xyloglucan, and elastin-like polypeptides have also been demonstrated to control cell adhesion [29–32]. These polymers show good biocompatibility and their grafted surfaces are useful for low toxic cell culture substrates.

Another successful application using a PNIPAAm-grafted surface is the thermoresponsive chromatography system [33]. In this system, separation is achieved by control of hydrophobic interaction between solute molecules and PNIPAAm-grafted silica beads through the temperature changes under a constant aqueous mobile phase (Fig. 5.5.1a). On the PNIPAAm-grafted surfaces, increase in the retention times of mixed solutes was observed with increasing temperature, particularly around the PNIPAAm's LCST. The extension of the retention time depends on their hydrophobicity, resulting in separation at high temperature. The elution behavior can be effectively modulated in the thermoresponsive chromatography by temperature gradient (Fig. 5.5.1b) [34]. Long retention time is required

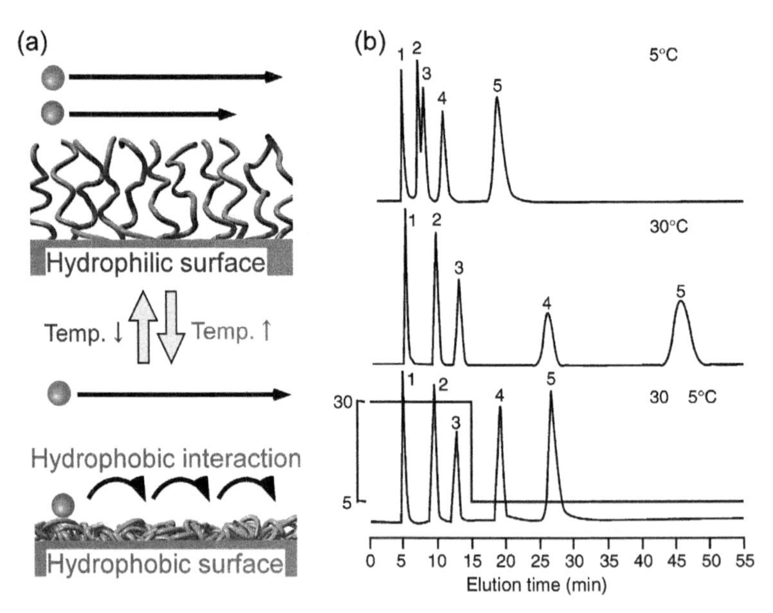

FIGURE 5.5.1 Thermoresponsive chromatography system. (a) Mechanism of elution control of solutes by changes in hydrophobic interaction with the PNIPAAm-grafted surfaces as a function of temperature. (b) Chromatograms of a mixture of four steroids and benzene by temperature gradient (peaks: 1, benzene; 2, cortisone; 3, prednisolone; 4, hydrocortisone acetate; and 5, testosterone) [34].

for the flowing out of all steroids from the thermoresponsive column at 30°C, while the separation was insufficient at 5°C. In order to obtain effective separation, column temperature was decreased to 5°C after the separation of low hydrophobic solutes at 30°C, resulting in an earlier separation time than at constant 30°C. In another conventional chromatography method, reverse-phase liquid chromatography (RPLC), the separation is based on the control of hydrophobic interactions by changes of the elution process. Although RPLC is useful in the field of analytical chemistry, the use of organic solvents as the mobile phase leads to the denaturation of bioactive molecules and therefore is a disadvantage in biomedical and pharmaceutical applications. In the thermoresponsive chromatography system, the hydrophobicity of the PNIPAAm-grafted stationary phases can be modulated by temperature changes under aqueous conditions, which is a similar effect to the use of organic solvents in RPLC. Thus, the separation under isocratic aqueous mobile phases is a powerful tool for bioactive compounds such as peptides, proteins, and metabolism of drugs [35].

As well as conventional chromatography, various modes of thermoresponsive chromatography have been demonstrated to be useful for separation of biomolecules depending on their properties. By incorporation of ionic comonomers into grafted PNIPAAm chains, hydrophobic and electrostatic interaction between solute molecules and the surfaces can be controlled simultaneously only by temperature changes, because thermoresponsive ionic copolymers exhibit apparent pK_a shifts depending on temperature changes [36]. Using this characteristic, ion-exchange chromatography in dual response to pH and temperature has been developed to separate cationic angiotensin subtype derivatives by surface modification with P(NIPAAm-*co*-acrylic acid (AA)-*co*-*t*-butyl acrylamide) [37]. The incorporation of cationic *N*-(2-dimethylaminoethyl)acrylamide into the PNIPAAm grafted onto the silica beads also allows separation of anionic oligonucleotides [38] in the same manner. Another feature of PNIPAAm chains is coil/globule transition of the polymer chains in response to external temperature, which has been used for switchable size-excluded chromatography (SEC) [39]. In common SEC mode, smaller molecules take a longer retention time to pass through the column by permeation into the packed matrices. While thermoreponsive SEC at low temperature behaves in the same manner as the conventional SEC, aggregation of grafted PNIPAAm at the temperature above its LCST expands the pore size of column matrices, resulting in elongation of the retention times for all samples. In contrast, the hydrophobilized PNIPAAm at high temperature easily interacts with hydrophobic molecules; thus, not only molecular weight but also hydrophobicity of samples should be considered in order to achieve successful separation in the thermoresponsive SEC system. Thermal-induced conformational changes of PNIPAAm chains also allow on/off switchable affinity chromatography. In this system, the access of biomolecules to specific ligands is controlled through the expansion/aggregation changes of the grafted PNIPAAm by temperature changes. There are mainly two types of surface modifications: binary grafting of free end PNIPAAm chains and ligands with spacer molecules [40], and grafting with NIPAAm copolymers having pendant functional groups of ligands [41]. In the case of binary grafting, the length of PNIPAAm and spacer molecules should be precisely controlled. Target molecules can bind to the ligand if the spacer length is longer than the aggregated PNIPAAm chains at higher temperatures above the LCST. On the other hand, lowering the temperature below the LCST leads to the expansion of grafted PNIPAAm and subsequently to the release of the target molecules from the surfaces by their size excluded effects. In contrast, grafted NIPAAm comopolymers with ligand groups allows access to target molecules at lower temperature than the LCST, and their shrinking behavior by an increase in temperature leads to dissociation between target molecules and ligands in polymer chains. Both switchable affinity chromatography methods are useful for separation of bioactive proteins because pH regulation of eluent and antagonist are not needed for the purification.

5.5.3.2 pH-Responsive Surfaces

Numerous polyelectrolytes exhibit reversible changes in their solubility and configuration in response to pH changes across its pK_a. The responsive properties are caused by the protonation/deprotonation of charge residues in polymers upon pH alteration of solution, and subsequently their hydration state and conformation can be controlled through the interaction between water molecules and the residues. Particularly, poly(meth)acrylate derivatives and polymers bearing tertiary amine groups are routinely used as typical pH-responsive polymers under acidic and basic conditions, respectively. The electrostatic interaction of charged pH-responsive polymer-grafted surfaces is noticed at relatively long distance from the surfaces. Kurihara et al. [42] investigated the distance-dependent interaction between anionic poly(methacrylic acid) (PMAA) layers on surfaces as a function of pH and added salt concentrations in order to obtain surface force measurement. When more carboxyl groups of PMAA were ionized at higher pH, repulsion was observed at longer range due to the extension of polyelectrolyte chains. Addition of a monovalent salt restrains the repulsion at longer separation distance as expected from the shielding effect of counterions, which is one to two orders of magnitude larger than the Debye lengths. The pH-dependent interaction must be associated with changes in the ionization state and the consequent conformation of the polyelectrolyte head groups.

pH-responsive polymers have been studied to prepare smart porous membranes with variable barrier properties [43]. In the surface grafting of pH-responsive polymers, porous membranes are used as modification substrates. The porous membranes allow control of permeability and selectivity by conformational changes in the polymer layers on the pore walls in response to pH and ionic strength. The graft density of pH-responsive polymers has significant influence on membrane permeability; lower density exhibits better permeation of buffer solution due to higher mobility of the polymer chains [44]. The pH-responsive membranes are an advance in the separation process for biomolecules and control of drug release for biomedical applications. The smart porous membranes coated with PAA allowed a reversible release/quench process for methylene blue as a model drug predominantly by pH change cycles [45]. By incorporation of glucose oxidase into the grafted PAA, pH changes can be used for controlled drug release through generation of glycolic acids in the enzymatic reaction. Modification with copolymer containing NIPAAm and MAA has also been practically used as a dual-responsive membrane for switchable drug delivery [46].

Another excellent application of pH-responsive surfaces is as an antibacterial material. The isoelectric point of most bacteria strains is known to be in the pH range of 1.5–4.5 [47], and the negative-charged bacterial cells can be attached on cationic materials under pH conditions above that, resulting in their extinction [48]. For instance, grafted surfaces with pH-sensitive polymer-bearing quaternary ammonium salts significantly reduce *Staphylococcus aureus* colonization under neutral conditions due to their positive charge tethered to the flexible polymer chains [49]. On the other hand, neutral charge surfaces are necessary to release the attached bacterial cells from the surfaces to keep the nonfouling properties [50]. From this perspective, a binary pH-responsive surface modified with a copolymer of (2-(acryloyloxy)ethyl)trimethyl ammonium chloride and 2-carboxy ethyl acrylate was prepared for tunable nonfouling properties by pH changes [51]. The surface shows charge transition between neutral and positive charge leading to switchable antifouling material, from adhesive to resistant, for *Staphylococcus epidermidis*. Although it is difficult to reuse the above-mentioned pH-responsive surfaces as antibacterial materials, Cao et al. developed a reversible surface between the killing and defending function against bacteria [52]. They used a smart polymer with cationic residues of *N,N*-dimethyl-2-morpholinone, which can reversibly change to zwitterionic carboxyl betaine by hydrolysis under wet conditions (Fig. 5.5.2a). The cationic charges in dried polymer chains can kill over 99.9% of *Escherichia coli* K12, followed by detachment from the zwitterionic surfaces by wetting the substrates (Fig. 5.5.2b). The functionalization triggered by this simple operation is an ideal and successful model in on/off switchable biomaterial surfaces.

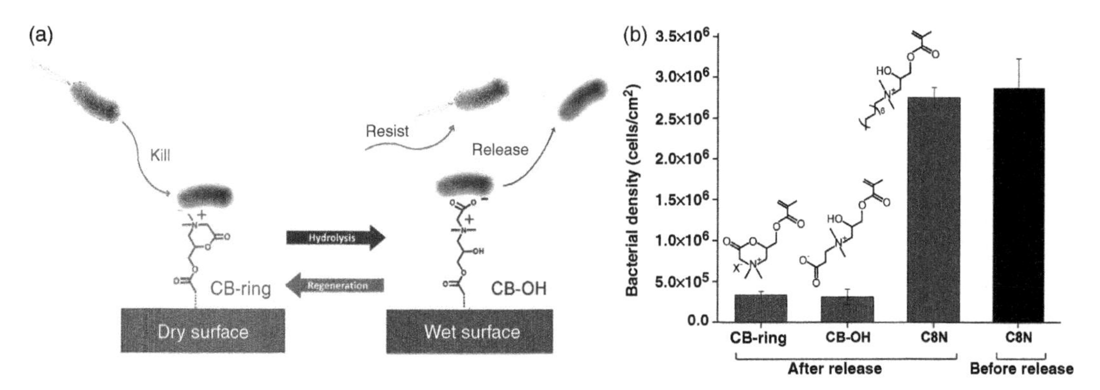

FIGURE 5.5.2 Switchable antibacterial surfaces [52]. (a) Mechanism of reversible cycles between attack and protect against bacterial cells using zwitterionic polymer-grafted surfaces. (b) Number of *Escherichia coli* K12 cells on the surfaces before and after the releasing procedure.

5.5.3.3 Photoresponsive Surfaces

Light exposure has advantages as a triggering stimulus in responsive polymers, such as easy and precise control of on/off switching and also positon control by using a photomask. Typical photoresponsive polymers are divided into two types by their pendant functional groups: cleavable and conformational changeable groups [53]. In this section, we focus on reversible conformational photoresponsive polymers since photocleavable polymers commonly show irreversible abilities.

The photoresponsive polymers bearing azobenzene residues have been used in various applications due to the good reversibility of the *trans–cis* isomerization. The azo chromophore isomerizes from stable *trans* to *cis* forms by UV exposure, and the irradiation with visible light induces the reverse *cis*-isomerization. This photoresponsive isomerization is useful in order to get conformational changes by switching between activation and deactivation of the incorporated biofunctional groups into the polymer chains. For example, cell adhesive Gly-Arg-Gly-Asp-Ser (GRGDS) peptide is bound to the free end of azobenzene-bearing PEG layers on the substrates, and cell adhesion can be controlled by tuning light exposure [54]. Although cells can interact with the terminated GRGDS peptides at the *trans* state of the azobenzene groups, the PEG chains at lower sides prevent cell adhesion because the *cis*-isomer masks the GRGDS into the layers (Fig. 5.5.3a). Dynamic switching of exposure with UV or visible lights allows detachment of the adhered cells from the surfaces for 30 min. As a similar strategy, phenylalanine-based trifluoromethyl ketone was used as the incorporated biofunctional group to modulate the binding of α-chymotrypsin enzymes to the surfaces [55].

Another typical photoresponsive material for preparation of switchable surfaces is the spiropyran–merocyanine system. The spiropyran isomerizes to zwitterionic merocyanine conformation by UV exposure, and the reverse reaction can be triggered by irradiation with visible light as well as azobenzene. The changes in hydrophilic/hydrophobic properties through the isomerization of spiropyran groups also enable the control of cell adhesion/detachment. Edahiro et al. reported photoresponsive cell culture substrates grafted

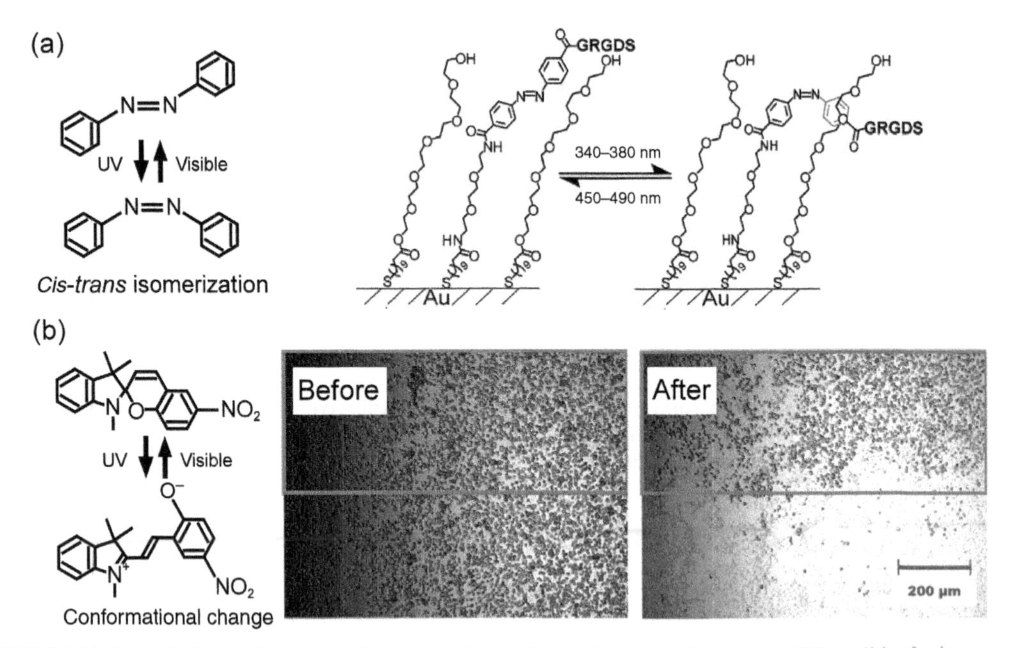

FIGURE 5.5.3 Control of cell adhesion on photoresponsive surfaces. (a) Access control of GRGDS peptides for biospecific cell adhesion by photoinduced *cis–trans* isomerization of terminal azobenzene residues in grafted polymers [54]. (b) Microscopic images of CHO-K1 cells on the surfaces grafted with *N*-isopropylacrylamide (NIPAAm)-based polymers having spiropyran resides (left) before and (right) after regional UV irradiation followed by the low-temperature washing [56].

with PNIPAAm having spiropyran chromophores [56]. The isomerization of spiropyran residues by irradiation with UV light can assist the cell detachment from the thermoresponsive surfaces after a cooling process (Fig. 5.5.3b). Remarkably, the photoinduced manipulation will provide a powerful tool for cocultured cell patterning. On the other hand, there is a possibility that, by repeating the operation, the extended UV exposure damages both the grafted polymer layers and adhered cells. Since the spiropyran derivative is well known as a photochromism dye, its surface grafting can also be useful for nanoparticles in order to show tunable fluorescence through the fluorescence resonance energy transfer process [57].

5.5.3.4 Electro-/Magnet-Responsive Surfaces

The properties of electroresponsive polymer-grafted surfaces can be precisely controlled because an electrical field can be applied specifically to the substrates. The electrical field is useful as a switching trigger as it is noninvasive for the surrounding environment. Therefore, applications using electroresponsive surfaces are attracting increasing interests. Polyelectrolytes and electrically conducting polymers, which are conjugated polymer chains with π electrons delocalized along the back bone, are mainly used for the responsive surfaces. In on/off switchable electroresponsive surfaces, polyelectrolytes exhibit conformational changes based on the voltage-induced motion of charged residues in the chains. When conductive metal materials are used as modification substrate, the changes in the surface charge are induced electrically to subsequently show electrostatic interaction between the surface charges and grafted polyelectrolytes. The conformational changes of grafted polymers depend on the graft density [58]. When a low density of end-charged polymer chains exists, they become fouling and eventually looping to the surfaces by applying an electrical field. This attractive behavior provides electrically switchable molecular capture/release on the surfaces [59]. The surfaces grafted with carboxyl group-terminated polymers allow the adsorption of positively charged proteins under a negative potential, and their release by applying the opposite electrical field. This system is also applicable to terminal amino-functionalized polymers for controlled capture/release of anionic biomolecules.

Among the candidates of electrically conducting polymers, polypyrrole (PPy) is a great candidate to use in biomedical applications due to its high stability and low cytotoxicity. Wong et al. reported a dynamic cell culture substrate using indium tin oxide glass coated with PPy (Fig. 5.5.4a) [60]. The oxidized PPy on the surfaces showed normal cell adhesion properties in terms of cell spreading and DNA synthesis. In contrast, the cell adhesion properties on the neutral PPy-coated surfaces were inhibited without effect of cell viability by applying an electrical potential. While the mechanism is not fully understood, the electroresponsive surfaces provide a noninvasive method to control cell adhesion behavior. In another example, amphipathic taurocholic acid (TCA) was doped into an array

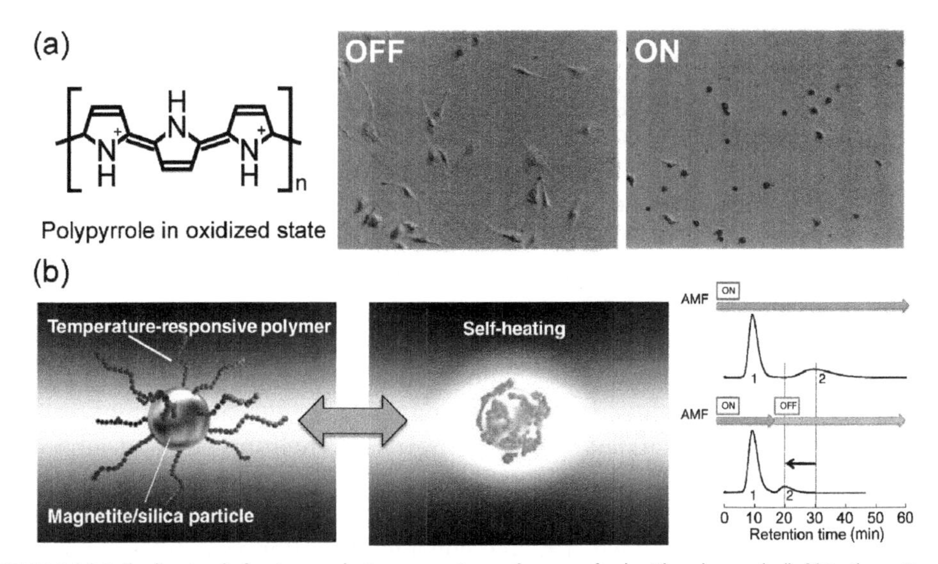

FIGURE 5.5.4 (a) Cell adhesion behavior on electroresponsive surfaces grafted with polypyrrole (left) in the native oxidized state and (right) after reduction by applying electrical potential [60]. (b) Modulation of steroid elution in magnetic-responsive column by self-heating through on/off switching of AMF (chromatogram peaks: 1, hydrocortisone; 2, testosterone) [63].

of nanoarchitectured PPy to control the wettability and cell adhesion response to potential [61]. The TCA molecules reversibly expose their hydrophilic β-face or hydrophobic α-face according to the on/off switching behavior depending on the applied potential, thus the molecular orientation allows the potential-induced wettability changes and subsequent reversible cell adhesion and spreading on the surfaces. Utilizing local application of electrical potential, stimulation of neurite outgrowth and guidance were also demonstrated for neural tissue engineering [62].

Similar to an electric field a magnetic field also has the advantage of remote control of the surface-grafted polymers. Generally, inorganic magnetic (nano)particles have been used for the preparation of magnet-responsive surfaces. Applying a magnetic field provides the grafted materials with the magnetic susceptibility that provides dispersion control and transportability, and these features have been widely used as drug carriers and for cell manipulation [64]. In addition, by applying an alternating magnetic field (AMF), magnetic nanoparticles can self-heat through magnetic hysteresis [65]. Aoyagi et al. showed a magnetic-responsive chromatography system using magnetite nanoparticles grafted with PNIPAAm as the stationary phase [63]. The retention time of steroids using their column was prolonged by hydrophobic interaction with hydrophobic PNIPAAm layers through AMF-mediated heat generation (Fig. 5.5.4b). It is notable that the temperature around the magnetic nanoparticles was estimated to be 48°C in spite of constant room temperature in the entire column and eluent. Thus, this smart chromatography system could be useful for the separation of bioactive compounds by locally controlling the temperature of the grafted surface by simply applying an AMF.

5.5.3.5 Biomolecule-Responsive Surfaces

In biomedical applications using on/off switchable surfaces, spontaneous appearance of their tunable function is desired in response to exposure to target biomolecules. In order to prepare the biomolecule-responsive surfaces, not only the introduction of affinity functional groups for target species is necessary but also the regulation of the biological process is required. A lot of biomolecules are known to dynamically change their conformation and physiological environment in response to specific biological species in the human body. Since the above-mentioned stimuli-responsive polymers are also sensitive to environmental alterations, there are now numerous examples of biomolecule-responsive surfaces that are typically based on a conventional responsive polymer bearing pendant affinity residues. Hence, conjugation between target molecules and affinity residues in grafted polymer chains induces changes in their external environment, and subsequently the responsive surfaces can show their functions.

Glucoses play an important role in various biological processes in the human body, and glucose-responsive polymers have attracted considerable attention for their potential as biomedical applications involving diagnostic sensing and drug delivery systems. Phenylboronic acid (PBA) is a typical example that shows specific binding to glucoses through reversible reaction with their diol groups, which accompanies changes in water solubility.

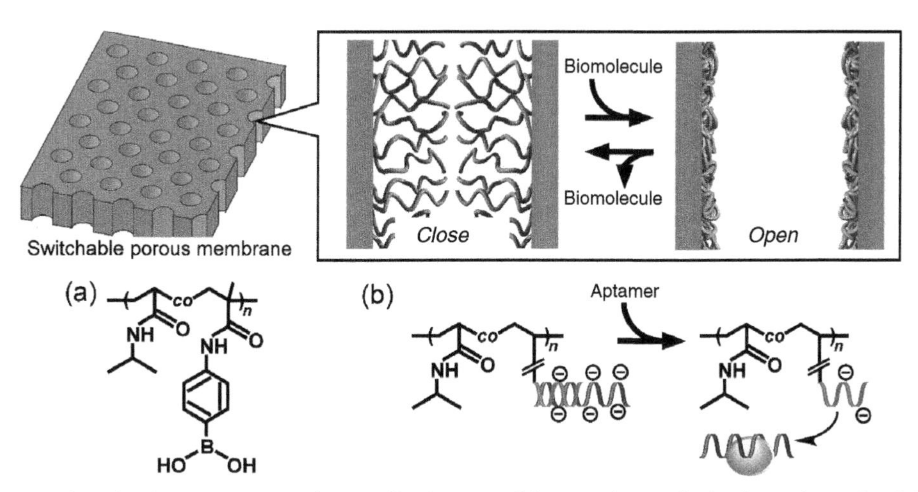

FIGURE 5.5.5 Biomolecule-responsive membranes allowing reversible open/close cycles by the conformational changes of grafted polymers. (a) Structure of copolymer comprising NIPAAm and phenylboronic acid (PBA) derivatives [66]. (b) Changes in negative charge density of DNA-conjugated PNIPAAm grafted on porous membranes by addition of DNA aptamers [70].

Graft copolymerization of NIPAAm and PBA derivatives (Fig. 5.5.5a) allows reversible changes in the surface wettability through the LCST shift of NIPAAm copolymer by the above-mentioned stimuli [66]. The P(NIPAAm-*co*-PBA) hydrogels coated on porous membrane were reported to act as a microvalve for drug release in response to glucose concentrations [67]. The shrunken hydrogels in the presence of glucoses allow solution to flow through an opened annular gap, while the swollen hydrogels block the flow completely by occupying the void space. The smart membrane represents an advantage in the controlled release of biologically important products involving insulin, as its liberation can be automatically triggered by an increase in blood glucose levels. Another glucose-specific molecule used as responsive polymers is glucose oxidase (GOx), whose function is based on the catalyzed reaction of glucose with oxygen. The enzymatic oxidation of glucose using GOx generates gluconic acid as a by-product, which produces a change in the pH and consequently switching of the responsive surfaces. The conformational change of PAA-based glucose-responsive polymers grafted on porous membranes allows reversible open/close cycles for the pores to insulin [68]. Concanavalin A, which competitively binds with carbohydrates depending on its concentration, was also used as an incorporated molecule into glucose-responsive surfaces for drug delivery [69].

Nucleotides in DNA consist of four types of deoxyriboses: cytosine, thymine, adenine, and guanine. These nucleotide units play critical roles in biological processes as most of DNA molecules form a double helix through specific binding with each other according to base pairing rules. The DNA hybridization plays an important role not only in biological processes but also in biomedical applications. Sunagawa et al. demonstrated molecular recognition gating using DNA-conjugated PNIPAAm grafted on porous membranes [70]. The pores in membranes are closed by a swollen polymer layer through electrostatic repulsion when the conjugated DNA forms a double-stranded state. In contrast, the addition of competitive aptamers allows the dissociation of the stranded DNA, resulting in pore opening by aggregation of PNIPAAm (Fig. 5.5.5b). On the other hand, the above-mentioned responsive surfaces comprising copolymers of NIPAAm and PBA also shows wettability changes in response to nucleotides by further incorporation of trifluoromethyl (CF_3)-substituted phenylthiourea [71]. In the grafted polymers, PBA and phenylthiourea derivatives can strongly bind the pentose ring and the phosphate of the nucleotides, respectively. Also CF_3 groups in the residues enhance the hydrophobicity, resulting in conformational changes in the PNIPAAm chains.

In other biomolecule-responsive surfaces, the incorporation of molecules with various functional groups in responsive polymers has been investigated, for example, benzo-18-crown-6 residue for ion selectivity [72], affinity binding between biotin and streptavidin [73], and oligopeptides for chiral recognition [74].

5.5.4 Conclusions and Future Trends

This chapter introduced the design of graft polymer architectonics on substrate surfaces for the development of switchable biomedical applications. A variety of stimuli-responsive polymers have been investigated, and their graft architectures on surfaces can be precisely controlled by CLRP techniques. Based on understanding the biomolecular and cellular adhesion, the on/off switchable surfaces can be used for versatile applications such as cell culture substrates, antifouling materials, chromatography matrices, and drug release carriers. Surface property is an essential factor in all biomaterials, thus surface design is expected to contribute to the advance in biomedical fields.

References

[1] B.D. Ratner, A.S. Hoffman, F.J. Schoen, J. Lemons, Biomaterials Science: An Introduction to Materials in Medicine, Academic Press, New York, (2013).

[2] J. Lee, H. Lee, J. Andrade, Prog. Polym. Sci. 20 (1995) 1043.

[3] T. Okano, S. Nishiyama, I. Shinohara, T. Akaike, Y. Sakurai, K. Kataoka, T. Tsuruta, J. Biomed. Mater. Res. 15 (1981) 393.

[4] K. Ishihara, R. Aragaki, T. Ueda, A. Watenabe, N. Nakabayashi, J. Biomed. Mater. Res. 24 (1990) 1069.

[5] D.G. Castner, B.D. Ratner, Surf. Sci. 500 (2002) 28.

[6] M. Ebara, Y. Kotsuchibashi, R. Narain, N. Idota, Y.-J. Kim, J.M. Hoffman, K. Uto, T. Aoyagi, Smart Biomaterials, Springer-Verlag, Berlin, (2014).

[7] M. Heskins, J.E. Guillet, J. Macromol. Sci. A 2 (1968) 1441.

[8] T. Sun, G. Qing, Adv. Mater. 23 (2011) H57.

[9] P.M. Mendes, Chem. Soc. Rev. 37 (2008) 2512.

[10] W. Norde, C.A. Haynes, Reversibility and the mechanism of protein adsorption, Proteins at Interfaces II: Fundamentals and Applications, American Chemical Society, Washington, DC, (1995).

[11] A. Kikuchi, T. Okano, J. Control. Release 101 (2005) 69.

[12] R. Barbey, L. Lavanant, D. Paripovic, N. Schüwer, C. Sugnaux, S. Tugulu, H.-A. Klok, Chem. Rev. 109 (2009) 5437.

[13] K. Matyjaszewski, J. Xia, Chem. Rev. 101 (2001) 2921.

[14] C.J. Hawker, A.W. Bosman, E. Harth, Chem. Rev. 101 (2001) 3661.

[15] J. Chiefari, Y.K. Chong, F. Ercole, J. Krstina, J. Jeffery, T.P.T. Le, R.T.A. Mayadunne, G.F. Meijs, C.L. Moad, G. Moad, E. Rizzardo, S.H. Thang, Macromolecules 31 (1998) 5559.

[16] J. Zasadzinski, R. Viswanathan, L. Madsen, J. Garnaes, D. Schwartz, Science 263 (1994) 1726.

[17] K. Ariga, J.P. Hill, Q. Ji, Phys. Chem. Chem. Phys. 9 (2007) 2319.

[18] J.C. Love, L.A. Estroff, J.K. Kriebel, R.G. Nuzzo, G.M. Whitesides, Chem. Rev. 105 (2005) 1103.

[19] H.C. Kolb, M.G. Finn, K.B. Sharpless, Angew. Chem. Int. Ed. 40 (2001) 2004.

[20] Y. Tsujii, K. Ohno, S. Yamamoto, A. Goto, T. Fukuda, Adv. Polym. Sci. 197 (2006) 1.

[21] A. Kikuchi, T. Okano, Prog. Polym. Sci. 27 (2002) 1165.

[22] A. Mizutani, A. Kikuchi, M. Yamato, H. Kanazawa, T. Okano, Biomaterials 29 (2008) 2073.

[23] T. Sun, G. Wang, L. Feng, B. Liu, Y. Ma, L. Jiang, D. Zhu, Angew. Chem. Int. Ed. 43 (2004) 357.

[24] Q. Yu, Y. Zhang, H. Chen, Z. Wu, H. Huang, C. Cheng, Colloids Surf. B 76 (2010) 468.

[25] C. Xue, N. Yonet-Tanyeri, N. Brouette, M. Sferrazza, P.V. Braun, D.E. Leckband, Langmuir 27 (2011) 8810.

[26] J.-F. Lutz, Adv. Mater. 23 (2011) 2237.

[27] J. Hyun, W.-K. Lee, N. Nath, A. Chilkoti, S. Zauscher, J. Am. Chem. Soc. 126 (2004) 7330.

[28] T. Okano, N. Yamada, H. Sakai, Y. Sakurai, J. Biomed. Mater. Res. 27 (1993) 1243.

[29] E. Wischerhoff, K. Uhlig, A. Lankenau, H.G. Börner, A. Laschewsky, C. Duschl, J.F. Lutz, Angew. Chem. Int. Ed. 47 (2008) 5666.

[30] A. Higuchi, N. Aoki, T. Yamamoto, T. Miyazaki, H. Fukushima, T.M. Tak, S. Jyujyoji, S. Egashira, Y. Matsuoka, S.H. Natori, J. Biomed. Mater. Res. A 79A (2006) 380.

[31] S.-J. Seo, I.-K. Park, M.-K. Yoo, M. Shirakawa, T. Akaike, C.-S. Cho, J. Biomater. Sci. Polym. Ed. 15 (2004) 1375.

[32] M. Mie, Y. Mizushima, E. Kobatake, J. Biomed. Mater. Res. B 86B (2008) 283.

[33] H. Kanazawa, K. Yamamoto, Y. Matsushima, N. Takai, A. Kikuchi, Y. Sakurai, T. Okano, Anal. Chem. 68 (1996) 100.

[34] H. Kanazawa, Y. Matsushima, T. Okano, Trends Anal. Chem. 17 (1998) 435.

[35] H. Kanazawa, J. Sep. Sci. 30 (2007) 1646.

[36] H. Feil, Y.H. Bae, J. Feijen, S.W. Kim, Macromolecules 25 (1992) 5528.

[37] J. Kobayashi, A. Kikuchi, K. Sakai, T. Okano, Anal. Chem. 75 (2003) 3244.

[38] E. Ayano, C. Sakamoto, H. Kanazawa, A. Kikuchi, T. Okano, Anal. Sci. 22 (2006) 539.

[39] M. Gewehr, K. Nakamura, N. Ise, H. Kitano, Die Makromol. Chem. 193 (1992) 249.

[40] K. Yoshizako, Y. Akiyama, H. Yamanaka, Y. Shinohara, Y. Hasegawa, E. Carredano, A. Kikuchi, T. Okano, Anal. Chem. 74 (2002) 4160.

[41] Z. Liu, K. Ullah, L. Su, F. Lv, Y. Deng, R. Dai, Y. Li, Y. Zhang, J. Mater. Chem. 22 (2012) 18753.

[42] K. Kurihara, T. Kunitake, N. Higashi, M. Niwa, Langmuir 8 (1992) 2087.

[43] C. Zhao, S. Nie, M. Tang, S. Sun, Prog. Polym. Sci. 36 (2011) 1499.

[44] F. Tomicki, D. Krix, H. Nienhaus, M. Ulbricht, J. Membr. Sci. 377 (2011) 124.

[45] I. Kaetsu, H. Nakayama, K. Uchida, K. Sutani, Rad. Phys. Chem. 60 (2001) 513.
[46] K. Zhang, X.Y. Wu, Biomaterials 25 (2004) 5281.
[47] V.P. Harden, J.O. Harris, J. Bacteriol. 65 (1953) 198.
[48] S.F. Rose, S. Okere, G.W. Hanlon, A.W. Lloyd, A.L. Lewis, J. Mater. Sci. 16 (2005) 1003.
[49] H.-S. Lee, D.M. Eckmann, D. Lee, N.J. Hickok, R.J. Composto, Langmuir 27 (2011) 12458.
[50] S. Chen, J. Zheng, L. Li, S. Jiang, J. Am. Chem. Soc. 127 (2005) 14473.
[51] L. Mi, M.T. Bernards, G. Cheng, Q. Yu, S. Jiang, Biomaterials 31 (2010) 2919.
[52] Z. Cao, L. Mi, J. Mendiola, J.-R. Ella-Menye, L. Zhang, H. Xue, S. Jiang, Angew. Chem. Int. Ed. 51 (2012) 2602.
[53] F. Ercole, T.P. Davis, R.A. Evans, Polym. Chem. 1 (2010) 37.
[54] D. Liu, Y. Xie, H. Shao, X. Jiang, Angew. Chem. Int. Ed. 48 (2009) 4406.
[55] D. Pearson, A.J. Downard, A. Muscroft-Taylor, A.D. Abell, J. Am. Chem. Soc. 129 (2007) 14862.
[56] J. Edahiro, K. Sumaru, Y. Tada, K. Ohi, T. Takagi, M. Kameda, T. Shinbo, T. Kanamori, Y. Yoshimi, Biomacromolecules 6 (2005) 970.
[57] T. Wu, G. Zou, J. Hu, S. Liu, Chem. Mater. 21 (2009) 3788.
[58] D. Heine, D.T. Wu, J. Chem. Phys. 114 (2001) 5313.
[59] L. Mu, Y. Liu, S. Cai, J. Kong, Chem. A Eur. J. 13 (2007) 5113.
[60] J.Y. Wong, R. Langer, D.E. Ingber, Proc. Natl. Acad. Sci. 91 (1994) 3201.
[61] J. Liao, Y. Zhu, Z. Zhou, J. Chen, G. Tan, C. Ning, C. Mao, Angew. Chem. Int. Ed. 53 (2014) 13068.
[62] C.E. Schmidt, V.R. Shastri, J.P. Vacanti, R. Langer, Proc. Natl. Acad. Sci. 94 (1997) 8948.
[63] P. Techawanitchai, K. Yamamoto, M. Ebara, T. Aoyagi, Sci. Technol. Adv. Mater. 12 (2011) 044609.
[64] S.F. Medeiros, A.M. Santos, H. Fessi, A. Elaissari, Int. J. Pharm. 403 (2011) 139.
[65] X. Wang, H. Gu, Z. Yang, J. Magnet. Magnet. Mater. 293 (2005) 334.
[66] F. Xia, H. Ge, Y. Hou, T. Sun, L. Chen, G. Zhang, L. Jiang, Adv. Mater. 19 (2007) 2520.
[67] A. Baldi, M. Lei, Y. Gu, R.A. Siegel, B. Ziaie, Sensors Actuat. B 114 (2006) 9.
[68] Y. Ito, M. Casolaro, K. Kono, Y. Imanishi, J. Control. Release 10 (1989) 195.
[69] L. Bromberg, L. Salvati, Bioconjug. Chem. 10 (1999) 678.
[70] Y. Sugawara, T. Tamaki, T. Yamaghchi, Polymer 62 (2015) 86.
[71] G. Qing, X. Wang, H. Fuchs, T. Sun, J. Am. Chem. Soc. 131 (2009) 8370.
[72] T. Yamaguchi, T. Ito, T. Sato, T. Shinbo, S.-I. Nakao, J. Am. Chem. Soc. 121 (1999) 4078.
[73] H. Kuroki, T. Ito, H. Ohashi, T. Tamaki, T. Yamaguchi, Anal. Chem. 83 (2011) 9226.
[74] G. Qing, T. Sun, Adv. Mater. 23 (2011) 1615.

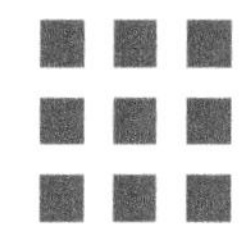

Author Index

L

N

O

Z

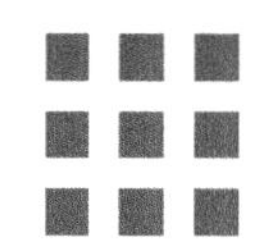

Subject Index

T

Edwards Brothers Malloy
Ann Arbor MI. USA
December 27, 2016

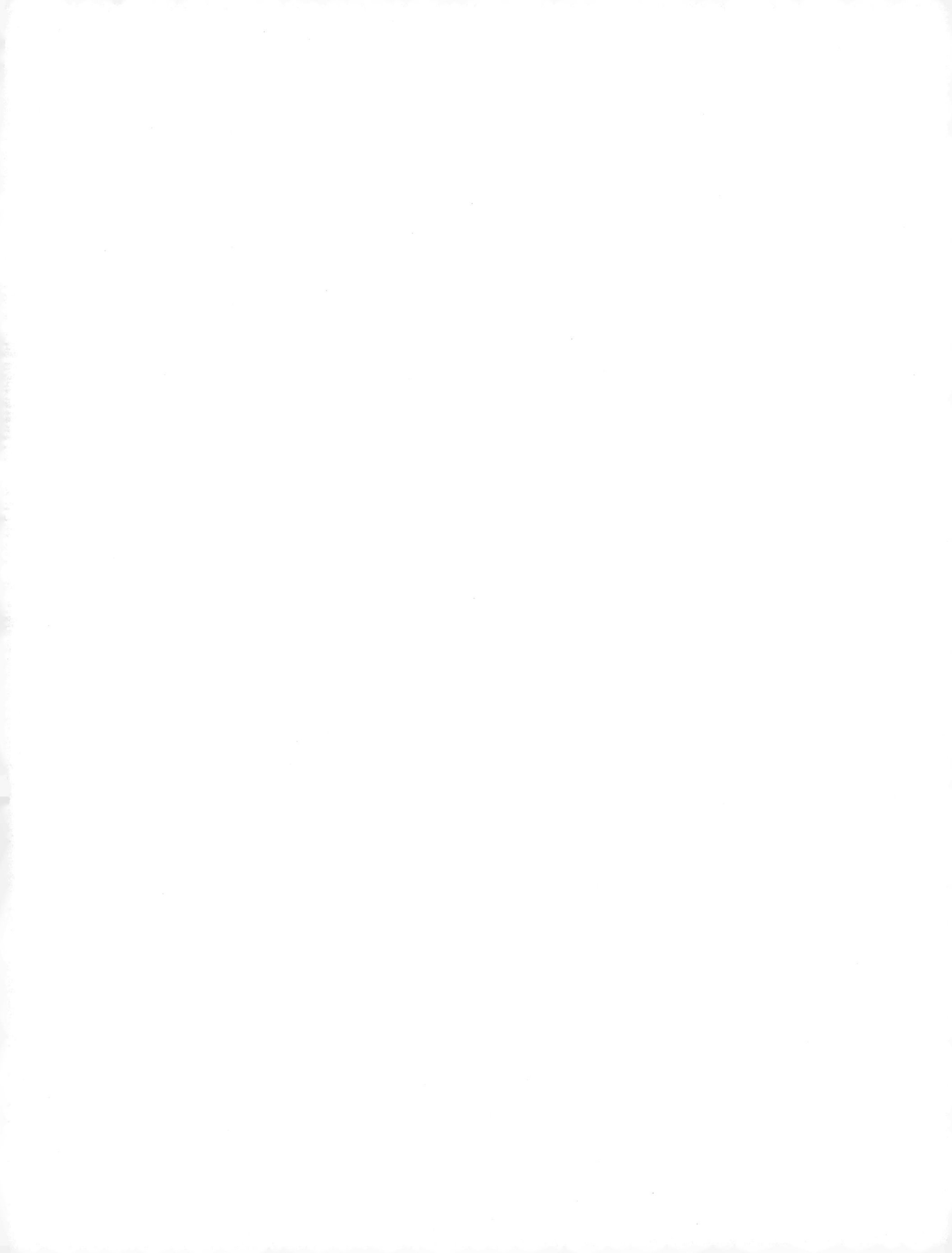